RECENT ADVANCES IN CANNABINOID RESEARCH

Edited by **Willard J Costain**
and **Robert B Laprairie**

Recent Advances in Cannabinoid Research
http://dx.doi.org/10.5772/intechopen.73801
Edited by Willard J Costain and Robert B Laprairie

Contributors

Lee Ellis, Lorane Hage-Melim, Jaderson Ferreira, Lenir Cabral Correia, Daniel Castro da Costa, Natalia Szejko, Kirsten Müller-Vahl, Ewgeni Jakubovski, Donald Simone, Megan Uhelski, Iryna Khasabova, Katrina Weston-Green, Patricia Reggio, Rufaida Al-Zoubi, Dow Hurst, Sara Panseri, Lorenzo Calvi, Radmila Pavlovic, Luca Giupponi, Valeria Leoni, Annamaria Giorgi, Jane Alcorn, Andrew Lyon, Fang Wu, Blair Seifert, Stephanie Vuong, Iris Balodis, James MacKillop, Richard Huntsman, Richard Tang-Wai, Jose Tellez-Zenteno, Willard James Costain, Robert Brad Laprairie

First published in London, United Kingdom, 2019 by IntechOpen
IntechOpen is the global imprint of INTECHOPEN LIMITED, registered in England and Wales, registration number: 11086078, The Shard, 25th floor, 32 London Bridge Street
London, SE19SG – United Kingdom
Printed in Croatia

British Library Cataloguing-in-Publication Data
A catalogue record for this book is available from the British Library

Additional hard copies can be obtained from orders@intechopen.com

Recent Advances in Cannabinoid Research, Edited by Willard J Costain and Robert B Laprairie
p. cm.
Print ISBN 978-1-83880-151-9
Online ISBN 978-1-83880-152-6
eBook (PDF) ISBN 978-1-83880-641-5

For EU product safety concerns:
IN TECH d.o.o., Prolaz Marije Krucifikse Kozulić 3, 51000 Rijeka, Croatia,
info@intechopen.com or visit our website at intechopen.com.

Meet the editors

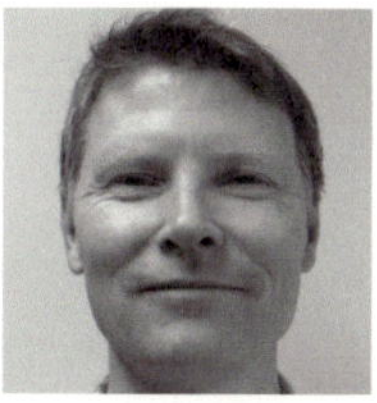

Dr. Willard J. Costain leads a team of researchers focused on developing biologic therapeutics for central nervous system diseases. His primary interest is in characterizing the pharmacology and signaling mechanisms of small and large molecule therapeutics. He studies G-protein-coupled receptor systems using a variety of techniques, with a recent focus on synthetic cannabinoid pharmacology.

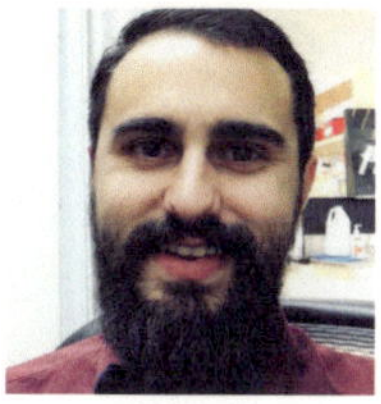

Dr. Robert B. Laprairie's research focuses on drug structure-activity relationships at the type 1 cannabinoid receptor (CB1R) and has published over 30 peer-reviewed publications in this area. He is cochair of the Cannabinoid Research Initiative of Saskatchewan and the Canadian Consortium for the Investigators of Cannabinoids.

Contents

Preface

Cannabis sativa has been used medicinally and recreationally for millennia by societies around the world; however, our comprehension of *Cannabis* and cannabinoids is still very much in its infancy. Although the field of cannabinoid research has seen incredible growth during the past three decades, many questions remain unanswered. With this book, we highlight the impressive work of some researchers in this field as they address what will become the critical scientific questions of our time concerning *Cannabis*. The book provides detailed and current reviews describing aspects of preclinical and clinical research written by experts in their respective fields. This book is highly relevant to scientists and clinicians who aim to understand cannabinoid pharmacology and exploit the therapeutic potential of *Cannabis*.

Dr. Willard J. Costain
Human Health Therapeutics
National Research Council
Ottawa, ON, Canada

Dr. Robert B. Laprairie
College of Pharmacy and Nutrition
University of Saskatchewan
Saskatoon, SK, Canada

Section 1

Introduction

Chapter 1

Introduction to Recent Advances in Cannabinoid Research

Robert B Laprairie and Will Costain

Additional information is available at the end of the chapter

http://dx.doi.org/10.5772/intechopen.85814

Abstract

On October 17, 2018, Canada became the first G20 nation to legalize the use of *Cannabis sativa* for both medicinal and recreational purposes. This change in legislation and end of prohibition are indicative of a larger global movement to understand *Cannabis*—and the bioactive chemicals present within *Cannabis* known as the cannabinoids—for its potential biomedical uses, harms, and economic values. Currently, interest in *Cannabis* and cannabinoid research is surging as the many knowledge gaps in basic biology, pharmacology, epidemiology, and clinical efficacy are identified. The purpose of this book is to summarize some leading areas of research in the cannabinoid field where knowledge gaps have been or are being actively addressed. The research described herein spans between basic biological and clinical research. As the editors of this text, we are grateful to the work of the chapter authors and their important contributions to this rapidly growing field.

Keywords: cannabinoids, *Cannabis sativa*, phytochemicals, cell signaling, animal models, clinical trials, pediatrics, epilepsy, crystallography, Tourette's syndrome

1. Introduction

Cannabis sativa has been used medicinally and recreationally for millennia by societies around the world, but our comprehension of *Cannabis* and cannabinoids from a modern perspective is still very much in its infancy [1]. The field of cannabinoid research has evolved from a curiosity following the first report of the medicinal properties of *Cannabis* in 1840 [2] to becoming a controlled product in 1925 following the signing of an international treaty controlling its trade [3] to ultimately becoming a highly active basic and clinical research discipline. The psychoactive and intoxicating constituent of *Cannabis sativa*, Δ^9-tetrahydrocannabinol (THC), was first isolated and described by Dr. Raphael Mechoulam in 1964 [4]. Following this discovery, it was not until 1991 that a human cannabinoid receptor—later named the type 1 cannabinoid receptor (CB1R)—was identified, isolated, and cloned [5]. Other components of the endogenous cannabinoid system (ECS) were subsequently identified in rapid succession, including the endogenous cannabinoid anandamide (AEA) and 2-arachidonoylglycerol (2-AG), the type 2 cannabinoid receptor (CB2R), and the anabolic and catabolic enzymes that synthesize and degrade the endogenous cannabinoids, respectively [6]. During this period there was also a rapid growth in tool compounds (synthetic cannabinoids) to study the ECS and a race to understand the physiological and behavioral effects cannabinoids evoke *in vivo* [7]. With this rapid growth came some of the first modern preclinical and clinical data to suggest clinical efficacy of cannabinoid-based medicines in the treatment of pain, anxiety, addiction, and metabolic disorders [8], as well as preclinical and clinical data that indicated the potential harms associated with *Cannabis* use, in particular the long-term use of THC in the context of the developing brain [9]. Our understanding of *Cannabis sativa* itself was also growing during the 1990s and 2000s, with the draft sequence of the genome published in 2011 [10] and more than 220 identified constituents (>100 cannabinoids and >120 terpenes) now identified in the plant [11, 12]. Most recently, several crystal structures of CB1R were solved in 2016 and 2017 by large interdisciplinary research groups [13–15]. These crystal structures will allow for rational drug design and comprehension of drug-receptor relationships for the first time in the cannabinoid field.

Although the field of cannabinoid research has seen incredible growth during the past three decades, many questions remain unanswered. As a demonstration of the cannabinoid field's infancy, the clinically relevant pharmacological effects of morphine have been documented since 1817 [16], and the crystal structure of the μ-opioid receptor was solved in 2012 [17]. The illegal status of *Cannabis* in most constituencies has represented a significant barrier to basic, epidemiological, and clinical research. However, interest in the potential applications of cannabinoids and their biology has grown tremendously since the discovery of the ECS. What was once a field with a single manuscript in 1964 has now grown to an area averaging 1500 studies per year in a veritable gold rush into a relatively poorly characterized system. With this book, our goal is to highlight the impressive work of some researchers in this field as they address what will become the critical scientific questions of our time concerning *Cannabis*.

2. Preclinical research

This book presents a collection of chapters addressing important preclinical topics, including the utility of the zebrafish model in cannabinoid research (Chapter 1), insights derived from the structural analysis of CB1R crystal structures (Chapter 2), and the analysis of medical *Cannabis* quality traits (Chapter 3). Dr. Ellis describes the historical usage of the zebrafish model and its applicability to studies of various aspects of vertebrate and mammalian biology, including neurobiology and neurological disorders, while focusing on the role of the endocannabinoid system. Dr. Al-Zoubi et al. provide an in-depth analysis of the unique aspects of cannabinoid receptors gleaned from studies of hCB1R crystal structures. These authors

http://dx.doi.org/10.5772/intechopen.85814

present an extensive review of studies using mutation and labeling of CB1R to characterize the orthostatic binding site and identify issues with crystal structures that could impact their utility in rational drug design. Dr. Calvi et al. provide a description of state-of-the-art analytical methods used to assess the quality attributes of medical *Cannabis* products. This is a particularly timely topic as the necessity to characterize *Cannabis* chemotypes has increased with the recent legalization and regulation of medicinal *Cannabis* in major markets around the world.

3. Clinical research

The clinical research described in this book focuses on the clinical effects of *Cannabis* and cannabinoids on cognition (Chapter 4), the treatment of pain (Chapter 5), Tourette's syndrome (Chapter 6), *Cannabis* use disorder and *Cannabis* withdrawal (Chapters 7 and 8), cannabinoid dosing considerations in pediatric populations (Chapter 9), and *Cannabis* use for treating pediatric and adult epilepsy (Chapter 10). Dr. Weston-Green provides a comprehensive overview of cannabinoid-dependent effects on cognition, including discussions about (1) the many "lesser-known" plant cannabinoids beyond THC and cannabidiol that have been under-assessed to date and (2) the potential "entourage effects" of cannabinoid combinations occurring in *Cannabis* products. Dr. Uhelski et al. review the anti-nociceptive properties of cannabinoids and the preclinical as well as clinical evidence for the use of cannabinoids as analgesics for peripheral pain. *Cannabis*-based medicines (CBM) are presently being examined for a wide array of psychiatric conditions for which the evidence base is small yet growing. Dr. Szejko provides a review of the clinical evidence for CBM in Tourette's syndrome and the potential mechanisms of action at work for cannabinoids in this disorder. *Cannabis* and the ECS are now recognized for their potential to treat substance abuse disorders, including opioid addiction and *Cannabis* use disorder itself. Dr. Balodis et al. provide a comprehensive review of *Cannabis* use disorder, its epidemiology, potential harms, and other important considerations. Dr. Ferreira et al. review the potential of cannabinoids—including novel bioligands—to treat substance use disorders. At long last, cannabidiol is now recognized and accepted as an anticonvulsant medication for the treatment of refractory pediatric epilepsies, such as Dravet and Lennox-Gastaut syndromes, with the recent FDA approval of Epidiolex® for these conditions. In the final chapters of this book, Dr. Huntsman et al. review the clinical evidence for high-cannabidiol *Cannabis* herbal extracts for the treatment of pediatric and adult epilepsies, while Dr. Alcorn et al. review critical dosing considerations and pharmacokinetic parameters for *Cannabis* in the pediatric population.

4. Looking forward

Basic and clinical cannabinoid research has recently become a greater priority due to the increasing number of jurisdictions where legalization of *Cannabis* use for both medical and recreational purposes has occurred. There have been numerous health claims attributed to *Cannabis*, and the evidence supporting some of the claims remains inconclusive. According to the conclusion of a report by a Committee On The Health Effects Of Marijuana, the therapeutic benefit of *Cannabis* on chronic pain, chemotherapy-induced nausea and vomiting, and multiple sclerosis spasticity has been deemed effective, whereas insufficient evidence was available to support a similar conclusion in the treatment of cancer, anorexia and weight loss, irritable bowel syndrome, epilepsy, spinal cord injury-induced spasticity, Tourette's syndrome, amyotrophic lateral sclerosis, Huntington's disease, Parkinson's disease, dystonia, dementia, glaucoma, traumatic brain injury or intracranial hemorrhage, addiction, anxiety, depression, sleep disorders, posttraumatic stress disorder, schizophrenia, and other psychoses [8]. Thus, while tremendous advances have been made in understanding the biology of the ECS and of *Cannabis sativa,* it is clear that many aspects of the medical use of *Cannabis* require further clarification. Additionally, there has been a marked increase in the generation of novel synthetic cannabinoids over the last decade [18], the general availability of which has prompted concern among regulatory agencies due to their unknown safety profiles [19, 20]. This is highlighted by the rapidly increasing number of case reports detailing the effects of acute synthetic cannabinoid intoxication [21–23]. The potential dangers of synthetic cannabinoid use are attributable to the intrinsic properties of these substances and their metabolites. The potential for harm is further exacerbated by the poor pharmacological and toxicological characterization of synthetic cannabinoids. Thus, intensified research efforts into the health benefits and harms of *Cannabis* and cannabinoids will hasten the positive exploitation of *Cannabis* and reduce the drawbacks of *Cannabis* and synthetic cannabinoids.

Author details

Robert B Laprairie[1,2] and Will Costain[3*]

*Address all correspondence to: will.costain@nrc-cnrc.gc.ca

1 College of Pharmacy and Nutrition, University of Saskatchewan, Saskatoon, SK, Canada

2 Department of Pharmacology, College of Medicine, Dalhousie University, Halifax, NS, Canada

3 Human Health Therapeutics, National Research Council, Ottawa, ON, Canada

References

[1] Pisanti S, Bifulco M. Modern history of medical cannabis: From widespread use to prohibitionism and back. Trends in Pharmacological Sciences. 2017;**38**:195-198. Available from: http://www.ncbi.nlm.nih.gov/pubmed/28095988

[2] O'Shaughnessy WB. On the preparations of the Indian Hemp, or Gunjah (*Cannabis indica*), their effects on the animal system in health, and their utility in the treatment of tetanus and other convulsive diseases. The British and Foreign Medical Review. 1840;**10**:225-228. Available from: http://www.ncbi.nlm.nih.gov/pubmed/30161735

[3] Pain S. A potted history. Nature. 2015;**525**:S10-S11

[4] Gaoni Y, Mechoulam R. Isolation, structure, and partial synthesis of an active constituent of Hashish. Journal of the American Chemical Society. 1964;**86**:1646-1647. Available from: http://pubs.acs.org/doi/abs/10.1021/ja01062a046

[5] Gérard CM, Mollereau C, Vassart G, Parmentier M. Molecular cloning of a human cannabinoid receptor which is also expressed in testis. The Biochemical Journal. 1991;**279**(1):129-134. Available from: http://www.ncbi.nlm.nih.gov/pubmed/1718258

[6] Di Marzo V, Piscitelli F. The endocannabinoid system and its modulation by phytocannabinoids. Neurotherapeutics. 2015;**12**:692-698. Available from: http://www.ncbi.nlm.nih.gov/pubmed/26271952

[7] Pertwee RG. Pharmacology of cannabinoid CB1 and CB2 receptors. Pharmacology & Therapeutics. 1997;**74**:129-180. Available from: http://www.ncbi.nlm.nih.gov/pubmed/9336020

[8] National Academies of Sciences and Medicine E. The Health Effects of Cannabis and Cannabinoids: The Current State of Evidence and Recommendations for Research. Washington, DC: The National Academies Press; 2017. Available from: https://www.nap.edu/catalog/24625/the-health-effects-of-cannabis-and-cannabinoids-the-current-state

[9] Broyd SJ, van Hell HH, Beale C, Yücel M, Solowij N. Acute and chronic effects of cannabinoids on human cognition-a systematic review. Biological Psychiatry. 2016;**79**:557-567. Available from: http://www.ncbi.nlm.nih.gov/pubmed/26858214

[10] van Bakel H, Stout JM, Cote AG, Tallon CM, Sharpe AG, Hughes TR, et al. The draft genome and transcriptome of *Cannabis sativa*. Genome Biology. 2011;**12**:R102. Available from: http://www.ncbi.nlm.nih.gov/pubmed/22014239

[11] ElSohly MA, Radwan MM, Gul W, Chandra S, Galal A. Phytochemistry of *Cannabis sativa* L. Progress in the Chemistry of Organic Natural Products. 2017;**103**:1-36. Available from: http://www.ncbi.nlm.nih.gov/pubmed/28120229

[12] Andre CM, Hausman J-F, Guerriero G. *Cannabis sativa*: The plant of the thousand and one molecules. Frontiers in Plant Science. 2016;**7**:19. Available from: http://www.ncbi.nlm.nih.gov/pubmed/26870049

[13] Shao Z, Yin J, Chapman K, Grzemska M, Clark L, Wang J, et al. High-resolution crystal structure of the human CB1 cannabinoid receptor. Nature. 2016;**540**(7634):602-606. Available from: http://www.ncbi.nlm.nih.gov/pubmed/27851727

[14] Hua T, Vemuri K, Nikas SP, Laprairie RB, Wu Y, Qu L, et al. Crystal structures of agonist-bound human cannabinoid receptor CB1. Nature. 2017;**547**:468-471. Available from: http://www.ncbi.nlm.nih.gov/pubmed/28678776

[15] Hua T, Vemuri K, Pu M, Qu L, Han GW, Wu Y, et al. Crystal structure of the human cannabinoid receptor CB1. Cell. 2016;**167**:750-762. e14. Available from: http://www.ncbi.nlm.nih.gov/pubmed/27768894

[16] Krishnamurti C, Rao SC. The isolation of morphine by Serturner. Indian Journal of Anaesthesia. 2016;**60**:861-862. Available from: http://www.ncbi.nlm.nih.gov/pubmed/27942064

[17] Manglik A, Kruse AC, Kobilka TS, Thian FS, Mathiesen JM, Sunahara RK, et al. Crystal structure of the μ-opioid receptor bound to a morphinan antagonist. Nature. 2012;**485**:321-326. Available from: http://www.ncbi.nlm.nih.gov/pubmed/22437502

[18] EMCDDA. Synthetic cannabinoids in Europe (Perspectives on drugs) | www.emcdda.europa.eu [Internet]. Lisbon; 2017. Available from: http://www.emcdda.europa.eu/publications/pods/synthetic-cannabinoids

[19] Costain WJ, Rasquinha I, Comas T, Hewitt M, Aylsworth A, Rouleau Y, et al. Analysis of the pharmacological properties of JWH-122 isomers and THJ-2201, RCS-4 and AB-CHMINACA in HEK293T cells and hippocampal neurons. European Journal of Pharmacology. 2018;**823**:96-104. Available from: http://www.ncbi.nlm.nih.gov/pubmed/29408093

[20] Costain WJ, Tauskela JS, Rasquinha I, Comas T, Hewitt M, Marleau V, et al. Pharmacological characterization of emerging synthetic cannabinoids in HEK293T cells and hippocampal neurons. European Journal of Pharmacology. 2016;**786**:234-245. Available from: http://www.ncbi.nlm.nih.gov/pubmed/27260125

[21] Brown GR, McLaughlin K, Vaughn K. Identifying and treating patients with synthetic psychoactive drug intoxication. Journal of the American Academy of Physician Assistants. 2018;**31**:1-5. Available from: http://www.ncbi.nlm.nih.gov/pubmed/30048361

[22] Hobbs M, Kalk NJ, Morrison PD, Stone JM. Spicing it up - synthetic cannabinoid receptor agonists and psychosis—a systematic review. European Neuropsychopharmacology. 2018;**28**:1289-1304. Available from: http://www.ncbi.nlm.nih.gov/pubmed/30454908

[23] Akram H, Mokrysz C, Curran HV. What are the psychological effects of using synthetic cannabinoids? A systematic review. Journal of Psychopharmacology. 2019;**33**:271-283. Available from: http://www.ncbi.nlm.nih.gov/pubmed/30789300

Section 2

Pre-Clinical Research

Chapter 2

Zebrafish as a High-Throughput In Vivo Model for Testing the Bioactivity of Cannabinoids

Lee Ellis

Additional information is available at the end of the chapter

http://dx.doi.org/10.5772/intechopen.79321

Abstract

Zebrafish represent an established vertebrate model system that helps to bridge the research gap between cell line/invertebrate studies and mammalian systems. While the initial testing of tetrahydrocannabinol (THC) using Zebrafish occurred in 1975, zebrafish are currently a burgeoning model for testing the bioactivity of cannabinoids. Zebrafish express both CB1 and CB2 receptors along with all of the other major endocannabinoid-related genes. Zebrafish endocannabinoid gene function has been associated with addiction, anxiety, development, energy homeostasis and food intake, immune system function, learning and memory. Both adult and larval zebrafish have been used to test the therapeutic potential of THC and cannabidiol (CBD) against various disease models such as models of nociception, epilepsy, stress/anxiety and addiction. This chapter will review recent studies that have used zebrafish as a model for testing the bioactivity of cannabinoids and provide insight on potential future work in this area.

Keywords: zebrafish, cannabinoid, pain, stress, addiction, epilepsy

1. Introduction

The use of zebrafish as a vertebrate model for biological research began in the late 1960s in the lab of George Streisinger at the University of Oregon. However, it was not until the middle of the 1980s that a community of researchers working on zebrafish began to emerge. Since that time the use of zebrafish as a model organism has continued to increase. Over the past 3 decades the use of zebrafish as a model species has contributed to our understanding of developmental biology, toxicology, drug efficacy and disease.

As a vertebrate, the zebrafish model provides more information than can be obtained from cell lines and invertebrate studies, while at the same time remaining low-cost and high-throughput compared with mammalian models. It has been estimated that screening 1 drug with rodent models costs approximately 50× more than through zebrafish assays and zebrafish testing can be done in days versus weeks to months for analogous rodent assays [1].

Another major advantage to using zebrafish as a model species is that they show high genetic homology to mammals. The sequencing of the zebrafish genome was begun in 2001 and the reference genome was published in 2013 [2]. This revealed that ~70% of human genes have at least 1 zebrafish ortholog and ~84% of genes known to be associated with human disease have a zebrafish counterpart. This then provides an important platform with which to begin to study genes linked to human disease. The initial studies that made use of zebrafish were largely entrenched in forward genetic screening, which revealed their genetic tractability and helped to lead the way to the generation of clonal lines [3]. While these original studies were begun nearly 40 years ago, since then an ever increasing number of genetic tools have been developed and used to alter the zebrafish genome such as zinc finger nucleases (ZFNs), transcription activator-like effector nucleases (TALENs) and clustered regularly interspaced short palindromic repeats (CRISPR) [4, 5]. These tools along with a fully sequenced genome provide a stage for the creation of any number of informative transgenic and knockdown/knockout lines. Along with this, zebrafish reach maturity by 90 days post fertilization and produce hundreds of eggs per clutch on a weekly basis. As screening for germline transmission is the general bottle neck in the generation of transgenic lines, the high fecundity of zebrafish allows for more rapid screening and development of transgenic lines compared with mammalian models. The use of transgenic models has a broad applicability and can potentially contribute to all facets of zebrafish research.

One of the major advantages of zebrafish as a model species is that their embryos are fertilized and develop externally providing easy access to embryos and larvae. Importantly, all major organs are formed by 1 day post fertilization (dpf) and larvae hatch from their chorion and become free swimming by 3 dpf. Larvae can live off of the nutrition provided by their yolk sac until 5 dpf, at which time they begin to feed. During this period, larvae are largely transparent making the development of organs and body patterning visible. Their rapid development and transparency provides an ideal setting for testing the effects of various compounds on normal development along with their potential acute toxicity. Standard toxicity testing models exist, including the OECD recognized fish embryo toxicity assay (FET) that tests the effects of compound exposure on normal development from 6 to 72 hpf (OECD guideline 236, adopted July 2013). The general and behavioral toxicity (GBT) assay tests the effects of compound exposure on larvae from 72 to 120 hpf [6]. Additionally, the effect of compounds on the larval heart rate has been shown to be a predictive indicator of potential bradycardia related cardiotoxicity [7]. This is important when screening neuroactive compounds as the blockage of numerous ion channels, often the target of neuroactives, can lead to arrhythmias [8]. The toxicity profiling of potential therapeutics at early stages of development allows for the identification of off-target side effects as well as the potential to calculate a therapeutic window when the toxicity profile is compared with the level of compound required to have a positive effect on disease models.

http://dx.doi.org/10.5772/intechopen.79321

The use of zebrafish in the field of neuroscience continues to increase and a number of recent reviews have highlighted both the strengths and weaknesses of using zebrafish to study neuroactive compounds and brain disorders [9–15]. The zebrafish brain has many analogous regions to those of higher vertebrates and the complexity of both juvenile and adult zebrafish brains has been well documented [16]. In addition to brain morphology, the neurochemistry and endocrine responses linked to zebrafish neuroactivity is highly homologous to other vertebrates including the same neurotransmitters, receptors, synthetic/metabolic enzymes and hypothalamo-pituitary hormones [9–11, 15, 17–19].

It has been demonstrated that zebrafish are sensitive to a large number of neurotropic drugs including: antipsychotics, mood stabilizers, anxiolytics, antidepressants, ethanol, hypnotics, stimulants, hallucinogens, antiepileptics, analgesics and cognitive enhancers [15, 16]. In addition, both adult and larval zebrafish can be used to model numerous neural disorders including pain/nociception, anxiety, stress, PTSD, ADHD, Autism, epilepsy, learning & memory deficits, psychiatric disorders, Alzheimer's disease, amyotrophic lateral sclerosis (ALS), Parkinson's disease, schizophrenia, bi-polar disorder, addiction and brain cancer [6, 9, 11, 14–16, 20–25]. This provides *in vivo* models with which to test not only the bioactivity of various neuroactive compounds, but also allows for the testing of their potential efficacy against numerous models of disease. Use of these models can provide an indication of the level of compound required to oppose a disease phenotype, which is required for the calculation of a therapeutic window for new drugs. The disease models also provide a platform for the testing and potential re-purposing of neuroactive compounds currently on the market. Finding an effective treatment for the disease models may help to provide clues to the etiology of human disease and insights into additional therapeutic targets.

Many of the neuronal disease models developed using zebrafish are centered on the assessment of aberrant behavior in both larvae and adults, which each provide their own distinct advantages [9, 11, 15, 16]. One of the major advantages of using larvae over adults stems from their reproducible patterns of behavior and potential to be screened in a high throughput fashion. Activity patterns can be assessed in multi-well plates allowing for up to 96 larvae to be tested simultaneously using benchtop tracking systems. As mentioned, larvae become free swimming between 3 and 5 dpf and develop stereotypical behavioral and stimulus response patterns. These include their response to startling stimuli such as noise, light–dark transitions and touch. Importantly the behavioral activity patterns are highly quantifiable and can be altered by neuroactive compounds with various targets. The assessment of adult behavior, while much lower throughput, does have some advantages over larval testing as it can often provide more intricate behavioral paradigms than can be obtained with larvae. Specifically, adult behavior can be tracked in 3 dimensions and various models of learning and memory, conspecific interactions and place preference exist that are not found for larvae. Many of these models are analogous to rodent behavioral models [16].

In addition to models of behavior, as previously mentioned, larval zebrafish are nearly transparent for their first week of development and a number of transgenic lines exist that completely lack pigment. This provides unparalleled access to an intact vertebrate brain. Numerous studies have used *in situ* hybridization and immunohistochemistry to map and profile neural activity using indicators such as *c-Fos*. Recent technical advances have allowed for a more in depth assessment of neuronal activity than is possible in mammalian systems. The assessment of neural activity has been accomplished using genetically encoded calcium indicators and whole brain imaging in immobilized larvae [26]. More recently the assessment of neural activity in freely behaving larvae at near cellular resolution has become possible [27]. The development of this new technology now allows for links to be made between localized brain activity and various behaviors and stimulus response patterns that is currently not possible with mammalian models.

While the original use of zebrafish as a model species was focused on genetics, they are currently contributing ever evolving models to the fields of developmental biology, neuroscience, molecular biology and pharmacology research.

2. Functions of the zebrafish endocannabinoid system

The initial use of zebrafish for testing the toxicity of THC occurred in 1975 [28]. However, it has only been the last 10–15 years that interest in the study of the zebrafish endocannabinoid system (ECS) has begun to grow. As outlined below, the zebrafish ECS shows genetic homology to mammalian systems and is involved in many of the same physiological processes. Importantly, the route of administration for cannabinoids to zebrafish is relatively straight forward as they can be added to the bath solution with either methanol or dimethyl sulfoxide (DMSO) as a solvent.

2.1. Gene expression patterns

The initial sequencing and mapping of the expression pattern of the CB1 receptor (CB1R) in both larvae and adults found that the zebrafish CB1R showed a 69% nucleotide identity and a 73.6% amino acid identity with the human CB1R [29]. Larvae begin to express the CB1R by the 3 somite stage of development [30] and, as expected, show a widespread and distinct expression pattern throughout the CNS (preoptic area, dorsal telencephalon, periventricular hypothalamus, tegmentum and anterior hindbrain) by 48 hpf that continues into adulthood [29, 31]. The general pattern of expression for the CB1R in the adult zebrafish brain appears to be homologous to that of mammals.

Shortly after the cloning of the CB1R zebrafish were found to express two CB2 receptor (CB2R) orthologs that showed 98% genetic identity with each other and a 39% amino acid identity with the human CB2R [32]. Importantly, similar to the CB1R, the expression patterns of the CB2R were homologous to those found in mammals with low levels in the brain and higher levels in the intestine, retina, gills, heart, muscle, pituitary and spleen.

Zebrafish also express the transient receptor potential vanilloid type 1 cation channel (TrpV1) and the G-protein coupled receptor 55 (Gpr55) early in development. Both receptors are known to bind endocannabinoids [33]. The cannabinoid receptor interacting protein (CRIP1A) is also expressed early in development [31].

In addition to the cannabinoid receptor genes, the genes responsible for the synthesis and catabolism of the endocannabinoids anandamide (AEA) and 2-arachidonoylglycerol (2-AG) begin to become expressed between 1 and 12 hpf and their expression levels continue to increase throughout development. These include the AEA biosynthetic enzymes *N*-acylphosphatidylethanolamine-selective phospholipase D (NAPE-pld) and $\alpha\beta$-hydrolase domain containing 4 (Abhd4), the AEA catabolic enzyme fatty acid amide hydrolase (faah), the 2-AG biosynthetic enzyme diacylglycerol lipase α (DAGL α) and the 2-AG catabolic enzymes monoglyceride lipase (mgll) and prostaglandin-endoperoxide synthase 2 (ptgs2b) [31, 33]. Importantly the expression of these biosynthetic enzymes is accompanied by an increase in the protein levels of AEA and 2-AG [33]. The tissue distribution pattern of these enzymes is vast with high levels found in the brain, muscle, heart, intestine, eyes and reproductive organs (ovary and testis) of adults (**Table 1**) [31]. In larvae mgll, dagla and cnr1 are expressed in different regions of the brain and all 3 show some overlap with the expression pattern of CB1R [31, 33].

2.2. Growth and development

The CB1 receptor is present at early developmental stages in mammals and it has been suggested that the ECS may contribute to CNS development, such as axonal elongation, myelination, migration, cell proliferation and synaptogenesis [34].

In zebrafish it has been shown that the developmental expression of the CB1R and Dagl2α occurs at the same time during larval development, suggesting that larvae are able to both synthesize and respond to 2-AG during development [35]. The same study demonstrated that morpholino knockdown of the CB1R expression lead to aberrant patterns of axonal growth. It was subsequently shown that knockdown of Dagl2 alters axon formation in the midbrain-hindbrain region and alters different patterns of behavior which suggests that 2-AG plays a role in axon formation which subsequently affects the control of vision and movement in larvae [33]. Additionally, the highest level of CB1R expression in the developing larvae occurs at the time of hatching, which may suggest that the proper expression of the CB1R is necessary for the increase in movement that is required for the hatching process [30].

In addition to neuronal development, it has also been shown that endocannabinoid signaling is required for normal embryonic liver development and function [36]. Alteration of this normal development appears to impact the structure and function of the adult liver and may impact metabolic homeostasis. It has also been shown that the CB2R plays a role in the production, expansion and migration of hematopoietic stem cells suggesting that it may play a role hematopoiesis during development [37].

2.3. Feeding and lipid metabolism

The consumption of *cannabis* is well known to stimulate appetite and numerous animal and human studies have detailed the role that the endocannabinoid system plays in appetite regulation, weight gain, energy balance, and lipid metabolism. Rodent models have shown that both the endocannabinoids as well as THC stimulate appetite and can produce hyperphagia [38–41], while CB1R antagonists can suppress appetite [42, 43]. In humans genetic variations in the CB1 receptor and a dysregulation of the endocannabinoid system have been linked to obesity [44, 45]. The first therapeutic targeting this system that was brought to market was the inverse agonist for the CB1 receptor rimonabant. It was shown to lead to weight loss in

Distribution			
Protein name	**Abbreviation**	**High levels**	**Low levels**
Cannabinoid receptor 1	CB1R	Brain	Eyes, testis
Cannabinoid receptor 2	CB2R	Intestine, eyes, gills, heart, muscle, pituitary, kidney, spleen	Brain, testis
Transient receptor potential vanilloid type 1 cation channel	TrpV1	Sensory neurons	
G protein-coupled receptor 55A	GPR55A	Brain, spleen, testis	
Cannabinoid receptor interacting protein	(CRIP1A)	Brain, eyes, testis	
N-acylphosphatidylethanolamine-selective phospholipase D	NAPE-pld	All organs	
αβ-Hydrolase domain containing 4	Abhd4	Spleen, testis	All organs
Fatty acid amide hydrolase	faah	Brain	Skin, testis
Fatty acid amide hydrolase 2a	faah2a	Brain	Intestine, eyes, testis
Diacylglycerol lipase α	DAGL α	Brain, muscle, kidney, eyes, testis, spleen	
Diacylglycerol lipase β	DAGL β	Brain, muscle, kidney, eyes, testis	Spleen
Monoglyceride lipase	mgll	Brain, kidney, spleen, eyes	
Prostaglandin-endoperoxide synthase 2	ptgs2a	Skin, spleen, eyes	
αβ-Hydrolase domain containing 6b	Abhd6b	Not detectable	
αβ-Hydrolase domain containing 6a	Abhd6a	Intestine, liver, testis	
αβ-Hydrolase domain containing 12	abhd12	Brain, muscles, eyes, reproductive organs	Kidney, heart, intestine
Glycerophosphodiester phosphodiesterase1	gde1	All organs	
N-acylspihingosine amidohydrolase 1a	naaa1a	Reproductive organs	
Peroxisome proliferator-activated receptor αβ	pparab	Muscles, spleen, brain, heart, eyes	
Peroxisome proliferator-activated receptor γ	pparg	Muscles, spleen, testis	

Adapted from Oltrabella et al. [31].

Table 1. Organ distribution patterns of cannabinoid related proteins in adult zebrafish

overweight subjects and was marketed as a therapeutic for the treatment of obesity [46]. In line with this, it has been shown that CB1 receptor knockout animals are thinner than controls and have less adipose tissue, which is thought to relate to both decreased caloric intake as well as changes in metabolic factors [47]. Less adipose tissue may also be linked to the therapeutic potential of targeting the CB1 receptor in the treatment of obesity, as obesity in humans is linked to hepatic stenosis, which was shown to be reduced by treatment with rimonabant [44]. Since the initial development of rimonabant, the endocannabinoid system has been of interest for the potential role its dysregulation may play in obesity [44]. Unfortunately, the side effect profile of rimonabant resulted in its withdrawal from the marketplace.

Zebrafish provide a model with which to study the role of the endocannabinoid system in appetite regulation and lipid bioaccumulation. Similar to what was found for mammals, rimonabant led to the suppression of feeding in juvenile fish [48]. In larvae it was found that rimonabant exposure led to larger yolk sacs during development, suggesting a decrease in the use of fat stores, which may be related to a decreased appetite. Exposure of adult zebrafish to melatonin, a known regulator of energy homeostasis, suppressed appetite through the downregulation of the CB1R gene expression [49]. It then appears that similar to rodents, modulation of the zebrafish endocannabinoid system can regulate appetite.

Zebrafish are also an established model for the study of lipid biology [50–52]. With respect to the endocannabinoid system, it has been shown that overexpression of the CB1R in liver leads to hepatic lipid accumulation, while suppression leads to a loss of lipid accumulation during hepatogenesis [53]. It has also been found that bisphenol A exposure produces hepatostenosis in adult zebrafish liver by increasing the liver levels of 2-AG and AEA [33]. Stimulation of the endocannabinoid system through CB1 and CB2 receptor activation can influence lipid deposition during embryogenesis through an up-regulation of the lipoprotein lipase gene [54]. Additionally, exposure to two non-psychoactive cannabinoids, namely CBD and tetrahydrocannabivarin (THCV), can lead to a decrease in intracellular lipid levels in zebrafish yolk along with human hepatocytes and adipocytes [55]. This activity does not appear to be linked to CB1R or TRPV1-R activation, but it may suggest a use for both cannabinoids in the treatment of obesity.

2.4. Learning and memory

The effects of cannabinoids on learning and memory in mammalian models is complex and often depends on the model employed and the neural pathways that are activated. However, cannabinoid exposure has been shown to lead to memory impairments for numerous rodent learning paradigms [56].

Zebrafish also have a number of different learning paradigms that include habituation learning, conditioned place preference, avoidance learning, associative learning and spatial memory tests. These learning paradigms are largely based on appetitive and/or fear conditioning [57]. Importantly, a number of these training models have been used to test the cognitive effects of various psychoactive drugs [58]. As many of these models involve the activation of different neuronal pathways, only some of which express cannabinoid receptors, the role of cannabinoid exposure on the development, retention and recall of memories can vary. One such example is a model of fear learning where adult fish were taught to associate the presentation of the alarm pheromone known as the Schreckstoff substance [59] with the presentation of a red light [60]. The response to Schreckstoff substance typically resulted in an increase in bottom dwelling and an increase in erratic movements, both of which are linked to stressful stimuli. Following training, the fish then respond to the red light stimulus, a previously inert stimulus, by showing a similar pattern of behavior. Pre-exposure to THC reduced, but did not eliminate the bottom dwelling and had only a minor effect on erratic movements

[60]. A previous study from the same group evaluating spatial memory and found that THC exposure did not affect associative memory but did impair spatial cognition and memory retrieval [60]. In addition to THC, high levels of CBD also appear to reduce memory retention in a spatial memory test [61]. While the number of studies testing the role of cannabinoids on learning and memory using zebrafish is currently limited, it appears the model has great potential in assessing the role of the endocannabinoid system in multiple aspects of learning and how this can be influenced by various cannabinoids.

3. Developing models

3.1. Pain

The treatment of chronic pain is the largest indication for medical cannabis [62–67]. This is not surprising given that endocannabinoids are known to act as retrograde transmitters blocking the transmission of pain signals at both GABAergic and glutamatergic synapses [68]. Unfortunately the etiology of pain is vast and thus there is not an all-encompassing treatment for pain. Often, an analgesic is only effective for a subset of patients or can only partially reduce pain, but cannot eliminate it [69, 70]. This often leads to multiple drugs being used in combination, which opens the door to various drug interactions that can lead to a number of potential adverse effects and an increased side effect profile.

It is now widely accepted that zebrafish have similar somatosensory systems to higher vertebrates and they can detect painful stimuli (nociception) [71–83]. The models that have been developed vary and include thermal and chemical stimuli that is either bath applied or focally by injection. The models also make use of both acute and chronic nociceptive stimuli and have been developed using larvae and adults. This then provides a number of platforms with which to test potential analgesics that may have links to different disease etiologies.

Recently, a novel model of nociception has been developed and used to test and compare a number of known therapeutics with THC and CBD. The model made use of a short-term exposure to acetic acid which led to tissue damage on the surface of zebrafish larvae and a distinct, reproducible, activity pattern that appears to indicate a multifaceted nociceptive response [83]. The study revealed that THC and CBD had different effects on the behavioral response pattern that varied from those of the known analgesics. Interestingly, of the compounds tested CBD had the most unique effect increasing the rate at which the larval activity pattern returned to that of controls. This would seem to suggest that CBD shortened the recovery from the nociceptive stimulus. This is consistent with literature that has suggested CBD is a strong candidate for pain management [84–86]. Importantly, this activity was found at a concentration of CBD that had no effect on baseline activity for controls, suggesting that there would be a low potential for side effects. One of the major issues surrounding the therapeutics currently used for pain management lies in their side effect profile, which is often vast and can range from relatively minor (constipation) to severe (addiction). This is especially evident for opioids, which are the most commonly used therapeutic for chronic pain, but have one of the highest addictive potentials [87]. While more work is required to test the effect of other cannabinoids and extracts on the various zebrafish models of nociception, the initial indications are that zebrafish will be valuable for assessing the efficacy of potential therapeutics for pain management.

3.2. Addiction

Recent data suggests that approximately 9% of individuals that use cannabis show symptoms associated with addiction, including tolerance and withdrawal [88]. Comparatively the rate of dependence for tobacco is 67.5% and for alcohol is 22.7% [89]. Zebrafish represent an underutilized model with which to study the addictive properties of cannabinoids. While it has been demonstrated that zebrafish can be used to study the pathology of addiction to numerous drugs of abuse, including, alcohol, cocaine, morphine, nicotine, amphetamine, diazepam and salvinorin A [90–95], thus far their use to study the addictive properties of cannabinoids has been minimal. Changes in both larval and adult zebrafish behavior can be linked to numerous phenotypes associated with addiction that include conditioned place preference for drugs of abuse, relapse, changes in social behavior, along with symptoms indicating the development of tolerance and withdrawal [90, 93, 96–99]. It has also been found that the genetic pathways linked to addiction are highly conserved in zebrafish [100]. Currently, with respect to cannabinoids, only one study has shown that zebrafish larvae develop tolerance to the effects of cannabinoids after chronic exposure [101]. As the levels of THC in cannabis plant strains is varied and the refinement and extraction processes allow for other cannabinoids to be used at higher levels both medicinally and recreationally, there is a need to develop models with which to test the addictive properties of both pure cannabinoids on their own, in combination and as part of a complex mixture or extract. Zebrafish have the potential to be such a model.

3.3. Stress and anxiety

One of the known difficulties in using cannabinoids as therapeutics lies in their effect on stress and anxiety. A sought after symptom of cannabis use is the euphoric feeling that often leads to it being considered an anxiolytic. However, it has been broadly shown that as the levels of cannabinoids (specifically THC) are elevated there can be an increase in anxiety-related effects [102]. This is important not only from a side effect perspective, but also becomes an issue when cannabinoids are used to treat anxiety related disorders such as PTSD.

Zebrafish provide numerous models with which to assess stress responses in both larvae and adults. Measurements such as scototaxis (light-dark preference), thigmotaxis (wall hugging), shoaling and the amount of time spent in the bottom of a tank are used as standard measures of stress. Induction of stress can occur by chemical means such as neuro-hyperactive compounds or exposure to the alarm substance. Stress can also be induced physically by touch or following the placement of a fish in a novel setting (novel tank response). Various visible stimuli can also lead to stress responses such as changes in back ground light/dark levels or the appearance of an image of prey. All of these models seem to activate both unique and overlapping neural pathways and thus could provide insight into the mechanism of action of any potential anxiolytic effect [103–105]. An example of the use of zebrafish stress models for testing cannabinoids was outlined in a recent paper that evaluated the acute effects of both THC and CBD on larval behavior [106]. Zebrafish larvae show a preference for light and a transition from a light to a dark setting results in an increase in activity in the form of darting type movements which are thought to be a stress response. It was found that while THC reduced the baseline activity in the light, the response to a light-dark transition was still evident. Exposure to CBD had a much different response with almost no effect on the baseline activity in the light accompanied by a concentration-dependant reduction in the light-dark transition until it was eliminated. This may suggest that CBD is showing anxiolytic effects at the levels tested [107].

It is currently felt that there is insufficient evidence to support the use of cannabis for the treatment more complex stress disorders such as PTSD [108]. Recently work has begun to establish zebrafish models of complex disorders such as PTSD [109, 110]. The development of these models will provide additional systems with which to test the efficacy of various cannabinoids and combinations thereof in the treatment of anxiety related disorders and may help provide insight into their etiology.

3.4. Uptake and metabolism

The adsorption and bioavailability of cannabinoids provides a challenge for their use as therapeutics. This is particularly true for orally ingested cannabinoids, which show low and, at times, unpredictable bioavailability [111]. The interaction between various cannabinoids along with their interaction with other therapeutics can affect their bioavailability. This is important since the effects of various cannabinoids can be bimodal (hyperactivity at low concentrations and sedation at higher concentrations). Having the ability to measure their uptake, bioaccumulation and excretion will provide insights into the exact levels found within the fish. Knowing the true concentration response profile based on the amount of compound found within zebrafish may also allow for comparisons to be made to the dose-response patterns found for mammals.

Previous work has shown that testing the uptake, metabolism and secretion of cannabinoids is possible using zebrafish larvae [106]. A number of important findings came from this study. First it was found that common pharmacokinetic cannabinoid metabolites are produced by the zebrafish larvae including the phase 1 and phase 2 metabolites hydroxylated THC (11-hyrdoxy-THC, 8-hydroxy-THC), 11-nor-9-carboxy THC, THC-glucuronide, hydroxyl-CBD and CBD-glucuronide. Both the cannabinoids and their metabolites were found to accumulate in the larvae with the metabolites eventually excreted into the bath. It was also shown that there appeared to be bioaccumulation of the cannabinoids in the larvae and a non-linear increase in the amount found in the larvae compared with the bath levels. The same study also revealed that when THC and CBD were co-administered the levels of metabolites that were produced was altered compared to when they were administered alone. This suggests that the complex chemical composition of various cannabis plant strains will also affect the normal metabolism of the individual cannabinoids. It then appears that it will be important to evaluate the uptake kinetics and metabolism of various cannabis derived compounds both alone and in combination.

3.5. Seizures

Approximately 1% of the world's population is purported to have epilepsy with 30% of those affected having multi-drug resistant epilepsy. This often leads to the requirement for strong anti-seizure medications or drug cocktails. In general this leads to an ever increasing side effect profile that is often debilitating in and of itself. The treatment of seizures is one of the oldest reported uses of cannabis and it has recently garnered attention along with the use of pure cannabinoids (CBD) for their ability to treat severe forms of refractory childhood epilepsy (i.e. Dravet syndrome [112]). However, to date there still remains some controversy regarding its efficacy, with some groups suggesting there is no concrete evidence that it is effective [113]. While it has been purported that cannabinoids, in particular CBD, can mitigate, to some degree, epileptic seizures, unfortunately, with the exception of the childhood epilepsy study [112], the numerous human studies that have evaluated the effect of cannabinoids on seizures have either been from small sample groups, had insufficient controls or were not blinded, which confounds any potential outcomes of the studies [114]. The study was able to show that there was a reduction in seizure frequency in patients with Dravet syndrome following the addition of CBD to their current prescription regime. The one question that does remain is whether the reduction in seizures was due to the direct effect of CBD or if the effect was due to the effect of CBD on the patient's current medication.

The lack of high-quality human trials for testing anti-epileptics stem from the difficulty in properly designing and/or interpreting the results of human studies. This is partially due to the fact that most study participants are already on another anti-epileptic drug, which often varies between participants in either the drug target or the dosage. During the course of the clinical trials often the levels of either the cannabinoid or the existing therapeutic have to be modified for an individual in order to resolve issues relating to side effects. This makes the proper grouping of different treatment regimens difficult.

There are currently a number of zebrafish models of epilepsy that have been generated to provide a platform for identifying new seizure medications and potentially to understand the etiology of the disease [115]. For instance, a number of small molecules that target different receptors or ion channels can be used to induce seizures or neural hyperactivity in larvae [103, 116, 117]. These platforms provide high throughput testing models with multiple etiologies. While CBD has been shown to be effective in the treatment of some forms of epilepsy, the mechanism of action is still largely unknown. The existing zebrafish seizure models provide multiple platforms with which to evaluate both the efficacy and potentially the mechanism of action for cannabinoids in the treatment of epilepsy. The further development of these models will be of great benefit for discerning the true therapeutic potential of various cannabinoids for the treatment of epilepsy.

3.6. Smoke toxicity

Currently the main delivery method for cannabinoids both medicinally and recreationally is by the inhalation of smoke from marijuana cigarettes. This is generally because of the rapid onset of effects compared with other delivery methods, which is beneficial from the perspective of symptom relief and also allows for a level of self-regulated dose control that is not possible with other delivery methods such as edibles, which can often take up to 90 min to reach peak effect [111]. Unfortunately, some of the major caveats to an inhaled product are that dosing is often inconsistent and difficult to titrate and they have the potential to have similar health risks as are found for smoked tobacco [118]. It has been suggested that high doses of THC containing products are associated with an increased risk of developing respiratory infections [119]. However, it has been difficult to establish a clear relationship between smoked cannabis and more severe lung disorders, such as cancer, since tobacco use is often co-morbid with cannabis. While in general the number of smoked cannabis cigarettes is lower on a per day basis, this risk cannot be overlooked. Additionally, the inhalation delivery methods for cannabis smoke are somewhat more diverse than for tobacco and include pipes, water pipes, burning on metal and vaporizers. All of these delivery methods produce smoke with its own set of chemical characteristics that depend on the temperature at which the smoke was created and any filtering that occurred before the smoke was inhaled. Processing of the plant material into oils or resins before combustion adds another level of complexity to the potential chemical diversity of the smoke that is inhaled.

Zebrafish larvae are an established model for testing vertebrate toxicity, teratogenicity and environmental risk assessment [120–122]. The use of these models has proven to be a valuable resource for testing the toxicity of various extracts and condensates obtained from tobacco cigarette smoke [6, 123, 124]. It was found that smoke from tobacco cigarettes was more toxic and produced different phenotypes than that of nicotine alone, suggesting, that the other toxic components found in tobacco smoke are having an effect. The use of the previously validated smoke testing models for testing cannabis smoke has the potential to provide information on developmental, cardiac, behavioral/neural and acute toxicity.

3.7. Multi-drug interactions and polypharmacology

One of the major complexities of working with cannabis is the fact that it is currently known to be comprised of 500+ constituents and more than 100 cannabinoid molecules [125]. The potential of interactions between many of these compounds is high and has been widely demonstrated for THC and CBD. It has been shown that the zebrafish can be used to assess the interaction of THC and CBD with respect to their effects on locomotor activity along with the uptake and metabolism of each compound [106]. Many of the aforementioned zebrafish models have the potential to be used to assess the potential interaction of THC and CBD and likely other cannabinoids. This is important as one of the next steps in the use of the zebrafish models for testing cannabinoids is to begin to test various extracts and isolates from cannabis for their bioactivity. Having an understanding of how the pure compounds interact in an *in vivo* system and how this relates to their activity in complex mixtures derived from plant material will be extremely valuable. In addition to the interaction of the various compounds found within cannabis, the use of cannabis or cannabinoids as therapeutics is also complicated by the fact that many patients are already taking a prescription drug for their particular indication. The zebrafish testing platforms appear to have the potential to characterize some of these interactions as well.

Understanding the pharmacokinetics and pharmacodynamics of cannabis is complicated by the fact that CBD (and potentially other cannabinoids) has numerous targets and mechanisms of action that contribute to its various biological effects. Similar to CBD a high percentage of neuroactive compounds have multiple targets and act on them within similar concentration ranges. This polypharmacology has both advantages and disadvantages. As many disease etiologies are not entirely known and may be multifactorial, there may be a substantial benefit of having activity on multiple targets. However, this may also increase the side effect potential and the potential of interacting with other therapeutics. It has been suggested that large-scale zebrafish behavioral testing models can be used to help discern the polypharmacological mechanisms of neuroactive compounds [126]. This provides an ideal platform with which to test cannabis derivatives.

4. Discussion

One of the unique characteristics of researching the effects of cannabis and cannabinoids using various models and for various disease indications is that often there is already clinical data on the effects in humans. While much of the data is often anecdotal in nature, it does allow for animal model testing to be used to back validate the findings of the clinical trials. By designing top-down translational research studies we can begin to elucidate the biological basis of the clinical findings and potentially provide information on the mechanism of action of therapeutic compounds. This is particularly true for cannabis uses where the cannabinoid mechanism of action is often difficult to discern. The use of animal models of disease may help to elucidate these mechanisms and further define the etiology of the disease.

As outlined in this chapter, zebrafish have an established endocannabinoid system that is highly analogous to that of humans. Additionally, as a model system both adults and larval zebrafish provide numerous models of disease that have been shown to be efficacious for testing the therapeutic potential of novel compounds. Importantly the response patterns in these various disease models following exposure to different cannabinoids reveal unique characteristics for each cannabinoid. Thus far, only a limited number of these models have been used to test the efficacy of cannabinoids. However, the framework is in place for an expansion of the use of zebrafish in this field.

Author details

Lee Ellis

Address all correspondence to: lee.ellis@nrc-cnrc.gc.ca

National Research Council of Canada, Halifax, Nova Scotia, Canada

References

[1] Steenbergen PJ, Richardson MK, Champagne DL. The use of the zebrafish model in stress research. Progress in Neuro-Psychopharmacology & Biological Psychiatry. 2011; **35**(6):1432-1451

[2] Howe K et al. The zebrafish reference genome sequence and its relationship to the human genome. Nature. 2013;**496**(7446):498-503

[3] Grunwald DJ, Eisen JS. Headwaters of the zebrafish—Emergence of a new model vertebrate. Nature Reviews. Genetics. 2002;**3**(9):717-724

[4] Hoshijima K, Jurynec MJ, Grunwald DJ. Precise editing of the Zebrafish genome made simple and efficient. Developmental Cell. 2016;**36**(6):654-667

[5] Sertori R et al. Genome editing in zebrafish: A practical overview. Briefings in Functional Genomics. 2016;**15**(4):322-330

[6] Ellis LD et al. Use of the zebrafish larvae as a model to study cigarette smoke condensate toxicity. PLoS One. 2014;**9**(12):e115305

[7] Park MJ et al. Predicted drug-induced bradycardia related cardio toxicity using a zebrafish in vivo model is highly correlated with results from in vitro tests. Toxicology Letters. 2013;**216**(1):9-15

[8] Langheinrich U, Vacun G, Wagner T. Zebrafish embryos express an orthologue of HERG and are sensitive toward a range of QT-prolonging drugs inducing severe arrhythmia. Toxicology and Applied Pharmacology. 2003;**193**(3):370-382

[9] Kalueff AV, Echevarria DJ, Stewart AM. Gaining translational momentum: More zebrafish models for neuroscience research. Progress in Neuro-Psychopharmacology & Biological Psychiatry. 2014;**55**:1-6

[10] Kalueff AV, Nguyen M. Testing anxiolytic drugs in the C57BL/6J mouse strain. Journal of Pharmacological and Toxicological Methods. 2014;**69**(2):205-207

[11] Stewart AM et al. Zebrafish models for translational neuroscience research: From tank to bedside. Trends in Neurosciences. 2014;**37**(5):264-278

[12] Gerlai R. Reproducibility and replicability in zebrafish behavioral neuroscience research. Pharmacology, Biochemistry, and Behavior. 23 Feb 2018; pii: S0091-3057(17)30608-1. DOI: 10.1016/j.pbb.2018.02.005

[13] Fontana BD et al. The developing utility of zebrafish models of neurological and neuropsychiatric disorders: A critical review. Experimental Neurology. 2018;**299**(Pt A):157-171

[14] Shams S et al. The zebrafish as a promising tool for modeling human brain disorders: A review based upon an IBNS symposium. Neuroscience and Biobehavioral Reviews. 2018;**85**:176-190

[15] Khan KM et al. Zebrafish models in neuropsychopharmacology and CNS drug discovery. British Journal of Pharmacology. 2017;**174**(13):1925-1944

[16] Kalueff AV, Stewart AM, Gerlai R. Zebrafish as an emerging model for studying complex brain disorders. Trends in Pharmacological Sciences. 2014;**35**(2):63-75

[17] Piato AL et al. Acute restraint stress in zebrafish: Behavioral parameters and purinergic signaling. Neurochemical Research. 2011;**36**(10):1876-1886

[18] Panula P et al. The comparative neuroanatomy and neurochemistry of zebrafish CNS systems of relevance to human neuropsychiatric diseases. Neurobiology of Disease. 2010;**40**(1):46-57

[19] Anichtchik O et al. Distinct structure and activity of monoamine oxidase in the brain of zebrafish (*Danio rerio*). The Journal of Comparative Neurology. 2006;**498**(5):593-610

[20] Baraban SC et al. Pentylenetetrazole induced changes in zebrafish behavior, neural activity and c-fos expression. Neuroscience. 2005;**131**(3):759-768

[21] Fonseka TM et al. Zebrafish models of major depressive disorders. Journal of Neuroscience Research. 2016;**94**(1):3-14

[22] Giacomotto J et al. Developmental suppression of schizophrenia-associated miR-137 alters sensorimotor function in zebrafish. Translational Psychiatry. 2016;**6**:e818

[23] Grone BP et al. Epilepsy, behavioral abnormalities, and physiological comorbidities in Syntaxin-binding protein 1 (STXBP1) mutant Zebrafish. PLoS One. 2016;**11**(3):e0151148

[24] Lee J, Freeman JL. Embryonic exposure to 10 mug L(−1) lead results in female-specific expression changes in genes associated with nervous system development and function and Alzheimer's disease in aged adult zebrafish brain. Metallomics. 2016;**8**(6):589-596

[25] Wood JD et al. Disrupted-in-schizophrenia 1 and neuregulin 1 are required for the specification of oligodendrocytes and neurones in the zebrafish brain. Human Molecular Genetics. 2009;**18**(3):391-404

[26] Ahrens MB et al. Whole-brain functional imaging at cellular resolution using light-sheet microscopy. Nature Methods. 2013;**10**(5):413-420

[27] Vanwalleghem GC, Ahrens MB, Scott EK. Integrative whole-brain neuroscience in larval zebrafish. Current Opinion in Neurobiology. 2018;**50**:136-145

[28] Thomas RJ. The toxicologic and teratologic effects of delta-9-tetrahydrocannabinol in the zebrafish embryo. Toxicology and Applied Pharmacology. 1975;**32**(1):184-190

[29] Lam CS, Rastegar S, Strahle U. Distribution of cannabinoid receptor 1 in the CNS of zebrafish. Neuroscience. 2006;**138**(1):83-95

[30] Migliarini B, Carnevali O. A novel role for the endocannabinoid system during zebrafish development. Molecular and Cellular Endocrinology. 2009;**299**(2):172-177

[31] Oltrabella F et al. Role of the endocannabinoid system in vertebrates: Emphasis on the zebrafish model. Development, Growth & Differentiation. 2017;**59**(4):194-210

[32] Rodriguez-Martin I et al. Characterization of two duplicate zebrafish Cb2-like cannabinoid receptors. Gene. 2007;**389**(1):36-44

[33] Martella A et al. Important role of endocannabinoid signaling in the development of functional vision and locomotion in zebrafish. The FASEB Journal. 2016;**30**(12):4275-4288

[34] Fernandez-Ruiz J et al. The endogenous cannabinoid system and brain development. Trends in Neurosciences. 2000;**23**(1):14-20

[35] Watson S et al. The endocannabinoid receptor, CB1, is required for normal axonal growth and fasciculation. Molecular and Cellular Neurosciences. 2008;**38**(1):89-97

[36] Liu LY et al. Cannabinoid receptor signaling regulates liver development and metabolism. Development. 2016;**143**(4):609-622

[37] Esain V et al. Cannabinoid receptor-2 regulates embryonic hematopoietic stem cell development via prostaglandin E2 and P-selectin activity. Stem Cells. 2015;**33**(8):2596-2612

[38] Kirkham TC et al. Endocannabinoid levels in rat limbic forebrain and hypothalamus in relation to fasting, feeding and satiation: Stimulation of eating by 2-arachidonoyl glycerol. British Journal of Pharmacology. 2002;**136**(4):550-557

[39] Williams CM, Kirkham TC. Anandamide induces overeating: Mediation by central cannabinoid (CB1) receptors. Psychopharmacology. 1999;**143**(3):315-317

[40] Williams CM, Kirkham TC. Reversal of delta 9-THC hyperphagia by SR141716 and naloxone but not dexfenfluramine. Pharmacology, Biochemistry, and Behavior. 2002; **71**(1-2):333-340

[41] Wiley JL et al. CB1 cannabinoid receptor-mediated modulation of food intake in mice. British Journal of Pharmacology. 2005;**145**(3):293-300

[42] Arias Horcajadas F. Cannabinoids in eating disorders and obesity. Molecular Neurobiology. 2007;**36**(1):113-128

[43] Ravinet Trillou C et al. Anti-obesity effect of SR141716, a CB1 receptor antagonist, in diet-induced obese mice. American Journal of Physiology. Regulatory, Integrative and Comparative Physiology. 2003;**284**(2):R345-R353

[44] Di Marzo V. CB(1) receptor antagonism: Biological basis for metabolic effects. Drug Discovery Today. 2008;**13**(23-24):1026-1041

[45] Russo P et al. Genetic variations at the endocannabinoid type 1 receptor gene (CNR1) are associated with obesity phenotypes in men. The Journal of Clinical Endocrinology and Metabolism. 2007;**92**(6):2382-2386

[46] Scheen AJ. CB1 receptor blockade and its impact on cardiometabolic risk factors: Overview of the RIO programme with rimonabant. Journal of Neuroendocrinology. 2008;**20**(Suppl 1):139-146

[47] Ravinet Trillou C et al. CB1 cannabinoid receptor knockout in mice leads to leanness, resistance to diet-induced obesity and enhanced leptin sensitivity. International Journal of Obesity and Related Metabolic Disorders. 2004;**28**(4):640-648

[48] Shimada Y et al. A high-throughput fluorescence-based assay system for appetite-regulating gene and drug screening. PLoS One. 2012;**7**(12):e52549

[49] Piccinetti CC et al. Appetite regulation: The central role of melatonin in *Danio rerio*. Hormones and Behavior. 2010;**58**(5):780-785

[50] Flynn EJ 3rd, Trent CM, Rawls JF. Ontogeny and nutritional control of adipogenesis in zebrafish (*Danio rerio*). Journal of Lipid Research. 2009;**50**(8):1641-1652

[51] Miyares RL, de Rezende VB, Farber SA. Zebrafish yolk lipid processing: A tractable tool for the study of vertebrate lipid transport and metabolism. Disease Models & Mechanisms. 2014;**7**(7):915-927

[52] Schlegel A, Stainier DY. Microsomal triglyceride transfer protein is required for yolk lipid utilization and absorption of dietary lipids in zebrafish larvae. Biochemistry. 2006; **45**(51):15179-15187

[53] Pai WY et al. Cannabinoid receptor 1 promotes hepatic lipid accumulation and lipotoxicity through the induction of SREBP-1c expression in zebrafish. Transgenic Research. 2013;**22**(4):823-838

[54] Fraher D et al. Lipid abundance in Zebrafish embryos is regulated by complementary actions of the endocannabinoid system and retinoic acid pathway. Endocrinology. 2015; **156**(10):3596-3609

[55] Silvestri C et al. Two non-psychoactive cannabinoids reduce intracellular lipid levels and inhibit hepatosteatosis. Journal of Hepatology. 2015;**62**(6):1382-1390

[56] Zanettini C et al. Effects of endocannabinoid system modulation on cognitive and emotional behavior. Frontiers in Behavioral Neuroscience. 2011;**5**:57

[57] Maximino C et al. Measuring anxiety in zebrafish: A critical review. Behavioural Brain Research. 2010;**214**(2):157-171

[58] Bailey JM, Oliveri AN, Levin ED. Pharmacological analyses of learning and memory in zebrafish (*Danio rerio*). Pharmacology, Biochemistry, and Behavior. 2015;**139**(Pt B):103-111

[59] K vF. Uber einen Schreckstoff der Fischhaut und seine biologisehe Bedeutung seine biologisehe Bedeutung. Zeitschrift für Vergleichende Physiologie. 1941;**29**:46-145

[60] Ruhl T et al. Acute administration of THC impairs spatial but not associative memory function in zebrafish. Psychopharmacology. 2014;**231**(19):3829-3842

[61] Nazario LR et al. Caffeine protects against memory loss induced by high and non-anxiolytic dose of cannabidiol in adult zebrafish (*Danio rerio*). Pharmacology, Biochemistry, and Behavior. 2015;**135**:210-216

[62] Lynch ME. Cannabinoids in the management of chronic pain: A front line clinical perspective. Journal of Basic and Clinical Physiology and Pharmacology. 2016;**27**(3):189-191

[63] Lynch ME, Ware MA. Cannabinoids for the treatment of chronic non-Cancer pain: An updated systematic review of randomized controlled trials. Journal of Neuroimmune Pharmacology. 2015;**10**(2):293-301

[64] Savage SR et al. Cannabis in pain treatment: Clinical and research considerations. The Journal of Pain. 2016;**17**(6):654-668

[65] Kondrad E. Medical marijuana for chronic pain. North Carolina Medical Journal. 2013; **74**(3):210-211

[66] Kondrad E, Reid A. Colorado family physicians' attitudes toward medical marijuana. Journal of American Board of Family Medicine. 2013;**26**(1):52-60

[67] Romero-Sandoval EA, Kolano AL, Alvarado-Vazquez PA. Cannabis and cannabinoids for chronic pain. Current Rheumatology Reports. 2017;**19**(11):67

[68] Zogopoulos P et al. The role of endocannabinoids in pain modulation. Fundamental & Clinical Pharmacology. 2013;**27**(1):64-80

[69] Finnerup NB et al. Pharmacotherapy for neuropathic pain in adults: A systematic review and meta-analysis. Lancet Neurology. 2015;**14**(2):162-173

[70] Volkow ND, McLellan AT. Opioid abuse in chronic pain—Misconceptions and mitigation strategies. The New England Journal of Medicine. 2016;**374**(13):1253-1263

[71] Malafoglia V et al. The zebrafish as a model for nociception studies. Journal of Cellular Physiology. 2013;**228**(10):1956-1966

[72] Correia AD et al. A novel behavioral fish model of nociception for testing analgesics. Pharmaceuticals (Basel, Switzerland). 2011;**4**(4):665-680

[73] Curtright A et al. Modeling nociception in zebrafish: A way forward for unbiased analgesic discovery. PLoS One. 2015;**10**(1):e0116766

[74] Gau P et al. The zebrafish ortholog of TRPV1 is required for heat-induced locomotion. The Journal of Neuroscience. 2013;**33**(12):5249-5260

[75] Malafoglia V et al. Extreme thermal noxious stimuli induce pain responses in zebrafish larvae. Journal of Cellular Physiology. 2014;**229**(3):300-308

[76] Maximino C. Modulation of nocicpetive-like behavior in zebrafish by environmental stressors. Psychology & Neuroscience. 2011;**4**(1):149-155

[77] Prober DA et al. Zebrafish TRPA1 channels are required for chemosensation but not for thermosensation or mechanosensory hair cell function. The Journal of Neuroscience. 2008;**28**(40):10102-10110

[78] Reilly SC et al. Behavioural analysis of a nociceptive event in fish: Comparisons between three species demonstrate specific responses. Applied Animal Behaviour Science. 2008; **114**(1-2):248-259

[79] Steenbergen PJ, Bardine N. Antinociceptive effects of buprenorphine in zebrafish larvae: An alternative for rodent models to study pain and nociception? Applied Animal Behaviour Science. 2014;**152**:92-99

[80] Lima MG et al. Nocifensive behavior in adult and larval zebrafish. In: Kalueff AV, Stewart AM, editors. Zebrafish Protocols for Neurobehavioral Research. Totowa, NJ: Humana Press; 2012. pp. 153-166

[81] Taylor JC et al. A novel zebrafish-based model of nociception. Physiology & Behavior. 2017;**174**:83-88

[82] Lopez-Luna J et al. Reduction in activity by noxious chemical stimulation is ameliorated by immersion in analgesic drugs in zebrafish. The Journal of Experimental Biology. 2017;**220**(Pt 8):1451-1458

[83] Ellis LD et al. Comparison of cannabinoids with known analgesics using a novel high throughput zebrafish larval model of nociception. Behavioural Brain Research. 30 Jan 2018;**337**:151-159

[84] Costa B et al. The non-psychoactive cannabis constituent cannabidiol is an orally effective therapeutic agent in rat chronic inflammatory and neuropathic pain. European Journal of Pharmacology. 2007;**556**(1-3):75-83

[85] Hammell DC et al. Transdermal cannabidiol reduces inflammation and pain-related behaviours in a rat model of arthritis. European Journal of Pain. 2016;**20**(6):936-948

[86] Boychuk DG et al. The effectiveness of cannabinoids in the management of chronic nonmalignant neuropathic pain: A systematic review. Journal of Oral & Facial Pain and Headache. 2015;**29**(1):7-14

[87] Voon P, Karamouzian M, Kerr T. Chronic pain and opioid misuse: A review of reviews. Substance Abuse Treatment, Prevention, and Policy. 2017;**12**(1):36

[88] Cressey D. The cannabis experiment. Nature. 2015;**524**(7565):280-283

[89] Lopez-Quintero C et al. Probability and predictors of transition from first use to dependence on nicotine, alcohol, cannabis, and cocaine: Results of the National Epidemiologic Survey on alcohol and related conditions (NESARC). Drug and Alcohol Dependence. 2011;**115**(1-2):120-130

[90] Mathur P, Guo S. Use of zebrafish as a model to understand mechanisms of addiction and complex neurobehavioral phenotypes. Neurobiology of Disease. 2010;**40**(1):66-72

[91] Gerlai R et al. Acute and chronic alcohol dose: Population differences in behavior and neurochemistry of zebrafish. Genes, Brain, and Behavior. 2009;**8**(6):586-599

[92] Petzold AM et al. Nicotine response genetics in the zebrafish. Proceedings of the National Academy of Sciences of the United States of America. 2009;**106**(44):18662-18667

[93] Cachat J et al. Modeling withdrawal syndrome in zebrafish. Behavioural Brain Research. 2010;**208**(2):371-376

[94] Braida D et al. Hallucinatory and rewarding effect of salvinorin a in zebrafish: Kappa-opioid and CB1-cannabinoid receptor involvement. Psychopharmacology. 2007;**190**(4):441-448

[95] Bretaud S et al. A choice behavior for morphine reveals experience-dependent drug preference and underlying neural substrates in developing larval zebrafish. Neuroscience. 2007;**146**(3):1109-1116

[96] Stewart AM et al. Molecular psychiatry of zebrafish. Molecular Psychiatry. 2015;**20**(1):2-17

[97] Kily LJ et al. Gene expression changes in a zebrafish model of drug dependency suggest conservation of neuro-adaptation pathways. The Journal of Experimental Biology. 2008;**211**(Pt 10):1623-1634

[98] Lopez Patino MA et al. Gender differences in zebrafish responses to cocaine withdrawal. Physiology & Behavior. 2008;**95**(1-2):36-47

[99] Mathur P, Lau B, Guo S. Conditioned place preference behavior in zebrafish. Nature Protocols. 2011;**6**(3):338-345

[100] Klee EW et al. Zebrafish: A model for the study of addiction genetics. Human Genetics. Jun 2012;**131**(6):977-1008

[101] Akhtar MT et al. Developmental effects of cannabinoids on zebrafish larvae. Zebrafish. 2013;**10**(3):283-293

[102] Viveros MP, Marco EM, File SE. Endocannabinoid system and stress and anxiety responses. Pharmacology, Biochemistry, and Behavior. 2005;**81**(2):331-342

[103] Ellis LD, Seibert J, Soanes KH. Distinct models of induced hyperactivity in zebrafish larvae. Brain Research. 17 Apr 2012;**1449**:46-59

[104] Stewart A et al. Modeling anxiety using adult zebrafish: A conceptual review. Neuropharmacology. 2012;**62**(1):135-143

[105] Stewart A et al. Pharmacological modulation of anxiety-like phenotypes in adult zebrafish behavioral models. Progress in Neuro-Psychopharmacology & Biological Psychiatry. 1 Aug 2011;**35**(6):1421-1431

[106] Achenbach JC et al. Analysis of the uptake, metabolism, and behavioral effects of cannabinoids on Zebrafish larvae. Zebrafish. 10 Apr 2018. DOI: 10.1089/zeb.2017.1541

[107] Maximino C et al. Scototaxis as anxiety-like behavior in fish. Nature Protocols. 2010; **5**(2):209-216

[108] O'Neil ME et al. Benefits and harms of plant-based Cannabis for posttraumatic stress disorder: A systematic review. Annals of Internal Medicine. 2017;**167**(5):332-340

[109] Caramillo EM et al. Modeling PTSD in the zebrafish: Are we there yet? Behavioural Brain Research. 2015;**276**:151-160

[110] Stewart AM et al. Developing zebrafish models relevant to PTSD and other trauma- and stressor-related disorders. Progress in Neuro-Psychopharmacology & Biological Psychiatry. 2014;**55**:67-79

[111] Grotenhermen F. Pharmacokinetics and pharmacodynamics of cannabinoids. Clinical Pharmacokinetics. 2003;**42**(4):327-360

[112] Devinsky O et al. Trial of Cannabidiol for drug-resistant seizures in the Dravet syndrome. The New England Journal of Medicine. 2017;**376**(21):2011-2020

[113] Abrams DI. The therapeutic effects of Cannabis and cannabinoids: An update from the National Academies of sciences, engineering and medicine report. European Journal of Internal Medicine. 2018;**49**:7-11

[114] Perucca E. Cannabinoids in the treatment of epilepsy: Hard evidence at last? Journal of Epilepsy Research. 2017;**7**(2):61-76

[115] Cunliffe VT. Building a zebrafish toolkit for investigating the pathobiology of epilepsy and identifying new treatments for epileptic seizures. Journal of Neuroscience Methods. 2016;**260**:91-95

[116] Burgess HA, Granato M. Modulation of locomotor activity in larval zebrafish during light adaptation. The Journal of Experimental Biology. 2007;**210**(Pt 14):2526-2539

[117] Kim YH et al. Reduced neuronal proliferation by proconvulsant drugs in the developing zebrafish brain. Neurotoxicology and Teratology. 2010;**32**(5):551-557

[118] Joshi M, Joshi A, Bartter T. Marijuana and lung diseases. Current Opinion in Pulmonary Medicine. 2014;**20**(2):173-179

[119] Ware MA et al. Cannabis for the management of pain: Assessment of safety study (COMPASS). The Journal of Pain. 2015;**16**(12):1233-1242

[120] Padilla S et al. Zebrafish developmental screening of the ToxCast phase I chemical library. Reproductive Toxicology. 2011;**33**(2):174-187

[121] Sipes NS, Padilla S, Knudsen TB. Zebrafish: As an integrative model for twenty-first century toxicity testing. Birth Defects Research. Part C, Embryo Today. 2011;**93**(3):256-267

[122] Peterson RT, Macrae CA. Systematic approaches to toxicology in the zebrafish. Annual Review of Pharmacology and Toxicology. 2012;**52**:433-453

[123] Massarsky A et al. Teratogenic, bioenergetic, and behavioral effects of exposure to total particulate matter on early development of zebrafish (*Danio rerio*) are not mimicked by nicotine. Neurotoxicology and Teratology. 2015;**51**:77-88

[124] Folkesson M et al. Differences in cardiovascular toxicities associated with cigarette smoking and snuff use revealed using novel zebrafish models. Biology Open. 2016; **5**(7):970-978

[125] Mehmedic Z et al. Potency trends of Delta9-THC and other cannabinoids in confiscated cannabis preparations from 1993 to 2008. Journal of Forensic Sciences. 2010; **55**(5):1209-1217

[126] McCarroll MN et al. Leveraging large-scale behavioral profiling in Zebrafish to explore neuroactive polypharmacology. ACS Chemical Biology. 2016;**11**(4):842-849

Chapter 3

Structural Insights from Recent CB1 X-Ray Crystal Structures

Rufaida Al-Zoubi, Dow P. Hurst and
Patricia H. Reggio

Additional information is available at the end of the chapter

http://dx.doi.org/10.5772/intechopen.80783

Abstract

Over the past 2 years, X-ray crystal structures of the antagonist- and agonist-bound CB1 receptor have been reported. Such structures are expected to accelerate progress in the understanding of CB1 and should provide an exceptional starting point for structure-based drug discovery. This chapter examines the consistency of these X-ray structures with the CB1 experimental literature, including mutation, NMR and covalent labeling studies. These comparisons reveal discrepancies between this literature and the TMH1-2-3 region of each CB1 crystal structure. The chapter also examines crystal packing issues with each X-ray structure and shows that the discrepancies with the experimental literature can be attributed to crystal packing problems that force the N-terminus deep in the binding pocket of the two inactive state structures and force TMH2 to bend at G2.53/S2.54 and invade the binding pocket in the activated state structure. Revision is advisable before these structures are used for structure-based drug discovery.

Keywords: cannabinoid CB1 receptor, CB1 mutation, CB1 cross-linking, CB1 nuclear magnetic resonance, crystal packing

1. Introduction

The cannabinoid receptor type 1 (CB1) belongs to the G-protein coupled receptors (GPCRs) superfamily. GPCRs comprise the largest group of integral membrane proteins that mediate cellular responses to a wide spectrum of signaling molecules including peptides, lipids, neurotransmitters, glycoproteins, as well as light, taste and odor substances. They act via coupling and activating intracellular effector proteins including G-proteins and arrestins leading to an array of intracellular signaling cascades.

GPCRs have a common architecture of seven transmembrane helices (TMHs) joined by extracellular (EC) and intracellular (IC) loops of varied lengths, in addition to an extracellularly extending N terminus, and an intracellular C terminus that begins with an amphipathic alpha helical segment (Helix 8) oriented parallel to the cell membrane. In Class A GPCRs, the binding site for the endogenous ligand is generally formed by the EC core within the TMH bundle, and may extend to EC loops, referred to as the orthosteric binding site. Ligands may also bind to distinct (allosteric) binding sites in the receptor.

Due to the various physiological functions mediated by GPCRs, they are considered major targets for drug discovery and design of novel therapeutics. However, understanding the structure-function relationship of these proteins and the design of high affinity, selective ligands that target these receptors requires a detailed knowledge of the three-dimensional structure of the receptor in general and of the ligand binding site in specific. However, structural characterization for membrane proteins in general has been a challenge due to their low expression in recombinant hosts and their inherent instability in surfactants. It was not until the year 2000 that the first high resolution GPCR structure was resolved by X-ray crystallography, Rhodopsin in its inactive state [1]. The following 10 years witnessed the release of other inactive state crystal structures of class A GPCRs (e.g. the Adenosine A2A, and the β1 and β2 adrenergic receptors [2–4]), in addition to the release of the active state crystal structure of Rhodopsin in complex with a synthetic peptide resembling the C-terminus of the G-alpha subunit of transducing [5]. Available structures during that time served as templates for homology modeling for other GPCRs including the CB1 receptor. And parallel with biophysical studies, available crystal structures provided structural insights for their activation mechanism. A breakthrough in GPCR structural characterization has been achieved in the last 8 years with more than 200 structures for different GPCRs being deposited in the Protein Data Bank, including the CB1 inactive and active state crystal structures which have been resolved in 2016, and in 2017 respectively [6–8]. Before that, structural characterization of CB1 orthosteric as well as allosteric binding domains have been extensively studied via mutations, site-directed labeling, mass spectrometry, SAR studies, and in-silico methods, and will be discussed in detail throughout this chapter.

2. Structural divergence of the cannabinoid receptors from class A GPCRs

The CB1 receptor is a class A (Rhodopsin-like) GPCR (**Figure 1**). Different phylogenetic studies and multidimensional scaling analysis of Class A GPCRs classify cannabinoid receptors (CB1/CB2) into one cluster along with the endothelial differentiation G-protein coupled receptors (EDGRs) (including Sphingosine 1-phosphate receptors (S1P) and Lysophosphatidic acid receptors (LPA)) [9–12]. Receptors from those families, except for the LPA_{4-6}, share common sequence divergence from other Class A GPCRs. Specifically, the absence of helix kinking proline residues in TMH2 and TMH5, and the absence of a disulfide bridge between the EC-2 loop and C3.25 at the EC end of TMH3. Instead, they share an internal disulfide bridge in the EC-2 loop, a conserved PxxGW motif at the EC end of TMH4, in addition to a Y5.39 that forms an aromatic pi-pi stack with W4.64 in that motif resulting in a similar shape of the EC2 loop as seen in the crystal structures for the CB1, $S1P_1$, and LPA_1 receptors [6, 7, 13, 14]. At the

http://dx.doi.org/10.5772/intechopen.80783

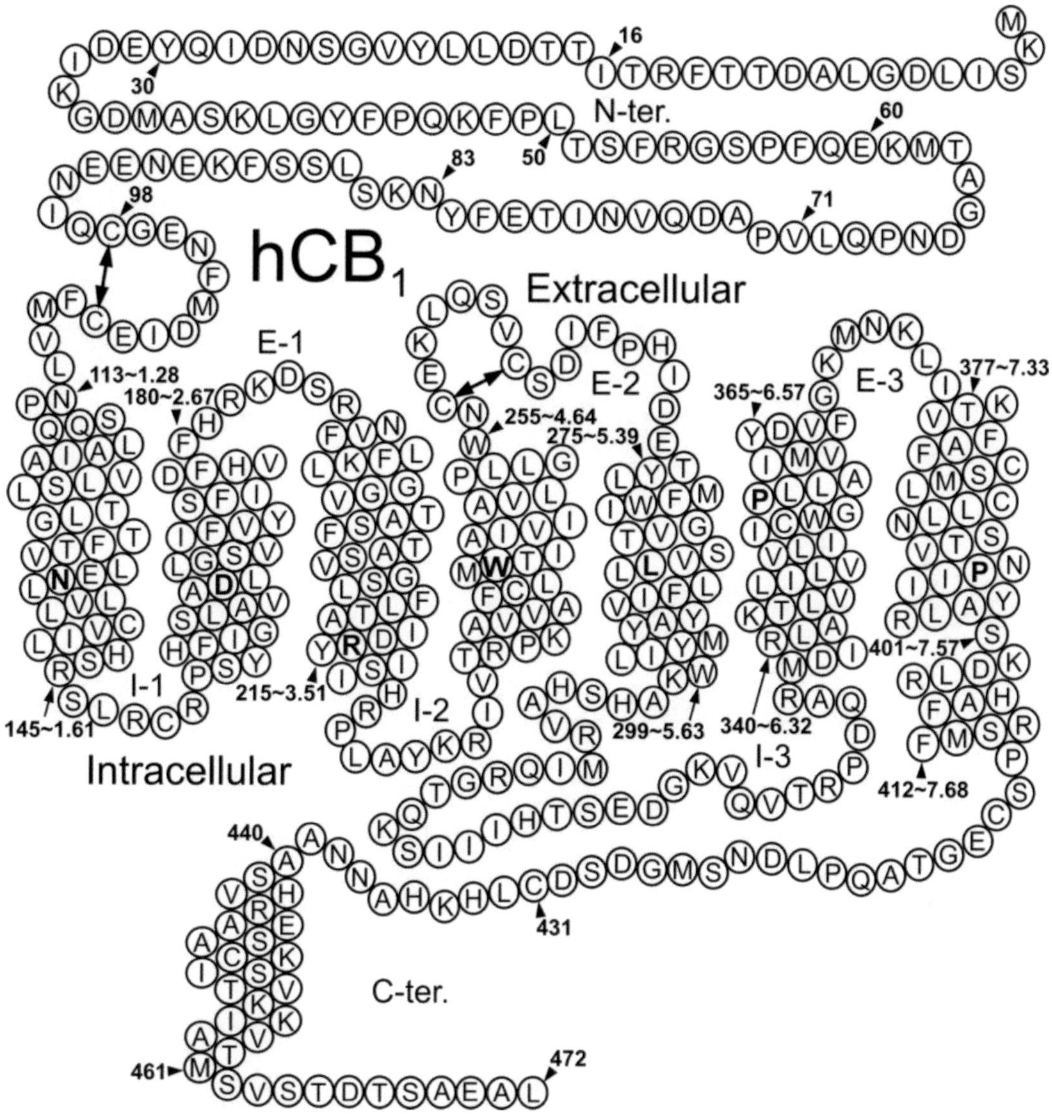

Figure 1. Helix net representation of the hCB1 receptor. The most highly conserved residue in each helix is shown in bold. Residues are numbered using the BW#: Ballesteros-Weinstein residue numbering system in GPCRs which uses the X.YY format; X denotes the transmembrane helix number and (YY) denotes residue position relative to the most conserved residue in the helix (X.50). Loop regions are numbered using absolute sequence numbers.

binding site, they share a common basic residue (K/R 3.28) on TMH3 and an aromatic residue (F/Y 2.57) on TMH2. In addition, the S1P receptors are like CB1/CB2 in the presence of E1.49 at TMH1. E1.49 has been reported to be a key interaction site for pregnenolone (an endogenous negative allosteric modulator that protects the brain from *cannabis* intoxication) with CB1 [15], while the LPA_{1-3} receptors share a W5.43 with CB1/CB2 that has been shown to affect antagonist binding to the cannabinoid receptors [16]. In addition, $S1P_1$, and the cannabinoid receptors recognize lipid-derived ligands that have been shown to bind to the receptor by diffusing from bulk lipid towards the binding site via a transmembrane portal [6, 7, 14, 17, 18].

3. CB1 receptor crystal structures

Two inactive state crystal structures for the hCB1 receptor have been resolved. The first structure (PDB ID: 5TGZ) was resolved at 2.8 Å; the receptor was truncated at both the N-terminus (1–98) and the C-terminus (415–472), with a flavodoxin protein fused into the IC3 loop (V306, P332), the receptor was crystalized in complex with a biaryl-pyrazole derivative (AM6358, **Figure 2**) and using thermo-stabilizing mutations (T3.46A, E5.37K, T5.47V, and R6.32E) [6]. The second structure was resolved at 2.6 Å (PDB ID: 5U09) in complex with an acyclic high affinity inverse agonist of the CB1 receptor, taranabant (**Figure 2**) [7]. In this structure, fewer amino acid residues were truncated from the N-terminus (1–76) and the C-terminus (422–472), and *P. abysii* glycogen synthase protein was fused into the IC3 loop (A301, D333) of a single point mutant (T3.46A) hCB1 receptor [7]. In both structures, resolved residues were from E100 at the N-terminus to F412 at the C-terminus of the receptor.

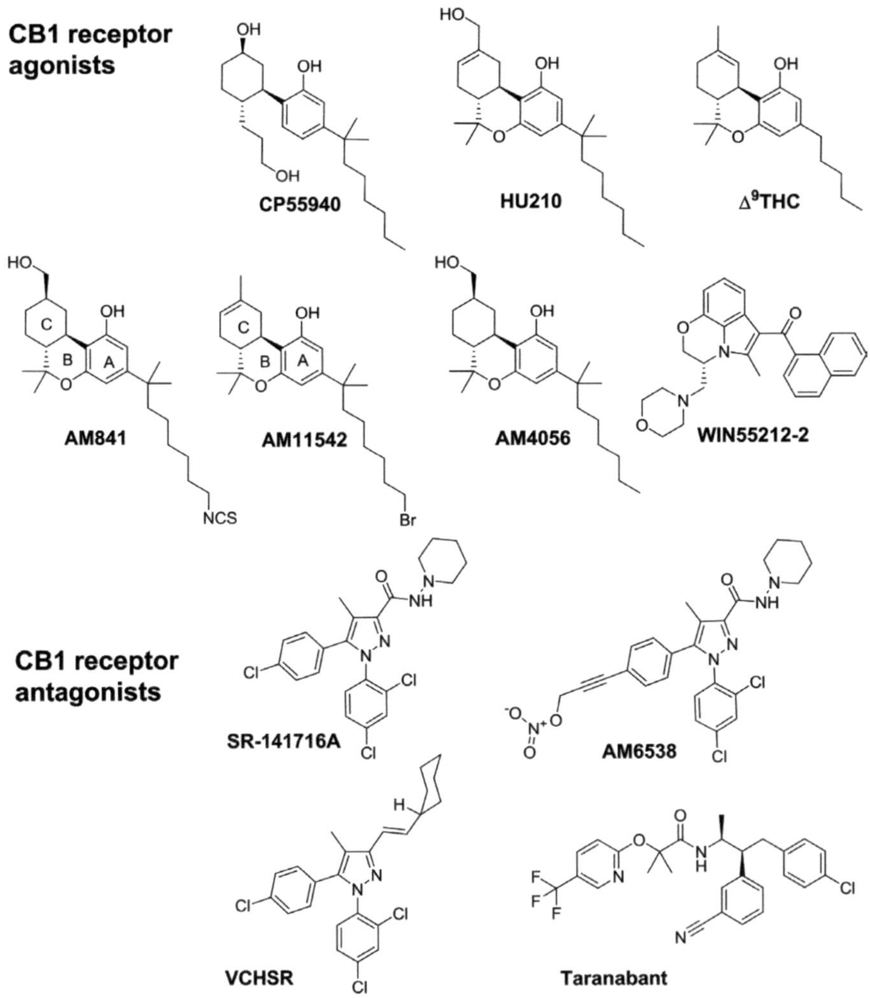

Figure 2. Compounds discussed in this chapter.

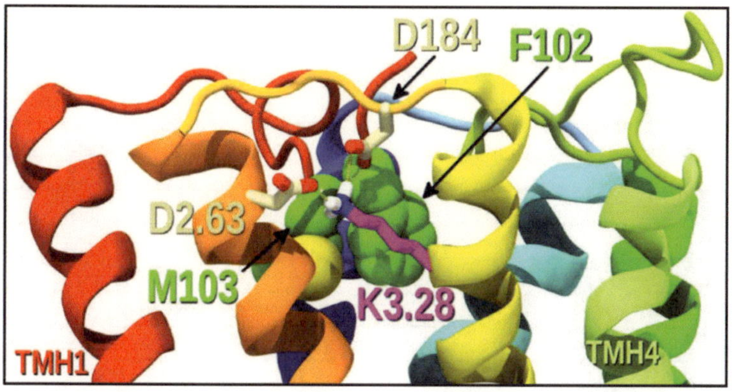

Figure 3. N-terminus residues F102 and M103 (green VdW) penetrate the binding crevice in the inactive state CB1 structure (PDB ID: 5U09. This influences the positions of K3.28 (magenta tube), D2.63 and D184 (wheat tube) which form an interaction with each other.

Agonist bound hCB1 crystal structures (PDB IDs: 5XRA, 5XR8) were resolved at 2.80 and 2.95 Å resolution and in complex with the classical cannabinoids (AM11542, AM841) respectively (**Figure 2**). The receptor was constructed in a similar way to the AM6358-bound crystal structure. Resolved residues included D104-S414 and F102-S414 in the 2.80 and 2.95 Å resolution structures respectively [8].

Inactive state CB1 structures show a transmembrane portal for antagonist entry between TMH1 and TMH7 that is similar to the $S1P_1$ structure. However, the membrane proximal region in the CB1 receptor forms a loop that extends towards the orthosteric binding site with two amino acid residues (F102, M103) invading unpredictably the binding site in the inactive state structures and forming Van der Waal (VDW) interactions with the antagonists (**Figure 3**) [6, 7].

Active state structures show characteristic conformational changes featuring class A GPCR activation including an outward movement and a counterclockwise rotation (EC view) of the IC end of TMH6, resulting in a break in the R3.50/D6.30 inactive state "ionic lock" [19, 20]. Unlike inactive state structures, a transmembrane portal is not present in active state structures due to the packing of the EC domain of TMH1 towards TMH7. In addition, the N-terminus resides at the top of the receptor with no invasion of the orthosteric binding site. On the other hand, the active state binding site displays a profound (53%) reduction in size that is resulting from an inward kink of the EC domain of TMH2 towards the orthosteric binding site, as well as, rotation of TMH3 towards TMH2 [8].

4. Mutation and labeling studies on CB1: consistency with CB1 crystal structures

Multiple mutation studies on either mCB1 or hCB1 were aimed to study the receptor's binding site and to identify key residues for CB1 receptor activation (**Figure 4**). While different ligands where used in functional and binding affinity assessment, WIN55212, SR141716A and CP55940, were used primarily, due to the availability of tritiated versions of these compounds.

ref.	residue	BW/#	mutation	CP55	HU210	THC	SR	TARA	AM841
38	P	1.29	GA	a			a		
38	S	1.30	A	a			a		
38	Q	1.31	A	a			a		
32	F	2.57	L					b	
64	S	2.60	A	b	b		b		
44, 45	F	2.61	A	a	a	a	a		
35	I	2.62	T	b	b		b		
35	D	2.63	N	b	b		b		
35	D	2.63	E	b					
37	D	2.63	A	a			a		
45	F	2.64	A	a	a	a			
38	H	181	A	a			a		
38	R	182	A	a			a		
38	K	183	A	a			a		
38	D	184	A	a			a		
38	V	3.24	A	a			a		
38, 46	F	3.25	A	a,b			a		
22	K	3.28	R	b					
22	K	3.28	Q	b					
22	K	3.28	E	b					
21, 29	K	3.28	A	c	c		a		
32	K	3.28	L				a	b	
44, 45	L	3.29	A	a	a	a	a		
44	T	3.33	A				a		
32, 46, 57, 58	F	3.36	A	b			b		
57	F	3.36	L	b			b	b	

ref.	residue	BW/#	mutation	CP55	HU210	THC	SR	TARA	AM841
60	N	256	A	b					
60	E	258	A	b					
60	K	259	A	b					
60	L	260	A	b					
60	Q	261	A	b					
60	S	262	A	b					
60	V	263	A	b					
60	S	265	A	b					
60	D	266	A	b					
60	I	267	A	b					
60	F	268	Y	b			a		
60	F	268	W	a,b	a		a		
60	F	268	A	b			a		
60	F	268	N	b			a		
60	P	269	A	a,b	a		a		
60	H	270	A	a,b	a		a		
60	I	271	A	a,b	a		a		
60	D	272	A	b					
47	Y	5.39	F	b		b	b		
47	Y	5.39	I	b					
46	W	5.43	A	b			b	b	
59, 61	C	6.47	A	b		b	a		b
61	C	6.47	S	b		b			b
61	C	6.47	L	b		b			b
46	W	6.48	A	b			b		
44, 45	M	6.55	A	a	a	a	a		
37	K	373	A	a			a		
44	F	7.35	A				a		
59	C	7.38	A	b			a		
32, 57, 64	S	7.39	A	b,c	c		c	a	
59	C	7.42	A	b			a		
59	C	7.42	M	b			a,b		

Key

- more than 100
- 50-100
- 25-50
- 10-25
- 5-10
- ≤5
- NS
- increased

- a,b different affinity results determined against SR or CP
- b no binding up to 75nM
- a,b different affinity results between species
- a against SR14176a
- b against CP55,940
- c against WIN55,212

Figure 4. Mutations in or near the binding crevice of the CB1 receptor. The key represents changes in binding affinities of ligands to mutant CB1 receptor compared to WT. Residues are numbered using Ballesteros-Weinstein numbers. See **Figure 1** for more details.

Other ligands characterized include HU210, Δ9-THC, taranabant, and AM251. The discussion here will be focused on mutation and labeling studies near the orthosteric binding site and those affecting crystalized ligands or closely related structures such as SR141716A, HU201, or CP55940 (**Figure 2**).

4.1. K3.28 residue

One of the earliest mutational studies on the CB1 receptor targeted K3.28 [21, 22]. The lipophilic nature of CB1 ligands and the fact that the third TMH in CB1 has a V3.32 instead of an acidic residue at that position (as being conserved in aminergic receptors), directed the attention towards K3.28 to investigate its role in ligand binding.

Song and Bonner first reported that the binding of CP55940, HU210, and anandamide to a K3.28A mutant hCB1 expressed in HEK293 cells resulted in severe impairment, with more than 100-fold decrease in their potencies in inhibiting cAMP accumulation. On the other hand, the binding and the potency of WIN55212 at the K3.28A mutant receptor were comparable to WT, suggesting that the receptor is still functioning [21]. Shortly afterwards, Kendall's Lab demonstrated retained binding affinity and potency for CP55940 in CHO cells expressing K3.28R hCB1 mutant, with no binding for up to 75 nM concentration in cells expressing K3.28Q or K3.28E mutants compared to cells expressing WT receptor (K_d = 7.7 ± 3.5 nM). In the same study, WIN55212 displayed comparable affinity for the three mutants with more than one order of magnitude decrease in potency in the K3.28E mutant, while its potency in K3.28Q mutant was not determined due to low receptor density [22]. A significant loss of CP55940's potency in stimulating [^{35}S]GTPγS binding in HEK293 cells expressing the K3.28A hCB1 mutant were also reported where the EC_{50} values for the WT and the mutant receptor were 1.3 and 225 nM respectively [23].

Results suggested that the loss of potencies of anandamide, and the classical and non-classical cannabinoids, but not WIN55212 at the K3.28A mutant is due to their low affinities to the receptor, and a basic residue at 3.28 is required for CP55940 binding. Based on mutation data, modeling studies suggested a hydrogen bond interaction between K3.28 and the amide oxygen of anandamide [16, 24], and with classical and non-classical cannabinoids [25–27]. While Shim argued later that K3.28 is important for stabilizing the binding site for the endocannabinoids and the classical and non-classical cannabinoids and not directly involved in their binding [28].

K3.28 mutations have also been demonstrated to affect affinities and deactivation profile of biaryl-pyrazole derivatives. The affinity of SR141716A to K3.28A hCB1 mutant has been reported to be 17-fold lower compared to the WT [29]. In addition, SR141716A was reported to act as neutral antagonist with loss of ability to turn off receptor's basal activity in inhibiting Ca^{2+} currents in SCG neurons microinjected with K3.28A hCB1 mutant cDNA [30]. This data prompted a mutant cycle study using an SR141716A analog (VCHSR) to test the hypothesis that an interaction between the carboxamide oxygen in SR141716A and K3.28 is essential for its inverse agonist activity. The results supported the hypothesis by demonstrating that VCHSR acts as neutral antagonist with comparable affinities to both K3.28A and WT receptor [29]. A set of SR141716A analogues were also designed later that support the hypothesis [31]. A K3.28L mutation at hCB1 has been also reported to lower the binding affinity of AM251 by 17-fold compared to the WT, while it had no effect on the affinity of the acyclic antagonist, taranabant, to the receptor [32]. The discriminatory effect of K3.28 mutants on different classes of antagonists may suggest different binding interactions within the receptor's binding site, especially that taranabant acts also as an inverse agonist [33].

CB1 crystal structures, on the other hand, do not support proposed hydrogen bonding of ligands to K3.28. In both inactive state and the active state structures of CB1, K3.28 orients its side chain towards the TMH2/3 interface forming salt bridges with D184 in the EC1 loop and D2.63 at the top of TMH2. The K3.28/D2.63 interaction is only noticeable in the inactive state crystal structures (**Figure 3**).

4.2. D2.63 mutations

As described above, this residue forms a salt bridge with K3.28 in the inactive state crystal structures (**Figure 4**). This K3.28/D2.63 salt bridge has been previously proposed to be essential for CB1 basal activity [34]. However, an earlier study on K3.28A mutant reported a comparable basal activity to the WT receptor in inhibiting Ca^{2+} currents which does not support the role of K3.28/D2.63 salt bridge in controlling receptor's basal activity [30]. Individual effects of D2.63 mutation on ligand binding and receptor activation have been also reported. In HEK293 cells expressing a D2.63N hCB1 mutant, binding affinities for the classical cannabinoid (HU210), non-classical cannabinoid (CP55940), and the amino alkyl indole (WIN55212) were not significantly different from WT, while the affinity for SR141716A was 5-fold decreased compared to the WT. In addition, the potencies of CP55940 and HU210 in stimulating [^{35}S] GTPγS binding were significantly different from WT with about 12-fold increase in their EC_{50} values, while the basal activity of the D2.63N mutant was not different from WT [35]. In a different study, a double hCB1 mutant (L3.43A/D2.63A) was shown to lower the affinity of CP55940 to the receptor by 7-fold, while increasing the affinity of SR141716A by 3-fold. The L3.43A single mutant had an opposite effect by increasing the affinity of CP55940 to the receptor by 6-fold and lowering the affinity of SR141716A by 7-fold. Knowing that L3.43A mutation has been shown to increase the basal signaling of CB1 receptor in stimulating [^{35}S] GTPγS binding, combining D2.63A with L3.43A mutation lowered the basal signaling below CB1 WT levels. Results suggest that D2.63 may be involved in receptor activation and that mutation into alanine stabilizes the inactive state of the receptor [34, 36]. A modeling and mutation study suggested that an ionic interaction between D2.63 and K373 in the EC-3 loop is important for receptor activation. In the study, a reciprocal mutant D2.63K/K373D resulted in similar potencies for CP55940 and WIN55212 in stimulation for [^{35}S]GTPγS compared to the WT receptor, while their potencies were more than 5-fold lower in the single and double alanine mutants [37]. Such an interaction is not present in the crystal structures.

4.3. Mutation studies on the CB1 N-terminus

The CB1 receptor is unique in having a relatively long (114 amino-acid residues) N-terminus compared to other class A GPCRs. Analysis of the amino acid sequence of the membrane proximal region (MPR) of the amino terminus reveals a remarkably high degree of conservation in that region (**Figure 5**).

Early studies on the N-terminus reported no effect on prolylglycine insertion in the N-terminus (at A73, L86, and E100) of hCB1 receptor expressed in HEK 293T cells on agonist (CP55940) and antagonist (SR141716A) binding. In addition, S1.30A and Q1.31A mutants at the N-terminal

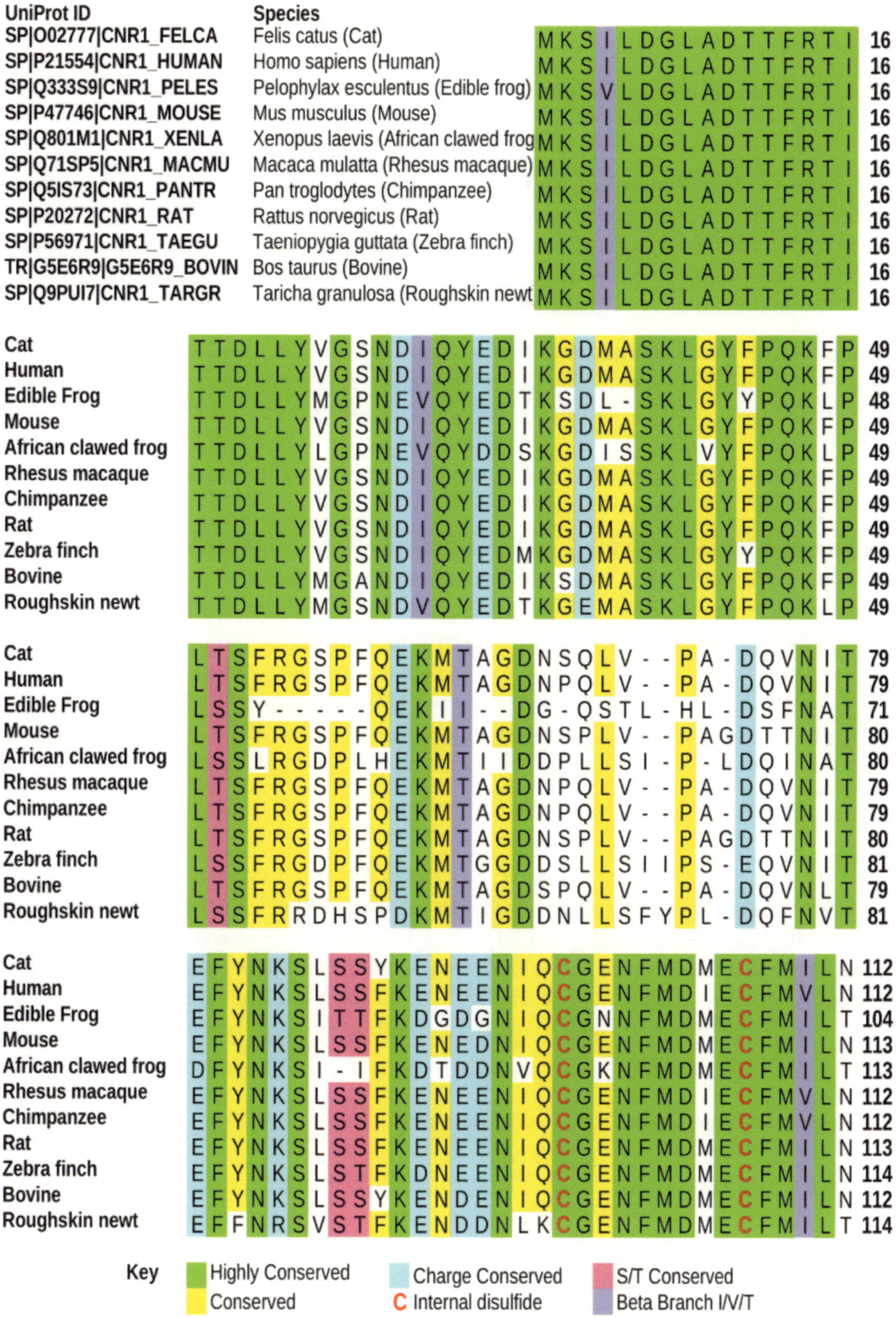

Figure 5. Sequence alignment of the CB1 N-terminus of 11 different species downloaded from the UniProt online database (www.uniprot.org).

end of TMH1 did not affect the binding affinity for SR141716A, while they reduced the binding affinity of CP55940 by 5- and 10-fold respectively [38].

In addition, CP55940 binding to truncated receptor at the N-terminal region (Δ64, Δ80, Δ89, Δ103 shCB1) was comparable to the WT receptor [39, 40]. On the other hand, the binding affinity of SR141716A to the Δ103 synthetic hCB1 (shCB1) truncation mutant was higher compared to the WT with retained ability to inhibit basal signaling of the truncated mutant [39]. As described earlier, in the (inactive state CB1 X-ray crystal structures, two amino acid residues from the N-terminus occupy the receptor's orthosteric binding site, forming strong VDW interactions with the antagonists, those are F102, M103. Affinity data of SR141716A to the Δ103 shCB1 truncation mutant is inconsistent with the inactive state crystal structures.

Reduction of the proposed disulfide bridge at the N-terminus C98/C107 reduces CP55940 potency in [^{35}S]GTPγS binding assay [39]. However, a previous study reported that a double mutant of the two cysteine residues into serine subtly affected CP55940 binding, but did not affect SR141716A binding [41]. It is worth-mentioning that the C98/C107 residues are conserved among all 11-CB1 species available from UniProt. This sulfide bridge is not apparent in crystal structures.

Interestingly, a recent mutational, and modeling study from the Kunos lab identified an N-terminal residue (M106 in rodent CB1 compared to I105 in hCB1) as the determinant of the species differential affinity of {5-(4-chlorophenyl)-N-{(1R,2R)-2-hydroxycyclohexyl}-6-(2-methoxyethoxy)-3-pyridinecarboxamide} (14 h) at the CB1 receptor [42]. The compound, has been described previously as a peripherally selective, high affinity CB1 receptor antagonist [43]. However, this compound has been shown to have higher affinity for the hCB1 receptor compared to mouse and rat CB1 receptor [42]. This residue faces the ligand binding site in crystal structures, but with a changed position in the different structures.

4.4. EC1 loop

Mutations of the EC1 loop negatively impacted CP55940 but not SR141716A binding, the K_i value of CP55940 was 26-fold higher in D184A hCB1 mutant compared to the WT receptor expressed in HEK293 cells. Here, the K_i was determined by competition binding against [^{3}H]SR141716A [38]. This aspartate residue forms an ionic interaction with K3.28 in both the active and inactive state CB1 crystal structures (**Figure 3**) [6–8]. H181A, R182A, and K183A have also lowered CP55940 affinity by 3–4-fold compared with the WT [38]. None of the EC1 loop residues forms direct contact with crystallized ligands.

4.5. Aromatic residues lining the orthosteric binding site

The orthosteric binding site of CB1 is lined with multiple aromatic residues located on TMH2/3/5/6/7, as well as, F286 in the EC2 loop.

4.5.1. F2.57, F2.61, and F2.64

F2.57 is two turns extracellular to the conserved D2.50, facing the orthosteric binding site. In the inactive state CB1 crystal structures, this residue has been shown to form an aromatic π-π stack with the 2,4-dichlorophenyl ring in AM6538 [6], and with the cyanophenyl ring in taranabant [7]. Mutation data show a reduced affinity for taranabant and AM251 (a diarylpyrazole antagonist) by 30- and 97-fold respectively in F2.57L hCB1 mutant [32]. In addition, both SR141716A and AM6538 failed to antagonize 100 nM CP55940-induced inhibition of cAMP in F2.57A hCB1 mutant while preserving their abilities in F2.57W hCB1 mutant [6]. Results indicate a major role for this residue in antagonist binding via aromatic interactions and in shaping the antagonist binding site. On the other hand, while this residue shows a major contact with the agonists (A-ring, **Figure 2**) in the AM11542 and the AM841 bound crystal structures, [8] CP55940 displayed similar potency for inhibition of cAMP in both F2.57A, and F2.57W mutants compared to WT [8].

Mutations on F2.61 revealed effects on antagonist and agonist binding and potencies. In the inactive state CB1 structures, this residue is rotated towards TMH1 and its side chain is at the TMH1/TMH2 interface, yet it forms moderate VDW interactions with the piperidine and with the trifluoro-methyl pyridine in AM6538 and taranabant respectively [6, 7]. While in the active state structures, this residue faces the binding site and forms strong VDW interactions with the agonists (AM11542 and AM841) B-ring (**Figure 2**) [8]. SR141716A displayed only 5-fold higher K_d value in F2.61A hCB1 mutant transiently expressed in HEK293 cells [44], but both SR141716A and AM6538 failed to antagonize 100 nM CP55940-induced inhibition of cAMP in F2.61A mutant while preserving their potencies in F2.61W mutant (mutations were on hCB1, and functional assays were done in stably transfected CHO cells) [6]. Also, CP55940 displayed similar potency in both F2.61A and F2.61W in inhibition of cAMP compared to the hCB1 WT stably transfected in CHO cells, [8] while the binding affinities for CP55940, HU210, and Δ9-THC determined against [^{3}H]SR141716A were severely affected by F2.61A mutation transiently transfected in HEK293 cells [45]. In the same study, the potency of HU210 in inducing [^{35}S]GTPγS binding has been reported to be 30-fold less in F2.61A hCB1 mutant compared to the WT [45].

The F2.64A mutation has also been shown to be detrimental for agonists (HU210, CP55940, and Δ9-THC) binding [45]. CP55940, AM841, and AM11542 displayed about an order of magnitude lower potency in inhibition of forskolin-stimulated cAMP in CHO cells expressing the mutant receptor [8]. In crystal structures, this residue forms major contacts with the agonists' (C-ring, **Figure 2**) [8], and does not display any contact with the antagonists due to the presence of the N-terminus [6, 7], and no mutation data are available to characterize antagonists binding or potency in this mutant.

4.5.2. F3.25

Different studies determined binding affinity of CP55940 to F3.25A mutant; in one study, the binding affinity of CP55940 determined by saturation binding against [^{3}H]SR141716A was 60-fold lower in F3.25A hCB1 stably transfected in CHO-K1 cells compared to WT [38]. In other studies, CP55940 affinity was not affected in F3.25A mCB1 mutant receptor stably transfected into HEK293 cells, affinity was determined using [^{3}H]CP55940 [16, 46]. The discrepancy in binding affinities here could be due to species differences. F3.25A did not affect SR141616A binding in those studies [16, 38, 46]. Basal [^{35}S]GTPγS binding was also determined for the F3.25A mCB1 mutant stably transfected in HEK293 cells and was not significant from WT, while the WIN55212-2 induced [^{35}S]GTPγS binding was lower in the mutant with EC_{50} value being 6-fold higher compared to the WT. In crystal structures, this residue shows moderate VDW interactions with the crystallized agonists (C-ring, **Figure 2**) [8], and no direct interactions with the antagonists [6, 7].

4.5.3. Y5.39, W5.43

Y5.39 is a conserved residue in many class A GPCRs. In the active state crystal structures, Y5.39 interacts with the agonists and forms a hydrogen bond interaction with the isothiocyanate moiety in AM841. Mutation data published along with the crystal structures show that mutation of this residue in hCB1 into phenylalanine or alanine results in significant reduction in the potencies of CP55940, AM841, and AM11542 in the inhibition of forskolin-induced cAMP, with pEC_{50} values for CP55940 being 8.3 ± 0.15 for the WT and 6.7 ± 0.13 and 5.4 ± 0.95 for the Y5.39F and Y5.39A mutants respectively [8]. Efficacy data for CP55940 are consistent with previous report from Abood's Lab [47]. In this report, WIN55212-2 has been shown to retain its WT potency in the Y5.39F mutant. In addition, the Y5.39F hCB1 mutant generally retained WT binding affinities for CP55940, Δ9-THC, WIN55212-2, and SR141716A and resulted in 17-fold lower K_i value for anandamide. On the other hand, Y5.39I hCB1 mutant resulted in loss of ligand binding. Authors concluded that aromaticity is required at this position [47]. Results from Abood's lab suggest that aromaticity is required for ligand binding generally, while the phenolic ring is required for signal transduction for classical and non-classical cannabinoids.

The W5.43A mutation in mCB1 was detrimental for the binding of SR141716A [16, 46], this mutation also negatively affected the binding affinity of AM251 to the mutant hCB1 with 54-fold lower affinity, while it resulted in only 7-fold lower affinity for taranabant [32]. This mutant resulted in 16-fold reduction in affinity of WIN55212-2, but did not affect either CP55940 or anandamide binding [16, 46]. The potency of CP55940 in stimulation of [^{35}S]GTPγS, however, was 66-fold lower in the mutant receptor compared to the WT, while the basal [^{35}S]GTPγS binding for the W5.43A mutant being comparable to WT [46]. In active state crystal structures, this residue forms strong VDW interaction with AM841 and AM11542 aliphatic tails. In inactive state structures, the residue forms moderate VDW interactions with the 4-chlorophenyl ring in taranabant and the aliphatic chain-substituted phenyl ring in AM6538, an interaction that is inconsistent with the mutation data which suggests that W5.43 stabilizes the binding site of the antagonists, rather than being a strong interaction site with the antagonists.

4.5.4. W6.48, F3.36: the rotamer toggle switch

W6.48 belongs to the conserved CWXP hinge motif in TMH6. A W6.48 $\chi 1$ rotameric state change from g+ to trans has been proposed to be the binding pocket trigger for the hinge motion of TMH6 that occurs during receptor activation. Here the IC end of TMH6 moves away from the TMH bundle, providing an opening into which the alpha-5 helix of the G-protein can insert [48–52]. This rotameric change is manifest for class A GPCRs in Molecular Dynamics (MD) simulations [18, 53–55], even though available active state crystal structures of class A GPCRs do not show evidence for this rotameric change. The W6.48A mCB1 mutation resulted in a 7-fold increase in binding affinity (K_i) of SR141716A compared to the WT receptor, while it had no effect on the dissociation constant of CP55940 [16, 46]. In the CB1 crystal structures, only antagonists show mild VDW interaction with W6.48.

Computational modeling and mutation studies targeting F3.36 in CB1 receptor suggested that the F3.36/W6.48 interaction represents a toggle switch that stabilizes the inactive state of the receptor [46, 56]. Consistent with the inactive and active state CB1 crystal structures, the modeling study suggested that F3.36/W6.48 contact is broken during activation with a rotameric change of the $\chi 1$ dihedral of F3.36 from trans in the inactive state to g+ upon activation. The F3.36A CB1 mutation resulted in increased basal signaling of the receptor and did not affect the CP55940 dissociation constant, but reduced the binding affinity of SR141716A [16, 46, 57, 58]. An F3.36L mutation generally restored the binding affinity of SR141716A to the receptor [57]. In a different study, the F3.36L mutation resulted in a 7- and 9-fold lower binding affinities for taranabant and AM251 respectively [32]. In the CB1 crystal structures, only agonists show mild VDW interaction with F3.36 via their dimethyl substituent. Thus, the reduction in the binding affinity of SR141716A to the F3.36A mutant could be a result of shifting the equilibrium towards active state.

While the rotameric change of F3.36 only and not W6.48 is evident in the CB1 crystal structures, it is essential to notice that this change requires a synchronized rotameric change in the $\chi 1$, as well as, the $\chi 2$ dihedrals of W6.48. Thus, it could be proposed that a transient rotameric change in $\chi 1$ dihedral of W6.48 from g+ to trans or vice-versa is required to permit conformational changes in F3.36. In addition, the major rotameric change in F3.36 is associated with a rotational movement of TMH3 towards TMH2. Agonists appear to stabilize this conformational change in TMH3 by blocking F3.36 in g+, thus stabilizing the active state of the receptor. While in the inactive state structures, it could be noticed that the antagonists seem to prohibit the rotameric change of W6.48 into trans, thus acting as inverse agonists at the CB1 receptor.

4.5.5. F7.35

This residue has been shown to mildly affect SR141716A binding with ~4-fold increase in K_d in F7.35A hCB1 mutant [44]. Potencies of SR141716A and AM6538 in inhibiting 100 nM CP55940 activity were also retained in F7.35A and F7.35W hCB1 mutations [6]. However, the potency of CP55940, AM841, and AM11542 in inhibition of forskolin-induced cAMP has been shown to be around one order of magnitude affected by F7.35W mutation which might be due to steric hindrance, while their potencies were majorly affected by a 7.35A mutation [6, 8]. This residue shows moderate VDW interactions with the gem dimethyl group at C1′ of agonists and very mild VDW interactions with the antagonists in the active and inactive state crystal structures respectively.

4.6. EC2 loop residues

The CB1 EC2 loop lines the binding site with five amino acid residues residing on top of the ligand binding site; 267-IFPHI-271. Mutations at the EC2 loop have been shown to affect CP55940 binding generally and have no effect on SR141716A binding. Replacement of the entire hCB1 EC2 loop (254-GWNCEKLQSVCSDIFPHIDETYL-276) by the hCB2 EC2 loop (GWTCCPRP - - CSELFPLIPNDYL) did not affect SR141716A binding but resulted in a complete loss of CP55940 binding, while replacing EKLQSV in CB1 by CPRP (CB2/EC2) resulted in receptor sequestration [41]. In addition, the C257/C264 internal disulfide bridge has been determined to be required for membrane expression [41, 59]. Single point alanine mutations were investigated for the majority of the EC2 loop. Among the residues that face the binding site, F268A/N hCB1 mutation impaired receptor membrane expression. F268Y hCB1 mutation had no effect on ligand binding, while F268W mutation drastically affected CP55940 binding with no effect on SR141716A binding. In addition, P267A, H270A, and I271A mutants showed no effect on SR141716A binding while drastically affecting CP55940 binding [60]. In crystal structures, F268 forms strong VDW interaction with both agonists and antagonists in addition to an aromatic stacking with the agonists. P267 and I271 form week VDW interaction with agonists while the H270 side chain points towards TMH3 and is packed against F3.25. In addition, due to closer packing of the EC end of TMH5/6 towards the ligand binding site in the active state compared to the inactive state, and the fact that agonists are cupping F268 compared to the antagonists, it could be interpreted that F268W mutation data regarding the binding of agonists versus the antagonists could be consistent with crystal structures.

4.7. Cysteine residues in the EC domain of CB1; labeling and mutation studies

Among the 13 cysteine residues in the CB1 receptor, C6.47, C7.38, and C7.42 reside in the EC transmembrane domain and are not engaged in a disulfide bond. C6.47 is only available in the binding pocket in the activated state of Class A GPCRs. Consistent with this, the earliest CB1 cysteine reactivity study using the isothiocyanate derivatized agonist, AM841, showed that AM841 labels C6.47 [61]. A subsequent study showed that AM841 also labels C6.47 in CB2 [62]. The isothiocyanate derivatized anandamide analog, AM3677, was also found to label C6.47 [63]. This has led to the hypothesis that cannabinoid agonists enter CB1 via a portal between TMH6 and TMH7 at the level of C6.47. The active state crystal structure, is not consistent with cysteine crosslinking studies of AM841, since the AM841 alkyl tail points towards Y5.39 in the crystal structure.

In another cysteine reactivity study, C7.42, was found reactive, suggesting that it faces the binding pocket. Mutation of C7.42 to a larger amino acid resulted in loss of SR141716A binding, but not CP55940 binding. In all reported crystal structures, C7.42 faces into the binding pocket. Further, if C7.42 is mutated to M in the active state structure, it does not affect the agonist binding pocket. However, a methionine residue at that position in the inactive state structures clashes severely with the antagonists and surrounding residues, such clashes are not relieved by rotameric changes for nearby residues.

4.8. Serine residues in CB1

Mutation of S7.39 in hCB1 to alanine in was generally detrimental for CP55940, HU201 and AM4056 binding to the CB1 receptor, while it had no effect on the binding affinities for SR141716A, AM251, as well as, WIN55212 [32, 57, 64]. On the other hand, it resulted in a profound reduction in the binding affinity of taranabant to the receptor [32]. In the inactive state crystal structure in complex with taranabant, as well as, the active state crystal structure, there is a hydrogen bond interaction between S7.39 and the ligand. The residue adopts a g− χ1 dihedral that allows this interaction. In the AM6358/inactive state crystal structure, this residue adopts a g+ χ1 dihedral. In this structure, the ligand is incapable of forming a hydrogen bond interaction with S7.39, since such an interaction requires a high energy conformation of the antagonist.

Mutation data show that the S2.60A mutation in hCB1 has no effect on the binding affinities of both CP55940 and SR141716A [64]. S2.60 does not seem to be involved in any interactions with ligands in the crystal structures. This is due to the rotation of TMH2 towards TMH3 caused by the G2.53/S2.54 motif in TMH2 allowing a wider turn in that region.

4.9. L3.29A, M6.55A, and T3.33A mutations

L3.29 faces the ligand binding site and has been shown to interact with both agonists and antagonists. Such interactions are stronger in the active state due to the rotation of TMH3 towards TMH2, allowing L3.29 to be more oriented towards the binding site. The L3.29A mutation in hCB1 has been shown to mildly affect the binding affinity of SR141716A to the receptor, while having a profound effect on the binding of CP55940, HU210 and Δ9-THC. The L3.29A mutations resulted in reduced efficacy of both HU210 in stimulation of $[^{35}S]GTP\gamma S$ binding and in the efficacy of CP55940 in the inhibition of forskolin-induced cAMP accumulation [8, 44, 45].

Both T3.33A and M6.55A mutations did not have any effect on the binding affinity of SR141716A which is consistent with the inactive state crystal structures [44]. M6.55A mutation in hCB1 resulted in a 15- and 4-fold reduction in the affinity of HU210 and CP55940 respectively while it did not affect the affinity of Δ9-THC [45]. This residue shows moderate VDW interactions with the agonists in the crystal structures.

5. NMR and circular dichroism (CD) studies on the C-terminus

Both NMR and CD studies have been performed on the C-terminus of CB1 employing peptide segments that correspond to that receptor region. Results show a helical segment resembling helix 8 that is parallel to the plane of the membrane [65–67]. Ahn et al., reported two amphipathic α-helical domains; S410-F412 that corresponds to helix 8, and a second helical segment (A440-M461) that is also parallel to the membrane, (**Figure 1**) [65].

6. Crystal contacts

In the inactive and active state CB1 crystal structures, crystal packing impinges on the ligand binding site (**Figure 6**). In the first published CB1 inactive state structure [6], receptor bundles are crystallized top-to-top, forcing the N-terminus to invade the binding pocket and flattening the EC loops. In the second inactive state CB1 structure [7], adjacent bundles impinge on receptor EC loops and N-terminus around the "rim" of the receptor's EC domain (**Figure 6**). The effect on CB1 structure is similar to that discussed above for the first inactive crystal structure. Crystal packing in the active state structure [8] also causes an impact on the CB1 binding pocket. Packing causes TMH2 to hinge at G2.53/S2.54 (S2.54 has a $\chi 1 = g-$) and invade the binding pocket. Packing also impacts the N-terminus, TMH1 above N1.50, the EC top of TMH3, the EC-2 loop and the EC end of TMH4.

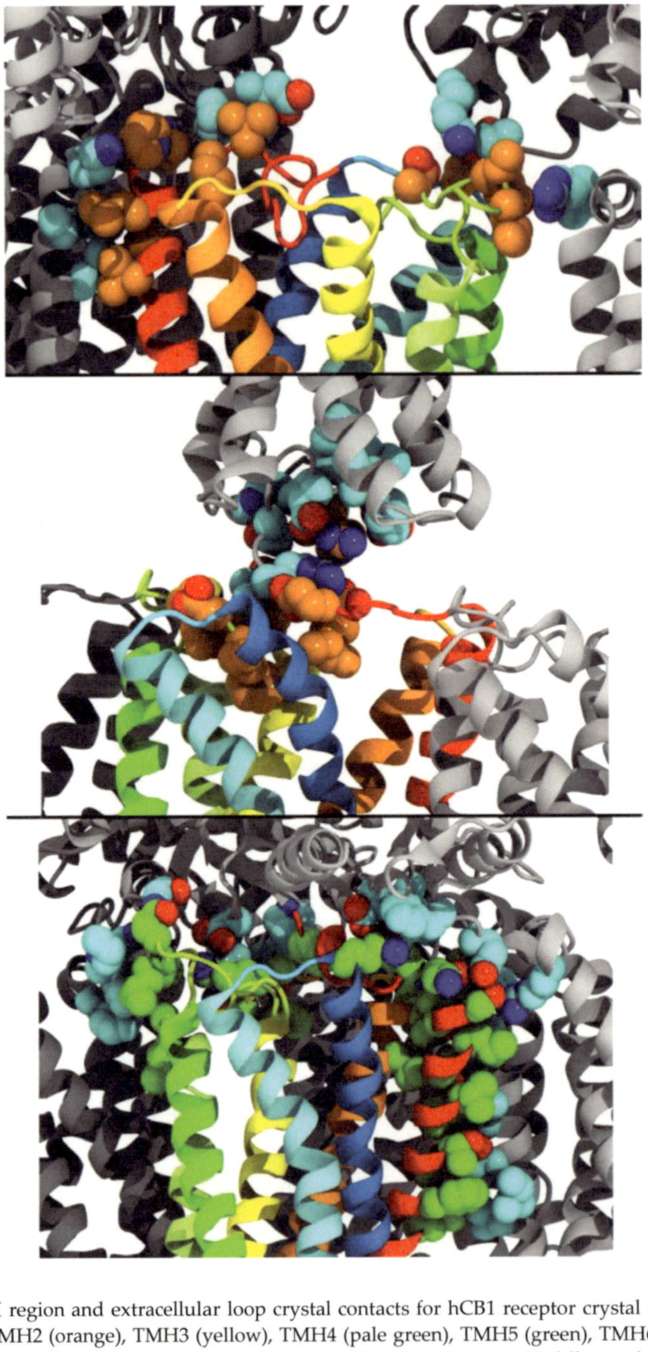

Figure 6. Unit cell TM region and extracellular loop crystal contacts for hCB1 receptor crystal structures. CB1 ribbon colors: TMH1 (red), TMH2 (orange), TMH3 (yellow), TMH4 (pale green), TMH5 (green), TMH6 (cyan), TMH7 (blue), crystal mate ribbons (white). Top panel: inactive state structure (PDB ID: 5TGZ) [6]. Middle panel: inactive state structure (PDB ID: 5U09) [7]. Bottom panel: active state structure (PDB ID: 5XRA) [8]. Amino acid residues for crystal mates are colored cyan, while inactive and active state structures are shown in orange and green respectively.

Such packing issues can promote non-genuine conformations in the structure that is promoted by the crystalline low energy state. A recently published crystal structure of the μ-opioid receptor (MOR) has revealed a histidine H54 residue in the N-terminus of the receptor that is positioned 2.6 Å from the secondary amine of the bound agonist. Mutation of this residue into alanine did not affect the affinity of the ligand to the receptor, suggesting that the resulting conformation of the N-terminus in MOR structure is a result of crystallization and not relevant in the real state [68].

7. Conclusions

Because X-ray crystal structures are used frequently for drug design projects, it is critical to identify any issues with these structures, such as crystal packing effects and to evaluate how consistent these structures are with the body of structural information in the literature for a given receptor, such as mutation, cross-linking and NMR studies. Results presented in this chapter show that crystal packing issues impact both of the CB1 inactive state crystal structures and the activated state CB1 crystal structures. Impacts include N-terminus insertions deep into the binding pocket seen in the CB1 inactive state structures, as well as, TMH1 and TMH2 bending into the binding pocket seen in the activated state structures. Not surprisingly, we find here that the CB1 structures have important inconsistencies with mutation data, particularly in their TMH1-2-3 regions. In addition, the CB1 crystal structures do not capture the movement of W6.48 during receptor activation, or the existence of a ligand portal in the activated state, however, X-ray structures by their very nature will not capture all transient changes. In conclusion, then, the CB1 crystal structures are an important contribution to the drug design field, but revisions are advisable before these structures are used for structure-based drug discovery.

Acknowledgements

This work was supported by NIDA RO1 DA003934 to PHR.

Author details

Rufaida Al-Zoubi[1], Dow P. Hurst[2] and Patricia H. Reggio[2]*

*Address all correspondence to: phreggio@uncg.edu

1 Department of Medicinal Chemistry and Pharmacognosy, Faculty of Pharmacy, Jordan University of Science and Technology, Irbid, Jordan

2 Department of Chemistry and Biochemistry, University of North Carolina at Greensboro, Greensboro, NC, USA

References

[1] Palczewski K et al. Crystal structure of rhodopsin: A G protein-coupled receptor. Science. 2000;**289**(5480):739

[2] Jaakola V-P et al. The 2.6 angstrom crystal structure of a human A2A adenosine receptor bound to an antagonist. Science. 2008;**322**(5905):1211-1217

[3] Warne T et al. Structure of a β1-adrenergic G-protein-coupled receptor. Nature. 2008;**454**: 486

[4] Hanson MA et al. A specific cholesterol binding site is established by the 2.8 Å structure of the human beta2 adrenergic receptor. Structure. 2008;**16**(6):897-905

[5] Scheerer P et al. Crystal structure of opsin in its G-protein-interacting conformation. Nature. 2008;**455**:497

[6] Hua T et al. Crystal structure of the human cannabinoid receptor CB1. Cell. 2016;**167**(3):750-762.e14

[7] Shao Z et al. High-resolution crystal structure of the human CB1 cannabinoid receptor. Nature. 2016;**540**:602

[8] Hua T et al. Crystal structures of agonist-bound human cannabinoid receptor CB1. Nature. 2017;**547**(7664):468-471

[9] Fredriksson R et al. The G-protein-coupled receptors in the human genome form five main families. Phylogenetic analysis, Paralogon groups, and fingerprints. Molecular Pharmacology. 2003;**63**(6):1256-1272

[10] Devillé J, Rey J, Chabbert M. An indel in transmembrane helix 2 helps to trace the molecular evolution of class A G-protein-coupled receptors. Journal of Molecular Evolution. 2009;**68**(5):475-489

[11] Pel J et al. Multidimensional scaling reveals the main evolutionary pathways of class A G-protein-coupled receptors. PLoS One. 2011;**6**(4):1-10

[12] Surgand JS et al. A chemogenomic analysis of the transmembrane binding cavity of human G-protein-coupled receptors. Proteins: Structure, Function and Genetics. 2006; **62**(2):509-538

[13] Chrencik JE et al. Crystal structure of antagonist bound human lysophosphatidic acid receptor 1. Cell. 2015;**161**(7):1633-1643

[14] Hanson MA et al. Crystal structure of a lipid G protein-coupled receptor. Science. 2012; **335**(6070):851

[15] Vallée M et al. Pregnenolone can protect the brain from Cannabis intoxication. Science. 2014;**343**(6166):94-98

[16] McAllister SD et al. An aromatic microdomain at the cannabinoid CB1 receptor constitutes an agonist/inverse agonist binding region. Journal of Medicinal Chemistry. 2003;**46**(24):5139-5152

[17] Stanley N, Pardo L, Fabritiis GD. The pathway of ligand entry from the membrane bilayer to a lipid G protein-coupled receptor. Scientific Reports. 2016;**6**:22639

[18] Hurst DP et al. A lipid pathway for ligand binding is necessary for a cannabinoid G protein-coupled receptor. Journal of Biological Chemistry. 2010;**285**(23):17954-17964

[19] Venkatakrishnan AJ et al. Diverse activation pathways in class A GPCRs converge near the G-protein-coupling region. Nature. 2016;**536**:484

[20] Carpenter B, Tate CG. Active state structures of G protein-coupled receptors highlight the similarities and differences in the G protein and arrestin coupling interfaces. Current Opinion in Structural Biology. 2017;**45**:124-132

[21] Bonner TI, Song ZH. A lysine residue of the cannabinoid receptor is critical for receptor recognition by several agonists but not WIN55212-2. Molecular Pharmacology. 1996; **49**(5):891-896

[22] Chin CN et al. Ligand binding and modulation of cyclic AMP levels depend on the chemical nature of residue 192 of the human cannabinoid receptor 1. Journal of Neurochemistry. 1998;**70**(1):366-373

[23] Shore DM et al. Allosteric modulation of a cannabinoid G protein-coupled receptor: Binding site elucidation and relationship to G protein signaling. Journal of Biological Chemistry. 2014;**289**(9):5828-5845

[24] Tuccinardi T et al. Cannabinoid CB2/CB1 selectivity. Receptor modeling and automated docking analysis. Journal of Medicinal Chemistry. 2006;**49**(3):984-994

[25] Salo OMH et al. 3D-QSAR studies on cannabinoid CB1 receptor agonists: G-protein activation as biological data. Journal of Medicinal Chemistry. 2006;**49**(2):554-566

[26] Salo OMH et al. Development of a 3D model for the human cannabinoid CB1 receptor. Journal of Medicinal Chemistry. 2004;**47**(12):3048-3057

[27] Shim JY, Welsh William J, Howlett Allyn C. Homology model of the CB1 cannabinoid receptor: Sites critical for nonclassical cannabinoid agonist interaction. Peptide Science. 2004; **71**(2):169-189

[28] Joong-Youn S. Understanding functional residues of the cannabinoid CB1 receptor for drug discovery. Current Topics in Medicinal Chemistry. 2010;**10**(8):779-798

[29] Hurst DP et al. N-(piperidin-1-yl)-5-(4-chlorophenyl)-1-(2,4-dichlorophenyl)-4-methyl-1H-pyrazole-3-carboxamide (SR141716A) interaction with LYS 3.28(192) is crucial for its inverse agonism at the cannabinoid CB1 receptor. Molecular Pharmacology. 2002;**62**(6):1274-1287

[30] Pan X, Ikeda SR, Lewis DL. SR 141716A acts as an inverse agonist to increase neuronal voltage-dependent Ca^{2+} currents by reversal of tonic CB1 cannabinoid receptor activity. Molecular Pharmacology. 1998;**1072**:1064-1072

[31] Hurst D et al. Biarylpyrazole inverse agonists at the cannabinoid CB1 receptor: Importance of the C-3 Carboxamide oxygen/lysine 3.28(192) interaction. Journal of Medicinal Chemistry. 2006;**49**(20):5969-5987

[32] Lin LS et al. Conformational analysis and receptor docking of N-[(1S,2S)-3-(4-chlorophenyl)-2-(3-cy-anophenyl)-1-methylpropyl]-2-methyl-2-\\{[5-(trifluoromethyl)pyridin-2-yl]oxy} propanamide (Taranabant, MK-0364), a novel , acyclic canna. Journal of Medicinal Chemistry. 2008;**51**:2108-2114

[33] Fong TM et al. Antiobesity efficacy of a novel cannabinoid-1 receptor inverse agonist, N-[(1S,2S)-3-(4-chlorophenyl)-2-(3-cyanophenyl)-1-methylpropyl]-2-methyl-2-[[5-(trifluoromethyl)pyridin-2-yl]oxy] propanamide (MK-0364), in rodents. Journal of Pharmacology and Experimental Therapeutics. 2007;**321**(3):1013

[34] Ahn KH et al. Computationally-predicted CB1 cannabinoid receptor mutants show distinct patterns of salt-bridges that correlate with their level of constitutive activity reflected in G protein coupling levels, thermal stability, and ligand binding. Proteins. 2013;**81**(8):1304-1317

[35] Kapur A et al. Mapping the structural requirements in the CB 1 cannabinoid receptor transmembrane Helix II for signal transduction. Journal of Pharmacology and Experimental Therapeutics. 2008;**325**(1):341-348

[36] D'Antona AM et al. A cannabinoid receptor 1 mutation proximal to the DRY motif results in constitutive activity and reveals intramolecular interactions involved in receptor activation. Brain Research. 2006;**1108**(1):1-11

[37] Marcu J et al. Novel insights into CB1 cannabinoid receptor signaling: A key interaction identified between the extracellular-3 loop and transmembrane helix 2. The Journal of Pharmacology and Experimental Therapeutics. 2013;**345**(2):189-197

[38] Murphy JW, Kendall DA. Integrity of extracellular loop 1 of the human cannabinoid receptor 1 is critical for high-affinity binding of the ligand CP 55,940 but not SR 141716A. Biochemical Pharmacology. 2003;**65**(10):1623-1631

[39] Fay JF, Farrens DL. The membrane proximal region of the cannabinoid receptor CB1 N-t erminus can Allosterically modulate ligand affinity. Biochemistry. 2013;**52**(46):8286-8294

[40] Andersson H et al. Membrane assembly of the cannabinoid receptor 1: Impact of a long N-terminal tail. Molecular Pharmacology. 2003;**64**(3):570

[41] Shire D et al. Structural features of the central cannabinoid CB1 receptor involved in the binding of the specific CB1 antagonist SR 141716A. Journal of Biological Chemistry. 1996; **271**(12):6941-6946

[42] Iyer MR et al. Structural basis of species-dependent differential affinity of 6-alkoxy-5-aryl-3-pyridinecarboxamide cannabinoid receptor 1 antagonists running title: Species-specific affinity of CB1 receptor antagonists. Molecular Pharmacology. 2015;**88**(2):238-244

[43] Rover S et al. 6-Alkoxy-5-aryl-3-pyridinecarboxamides, a new series of bioavailable cannabinoid receptor type 1 (CB1) antagonists including peripherally selective compounds. Journal of Medicinal Chemistry. 2013;**56**(24):9874-9896

[44] Shim JY, Bertalovitz AC, Kendall DA. Probing the interaction of SR141716A with the CB1 receptor. Journal of Biological Chemistry. 2012;**287**(46):38741-38754

[45] Shim J-Y, Bertalovitz AC, Kendall DA. Identification of essential cannabinoid-binding domains: Structural insights into early dynamic events in receptor activation. Journal of Biological Chemistry. 2011;**286**(38):33422-33435

[46] McAllister SD et al. Structural mimicry in class A G protein-coupled receptor rotamer toggle switches: The Importance of the F3.36(201)/W6.48(357) interaction in cannabinoid CB1 receptor activation. Journal of Biological Chemistry. 2004;**279**(46):48024-48037

[47] McAllister SD et al. A critical role for a tyrosine residue in the cannabinoid receptors for ligand recognition. Biochemical Pharmacology. 2002;**63**(12):2121-2136

[48] Klein-Seetharaman J et al. Differential dynamics in the G protein-coupled receptor rhodopsin revealed by solution NMR. Proceedings of the National Academy of Sciences of the United States of America. 2004;**101**(10):3409-3413

[49] Holst B et al. A conserved aromatic lock for the tryptophan rotameric switch in TM-VI of seven-transmembrane receptors. Journal of Biological Chemistry. 2010;**285**(6):3973-3985

[50] Lin SW, Sakmar TP. Specific tryptophan UV-absorbance changes are probes of the transition of rhodopsin to its active state. Biochemistry. 1996;**35**(34):11149-11159

[51] Borhan B et al. Movement of retinal along the visual transduction path. Science. 2000;**288**(5474):2209-2212

[52] Trzaskowski B et al. Action of molecular switches in GPCRs—Theoretical and experimental studies. Current Medicinal Chemistry. 2012;**19**(8):1090-1109

[53] Yuan S et al. Activation of G-protein-coupled receptors correlates with the formation of a continuous internal water pathway. Nature Communications. 2014;**5**(May):4733-4733

[54] Yuan S, Vogel H, Filipek S. The role of water and sodium ions in the activation of the μ-opioid receptor. Angewandte Chemie—International Edition. 2013;**52**(38):10112-10115

[55] Nygaard R et al. Conserved water-mediated hydrogen bond network between TM-I, -II, -VI, and -VII in 7TM receptor activation. Journal of Biological Chemistry. 2010; **285**(25):19625-19636

[56] Singh R et al. Activation of the cannabinoid CB1 receptor may involve a W6.48/F3.36 rotamer toggle switch. The Journal of Peptide Research. 2002;**60**(6):357-370

[57] Sitkoff DF et al. Cannabinoid CB1 receptor ligand binding and function examined through mutagenesis studies of F200 and S383. European Journal of Pharmacology. 2011;**651**(1):9-17

[58] Shen C-P et al. F200A substitution in the third transmembrane helix of human cannabinoid CB1 receptor converts AM2233 from receptor agonist to inverse agonist. European Journal of Pharmacology. 2006;**531**(1):41-46

[59] Fay JF, Dunham TD, Farrens DL. Cysteine residues in the human cannabinoid receptor: Only C257 and C264 are required for a functional receptor, and steric bulk at C386 impairs antagonist SR141716A binding. Biochemistry. 2005;**44**(24):8757-8769

[60] Ahn KH et al. Dual role of the second extracellular loop of the cannabinoid receptor 1: Ligand binding and receptor localization. Molecular Pharmacology. 2009;**76**(4):833-842

[61] Picone RP et al. (−)-7'-Isothiocyanato-11-hydroxy-1′,1′-dimethylheptylhexahydrocanna binol (AM841), a high-affinity electrophilic ligand, interacts covalently with a cysteine in Helix six and activates the CB1 cannabinoid receptor. Molecular Pharmacology. 2005; **68**(6):1623-1635

[62] Pei Y et al. Ligand-binding architecture of human CB2 cannabinoid receptor: Evidence for receptor subtype-specific binding motif and modeling GPCR activation. Chemistry & Biology. 2008;**15**(11):1207-1219

[63] Janero DR et al. Molecular-interaction and signaling profiles of AM3677, a novel covalent agonist selective for the cannabinoid 1 receptor. ACS Chemical Neuroscience. 2015;**6**(8): 1400-1410

[64] Kapur A et al. Mutation studies of Ser7.39 and Ser2.60 in the human CB1 cannabinoid receptor: Evidence for a serine-induced bend in CB1 transmembrane Helix 7. Molecular Pharmacology. 2007;**71**(6):1512

[65] Ahn KH et al. Structural analysis of the human cannabinoid receptor one carboxyl-terminus identifies two amphipathic helices. Biopolymers. 2009;**91**(7):565-573

[66] Choi G, Guo J, Makriyannis A. The conformation of the cytoplasmic helix 8 of the CB1 cannabinoid receptor using NMR and circular dichroism. Biochimica et Biophysica Acta (BBA)—Biomembranes. 2005;**1668**(1):1-9

[67] Tyukhtenko S et al. NMR solution structure of human cannabinoid receptor-1 helix 7/8 peptide: Candidate electrostatic interactions and microdomain formation. Biochemical and Biophysical Research Communications. 2009;**390**(3):441-446

[68] Huang W et al. Structural insights into μ-opioid receptor activation. Nature. 2015;**524**:315

Chapter 4

Quality Traits of Medical *Cannabis sativa* L. Inflorescences and Derived Products Based on Comprehensive Mass-Spectrometry Analytical Investigation

Lorenzo Calvi, Radmila Pavlovic, Sara Panseri,
Luca Giupponi, Valeria Leoni and Annamaria Giorgi

Additional information is available at the end of the chapter

http://dx.doi.org/10.5772/intechopen.79539

Abstract

Cannabis sativa L. has been cultivated throughout the world for industrial and medical purposes and is the most controversial plant ever exploited, with considerable discrepancies in the praise and disapproval it receives. Medical Cannabis prescriptions are on the increase in several countries where its therapeutic use is authorised due to its positive role in treating several pathologies even if it represents a multifaceted reality in terms of application. There at least 550 identified compounds in *C. sativa* L., including more than 100 phytocannabinoids and 120 terpenes. The chemical complexity of its bioactive constituents highlights the need for standardised and well-defined analytical approaches able to characterise plant chemotype and herbal drug quality as well as to monitor the quality of pharmaceutical cannabis extracts and preparations. This research highlights the potential of using different analytical procedures involving the combination of headspace-solid-phase microextraction (HS-SPME) coupled to GC–MS and accelerated solvent extraction (ASE) coupled to high resolution mass-spectrometry (HPLC-Q Orbitrap®) for the in-depth profiling of quality traits in authorised medical varieties of *Cannabis sativa* L. flos (Bediol®) and corresponding macerated oil preparations. This approach could add new knowledge to the field of "*omic*" analytical applications which are fundamental nowadays for Cannabis used for therapeutic remedies.

Keywords: Bediol®, terpenes, cannabinoids, GC-MS, HS-SPME, HPLC-Q-Exactive-Orbitrap-MS, *Cannabis sativa* L

IntechOpen

1. Introduction

Cannabis (*Cannabis sativa L.*) is the most controversial plant ever exploited, with considerable discrepancy in the praise and disapproval it receives. It is intriguing that cannabis produces the natural substances that appear to target key protein receptors of important physiological systems quite selectively [1]. Plants containing such secondary metabolites usually belong to unique chemotaxa that induce potent pharmacological effects and have typically been used for recreational and medicinal purposes. *Cannabis sativa* L. has a long history as a medicinal plant and was fundamental in the discovery of the endocannabinoid system.

Over the past decades, considerable research has been carried out to enable a clear distinction to be made between cannabis as a hazardous drug and as a beneficial medicine [2, 3].The authorised medicinal use of cannabis is still associated with doubts on its safe use due to a few ambiguous issues including quantity, dynamics and way of administration [4].

Medications based on cannabis have been used for therapeutic purposes in many cultures for centuries. In Europe, they were used at the end of the nineteenth century to treat pain, spasms, asthma, sleep disorders, depression, and loss of appetite. In the first half of the twentieth century, cannabinoid medications fell into almost complete disuse, partly because scientists were unable to establish the chemical structure of the main cannabis plant ingredients. The emergence of interest in botanical medicinal cannabis is thought by many to be a collateral effect of the opioid abuse epidemic; public perception surrounding the use of medicinal cannabis suggests that this plant-based therapy is viewed as not very different from a botanical drug product or supplement used for health or relief of symptoms if disease persists. Like some herbal preparations or supplements, however, medicinal cannabis may similarly pose health risks associated with its use, including psychoactive, intoxicating, and impairing effects, which have not been completely elucidated through clinical trials.

The method of its application for therapeutic purposes certainly depends on its phytocannabinoid profile: over 70 cannabinoids are defined in *Cannabis sativa L.* They are classified chemically into 10 most important categories where the THC, cannabidiol (CBD), cannabigerol (CBG), cannabichromene (CBC), and cannabinol (CBN)-types are recognised as the most relevant [5].

The main constituent of cannabis is THC, which is responsible for the psychoactive features of cannabis due to its high affinity to cannabinoid receptors. Most of the effects of cannabis preparations are based on the agonistic action of THC on the various cannabinoid receptors. Two primary endocannabinoid receptors have been identified: CB1 and CB2 [6]. CB1 receptors are found predominantly in the brain and nervous system, as well as in peripheral organs and tissues, and are the main molecular target of the endocannabinoid binding molecule, anandamide, as well as its mimetic phytocannabinoid, THC.

Another important component is cannabidiol (CBD) which was proven to possess several pharmacological properties (analgesic, antioxidant and antiepileptic), but not psychotropic activity as THC [7]. The presence and amount of CBD is essential in the therapeutic usage of cannabis, because it reduces THC collateral effects. Furthermore, minor constituents such as CBC and CBG exhibit anti-inflammatory, antibacterial and antifungal activity, while CBN has strong sedative properties [5, 7]. As regards cannabidiol (CBD)-based preparations that are becoming extremely popular as CBD has been shown to have beneficial effects on human health, a recent work highlighted a wide variability in the cannabinoid profile that justifies the need for strict and standardised regulations [8].

Although CBD and THC are the key molecules, the plant itself is capable of producing only their acid counterparts: cannabidiolic acid (CBDA) and tetrahydrocannabinolic acid (THCA) [9]. Decarboxylation of these forms leads to the formation of bioactive chemical species, CBD and THC, respectively. CBDA and THCA are the major components of cannabis inflorescence while among other cannabinoid acids, cannabigerolic acid (CBGA) is shown to be essential due to the fact that it is a precursor of all the other cannabinoid acids. It is worth mentioning the other minor acidic cannabinoids such as cannabichromenic acid (CBCA) which also gives corresponding neutral analogues upon decarboxylation.

At present, the international medical and scientific community has widely recognised *Cannabis sativa* L. as a promising source of therapeutic agents for the treatment of certain diseases such as multiple sclerosis, HIV, epilepsy, glaucoma, chemotherapy, chronic pain, nausea/vomiting [10, 11].

Unfortunately, despite the emergence of a huge amount of preclinical literature that describes the actions and effects of some cannabinoids, there have, as yet, been relatively few publications describing the effects produced by cannabinoids in clinical studies performed with human subjects. Importantly, a cannabis-based medication, Sativex®, approved by the European medical association (EMA), was recently licenced in 18 European countries for the treatment of tremor and spasticity symptoms associated with multiple sclerosis [12]. Besides, other cannabinoid drugs, Cesamet® (Nabilone) and Marinol® (synthetic tetrahydrocannabinol (THC)) were successfully applied for the treatment of vomiting and nausea caused by cancer therapy. Some other cannabis-derived substances seem to be on hold. For example, Epidolex®, an experimental drug derived from cannabis-based medicine for the treatment of child epilepsy is on the brink of becoming the first of its kind to obtain FDA government approval [13].

Capsules, cannabis extracts such as mouth spray or oils, dry cannabis for inhalation or as tea are the main medical products approved by the EU, according to the European Monitoring Center for Drugs and Drug Addiction (EMCDDA) 2017 [14].

Within the EU there is no agreement on the legalisation of medical cannabis, but it appears to be moving toward greater use faster than in the past [15, 16]. For the time being, only Austria, the Czech Republic, Finland, Germany, Italy, Portugal, Poland, Spain and Croatia have allowed the use of cannabis in medicine in the EU, while other countries are planning to legalise it. As a confirmation of the blurred legal status of *Cannabis sativa* L. within the EU community, it took a 4-year trial before the Danish Parliament approved the use of medical cannabis for patients suffering from various diseases starting from January 1, 2018. Moreover, in 2017, an increasing number of EU members, such as Greece and Ireland, announced or proposed changes in legislation and the use of medical cannabis. Since November 2017, cannabis-based medicines in Poland can be sold if they are made in pharmacies with the use of an imported substance.

The current status of cannabis highlights that, since it causes "psychoactive activity," its use in medicine should follow the legal provisions of member states, including "control of the use of narcotics and psychotropic substances" [17]. European countries have an obligation to control cannabis according to the three UN Conventions on Drug Control that require them to restrict drug supplies and use it exclusively for medical and scientific purposes.

At an EU level there are no harmonised laws on the recreational and medical use of cannabis and the member states themselves decide whether to legalise them.

As an example, medical cannabis in Italy represents a multifaceted reality [16, 18]. At present varieties Bedrocan, Bediol, Bedica and Bedrolite produced by company Bedrocan from Netherlands [19] and the new strain FM2 produced by the Military Pharmaceutical Chemical Works of Florence, Italy (authorised in November 2015 with a Ministerial Decree) can be prescribed to treat a wide range of pathological conditions [16]. In relation to this, Italian galenic pharmacies are authorised to prepare precise cannabis doses for vaping, herbal teas, resins, micronised capsules and oils [20]. The latter, prepared by using European Pharmacopoeia olive oil (FU) as extraction solvent has received great attention due to the easiness with which dosage can be modulated or titrated during the treatment period. Also, oil formulations are high-steamed because of the extended bioavailability of the active compounds contained.

As regards *Cannabis sativa* composition, beyond and besides cannabinoids, a substantial amount of the approximately 500 compounds (terpenes, flavonoids, stilbenoids, fatty acids, alkaloids, carbohydrates, and phenols) are described [21]. Terpenes represent the volatile component of the plant and have been proven to have a synergic action with cannabinoids [19]. Cannabis plants produce and accumulate a terpene-rich resin in glandular trichomes, which are abundant on the surface of the female inflorescence [22]. Bouquets of different monoterpenes and sesquiterpenes are important components of cannabis resin as they define some of the unique organoleptic properties and may also influence medicinal qualities of different cannabis strains and varieties [23]. Differences between the pharmaceutical properties of different cannabis strains have been attributed to interactions (or an 'entourage effect') between cannabinoids and terpenes [24]. Terpenes themselves exhibit a wide array of pharmacological properties, including interaction with the mammalian endocannabinoid system: sesquiterpene β-caryophyllene interacts with mammalian cannabinoid receptors [25, 26]. Some terpenes like β-myrcene, limonene and linalool display anxiolytic, antibacterial, anti-inflammatory, and sedative effects, too [27].

The chemical complexity of cannabis makes its pharmaceutical standardisation challenging and must include well-defined methodologies that would characterise the plant chemotype and the herbal drug as well as extraction procedures. As a matter of fact, it was found that the concentrations of target cannabinoids obtained for the same plant chemotype originating from different suppliers varied by more than 25% [28]. This lack of standardisation could be overcome with two distinct approaches.

The first is a botanical issue and points toward strict control of varieties and strains during cultivation in order to assure the highest homogeneity in the final plants, especially if the cannabis inflorescence is the final product. The other tactic is focused on extraction and purification procedures, which are fundamental if cannabis-derived formulations such as oils or tinctures are targeted. As recently reviewed by Citti et al. [29] and Calvi et al. [30], the choice of the analytical approach(es) employed represents a pivotal task, with particular emphasis on the need for a comprehensive chemical characterisation of the composition of cannabis and derived products. Nowadays, analytical methods based on gas chromatography-mass spectrometry (GC-MS) and/or high pressure liquid chromatography (HPLC) coupled to the recently introduced high resolution mass spectrometer HRMS-Orbitrap, represent the gold standard techniques for the investigation of the highly complex cannabis composition due to their excellent resolution, precision and sensitivity. Consequently, it is now crucial to complete the chemical and pharmacological characterisation of all phytocannabinoids known to be present in cannabis.

Based on the above-mentioned considerations, in the first part of the here presented research project different analytical procedures involving the combination of headspace-solid-phase microextraction (HS-SPME) coupled to GC-MS and accelerated solvent extraction (ASE) coupled to high resolution mass-spectrometry (HPLC-Q Orbitrap®) were applied for the in-depth profiling and fingerprinting of cannabinoids and terpenes in authorised medical grade varieties of *Cannabis sativa* L. *flos* (Bediol®) and in corresponding macerated oil preparation. Particular emphasis was given to the study of *untargeted* cannabinoids so as to investigate and obtain an exhaustive and realistic profile of medical Bediol® inflorescences and derived macerated oil preparations, since they have so far received less attention compared to target compounds (THC, THC-A, CBD, CBD-A). This approach could add new knowledge to the field of "*omic*" analytical applications as well.

2. Materials and methods

2.1. Chemical and reagents

All HPLC or analytical grade chemicals were from Sigma (Sigma-Aldrich, St. Louis, MO, USA). Formic acid 98–100% was from Fluka (Sigma-Aldrich, St. Louis, MO, USA). Ultrapure water was obtained through a Milli-Q system (Millipore, Merck KGaA, Darmstadt, Germany). For headspace (HS) analysis, the SPME coating fibre (DVB/CAR/PDMS, 50/30 μm) was from Supelco (Bellefonte, PA, USA). Acetonitrile, 2-propanol, formic acid LC-MS grade were purchased from Carlo Erba (Milan, Italy). CBD, THC, CBN, CBG, CBNA, THCA, CBGA were purchased from Sigma Aldrich (Round Rock, Texas). High intensity planetary mill Retsch (model MM 400, Retsch, GmbH, Retsch-Allee, Haan) was used to obtain representative aliquots of cannabis flos samples powder.

2.2. Cannabis plant material and superfine grinding (SFG) sample preparation

Bediol® medical Cannabis chemotype that contains 6.5% THC and 8% CBD as standardised and certified by the company Bedrocan was used for all analyses. It was selected as representative because it represents the most common medical variety actually prescribed alone or in combination for several pathologies. Superfine cannabis inflorescence powder was prepared using mechanical grinding-activation in an energy intensive vibrational mill. Different samples (1.0 g each) were ground in a high intensity planetary mill. The mill was vibrating at a frequency of 25 Hz for 1 min, using two 50 mL jars with 20 mm stainless steel balls. Prior to use, jars were precooled with liquid nitrogen. The speed differences between balls and jar result in the interaction of frictional and impact forces, releasing high dynamic energies. The interplay of all these forces results in the very effective energy input of planetary ball mills. Mechano-chemical technology has been developed and successfully adopted in different fields (synthesis of superfine powder, surface modification, drug and pharmaceutical applications) and could represent a novel research tool.

2.3. Accelerated Solvent Extraction (ASE) for cannabinoid analysis

All extractions to define the cannabinoid profile of Bediol® medical chemotype were executed using an ASE 350 (Thermo-Fisher Scientific, Waltham, MA, USA). 34-mL stain steel cells were used for the extraction. 100 mg of Cannabis flos powder obtained by using SFG was weighed and then homogenised with an equal weight of diatomaceous earth and transferred into the cell. Then, 100 μL of extraction solution containing the IS (diazepam 1 mg mL^{-1}) was added. Different extraction solvents were tested and were: methanol, methanol:CH_3Cl (9:1), hexane, acetonitrile and ethanol. Diatomaceous earths were added in order to fill the remaining empty part of the cell. Room temperature of 25°C, pressure (1500 psi), number of static cycles (2 cycles, 5 min each), purging time (60 s with nitrogen) and rinse volume (90%) were used for the study. Organic extracts were finally collected in 66 mL vials and treated with sodium sulphate to remove any possible humidity. Afterwards, the extract was collected and dried under vacuum in a centrifugal evaporator. The residue was dissolved in 1 mL of acetonitrile and after proper dilution, 2 μL were submitted to analysis by HPLC-Q-Exactive-Orbitrap-MS. Validation was performed according to the European Union SANTE/2015 guidelines usually adopted to test ASE performance especially for trace residue analysis [31].

The method was completely optimised investigating the typologies of extraction solvents, number of extraction cycles and extraction temperature to define the optimum analytical conditions as well. To realise the matrix-matched calibration curves (MMCs) blank samples (100 mg officinal plant previously analysed for the absences of cannabinoids) were used and spiked with appropriate standard solution of THC, THC-A, CBD, CBD-A and CBN covering the concentration range from 0.1 to 10 μg g^{-1}. Recoveries were calculated by comparing the concentrations of the extracted compounds with those from the MMC calibration curves at two different fortification levels (1.0 and 10 μg g^{-1}).

2.4. HS-SPME and GC-MS analysis for terpenes investigation

One gram of oil or 100 mg of inflorescence previously grinded were weighed and put into 20 mL glass vials along with 100 μL of the IS (4-nonylphenol, 2000 μg/mL in 2-propanol). Each vial was fitted with a cap equipped with a silicon/PTFE septum (Supelco, Bellefonte, PA, USA). A temperature of 37°C was selected as both the extraction and equilibration temperature according to previous published research, in order to prevent possible matrix alterations ensuring the most efficient adsorption of volatile compounds onto the SPME fibre [15, 16]. To keep the temperature constant during analysis, the vials were maintained in a cooling block (CTC Analytics, Zwingen, Switzerland). At the end of the sample equilibration time (30 min), a conditioned (60 min at 280°C) SPME fibre was exposed to the headspace of the sample for 120 min using a CombiPAL system injector autosampler (CTC Analytics, Zwingen, Switzerland). All analytical parameters had already been validated in our previous research [32].

Analyses were performed with a Trace GC Ultra coupled to a Trace DSQII quadrupole mass spectrometer (MS) (Thermo-Fisher Scientific, Waltham, MA, USA) equipped with an Rtx-Wax column (30 m × 0.25 mm i.d. × 0.25 μm film thickness) (Restek, Bellefonte, PA, USA). The oven temperature program was: from 35°C, held for 8 min, to 60°C at 4°C/min, then from 60 to 160°C at 6°C/min and finally from 160 to 200 at 20°C/min. Helium was the carrier gas, at a flow rate of 1 mL/min. Carry over and peaks originating from the fibres were regularly assessed by running blank samples. After each analysis fibres were immediately thermally desorbed in the GC injector for 5 min at 250°C to prevent contamination. The MS was operated in electron impact (EI) ionisation mode at 70 eV. An alkane mixture (C8-C22, Sigma R 8769, Saint Louis, MO, USA) was run under the same chromatographic conditions as the samples to calculate the Kovats retention indices (RI) of the detected compounds. The mass spectra were obtained by using a mass selective detector, a multiplier voltage of 1456 V, and by collecting the data at a rate of 1 scan/s over the *m/z* range of 35–350. Compounds were identified by comparing the retention times of the chromatographic peaks with those of authentic compounds analysed under the same conditions when available, by comparing the Kovats retention indices with the literature data and through the National Institute of Standards and Technology (NIST) MS spectral database. The quantitative evaluation was performed using the internal standard procedure and the results were finally expressed as μg/g or mg/g IS equivalents of each volatile compound. All analyses were done in triplicate.

2.5. Cannabis macerated oil preparations

Three different methods for oil preparation were performed and evaluated. The preparation conditions were selected on the basis of previously published methods [31]. Briefly, common issues for all three methods were the amount of Bediol® inflorescence used (1 g) and the European Pharmacopoeia (FU) olive oil volume (10 mL) that served as extraction matrix. The crucial differences concerning the preheating temperature of the inflorescence to perform the decarboxylation step and extraction process are highlighted in **Table 1.** After extraction and cooling down (methods 1 and 2) the oils were filtrated and subsequently prepared for LC-Q-Exactive-Orbitrap-MS analysis.

2.6. Cannabinoids LC-Q-Exactive-Orbitrap-MS analysis

The cannabinoid profile in plants and the corresponding oil were assessed applying the method recently published with particular emphasis on method development [31]. In order to perform HPLC-Q-Exactive-Orbitrap®-MS analysis, samples extracted with ASE were prepared as indicated in Section 2.4, while oil samples were prepared by dissolving 100 mg of

Preparation's step	Preparation method		
	Romano and Hazekamp [32]	Pacifici et al. [33]	Calvi et al. [30]
	(1)	(2)	(3)
Decarboxylation step (conversion acid form in neutral form of cannabinoids)	No	Yes/145°C, 30 min static oven	Yes/145°C, 30 min static oven
Amount inflorescence/FU oil volume	1 g:10 mL	1 g:10 mL	1 g:10 mL
Extraction process	Heating in water bath (98°C 120 min)	Heating in water bath (98°C 60 min)	Ultrasound (35 KHz 30 min)
Filtration	Yes/filter paper	Yes/filter paper	Yes/filter paper
Preparation time (min)	150	120	90

Table 1. Preparation procedures details for Bediol® macerated oils.

each oil in 10 mL of isopropanol. After adding 1 μg/mL of IS, 10 μL of each sample were diluted in 890 μL of initial mobile phase from which 2 μL was injected.

Chromatography was accomplished on an HPLC system (Thermo Fisher Scientific, San Jose, CA, USA) that was made up of a Surveyor MS quaternary pump with a degasser, a Surveyor AS autosampler with a column oven and a Rheodyne valve with a 20 μL loop. Analytical separation was carried out using a reverse-phase HPLC column 150 × 2 mm i.d., 4 μm, Synergi Hydro RP, with a 4 × 3 mm i.d. C18 guard column (Phenomenex, Torrance, CA, USA). The mobile phase contained a binary combination of 0.1% aqueous formic acid and acetonitrile. The gradient was initiated with 60% eluent 0.1% aqueous formic acid with a linear decrease up to 95% in 10 min. This condition was maintained for 4 min. The mobile phase was returned to initial conditions at 14 min, followed by a 6-min re-equilibration period. The flow rate was 0.3 mL/min. The column and sample temperatures were 30 and 5°C, respectively. The mass spectrometer Thermo Q-Exactive Plus (Thermo Scientific, San Jose, CA, USA) was equipped with a heated electrospray ionisation (HESI) source. Capillary temperature and vaporiser temperature were set at 330 and 280°C, respectively, while the electrospray voltage was adjusted at 3.50 kV (operating in both positive and negative mode). Sheath and auxiliary gas were 35 and 15 arbitrary units, with S lens RF level of 60. The mass spectrometer was controlled by Xcalibur 3.0 software (Thermo Fisher Scientific, San Jose, CA, USA). The exact mass of the compounds was calculated using Qualbrowser in Xcalibur 3.0 software. The FS-dd-MS^2 (full scan data-dependent acquisition) in both positive and negative mode was used for both screening and quantification purposes. Resolving power of FS adjusted on 140,000 FWHM at m/z 200, with scan range of *m/z* 215-500. Automatic gain control (AGC) was set at $3e^6$, with an injection time of 200 ms. A targeted MS/MS (dd-MS^2) analysis operated in both positive and negative mode at 35,000 FWHM (*m/z* 200). The AGC target was set to $2e^5$, with the maximum injection time of 100 ms. Fragmentation of precursors was optimised as two-stepped normalised collision energy (NCE) (25 and 40 eV). Detection was based on calculated exact mass of the protonated/deprotonated molecular ions, at least one corresponding fragment and on retention time of target compounds [12]. Extracted ion chromatograms (EICs) were obtained with an accuracy of 2 ppm *m/z* from total ion chromatogram (TIC) engaging the *m/z* corresponding to the molecular ions [M+H]+ 315,23145 for CBD and THC, 311,20020 for CBN. 317,24716 for CBG and 311,2024 for CBN. In ESI_ the molecular ions [M_H]_ considered were 357,2164 for CBDA and THCA, while CBGA was detected by 359,22269.

3. Results and discussion

3.1. Quality analysis of Cannabis inflorescences

3.1.1. ASE Cannabis sample preparations from Bediol® medical chemotype

The choice of the appropriate analytical approach for cannabinoid profiling in cannabis inflorescences is extremely important, considering the need for a comprehensive chemical characterisation of cannabis and derived products [34]. For these reasons, analytical techniques based on high resolution mass spectrometer (HRMS-Orbitrap), due to their excellent resolution, precision and sensitivity [35], nowadays represent the gold standard techniques for the investigation of the highly complex cannabis composition. Proper purification and extraction methodology must also be implemented and is considered crucial in order to achieve an in-depth screening of the cannabinoids in *Cannabis sativa L.* inflorescence [32, 33].

The traditional solvent extraction methods often used for the extraction of different bioactive compounds from plants carry certain drawbacks [30]. Often, they are time consuming, laborious, have low selectivity or low extraction yields and usually large amounts of toxic solvents are required. Emphasis has currently shifted toward the use of sub- and supercritical fluids and generally-recognised-as-safe (GRAS) solvents as also detailed elsewhere [34]. Recent advances using accelerated solvent extraction (ASE) systems, as described in several publications [35, 36] include procedures for selective removal of interferences during sample extraction, thus combining extraction and purification into a single step. ASE is considered one of the most promising extraction process because, unlike standard extraction methods, it utilises high temperature and pressure to improve the extraction of the analyte from the solid sample. These conditions enhance the diffusion of the extraction solvent throughout the sample matrix which result in the more complete dissolution and recovery of the investigated compounds. The sample to be extracted is placed in a sealed metal cell that is then allocated automatically in a heated oven chamber and filled with the extraction solvent. The extraction cell is then pressurised, allowing for an increase in the boiling point of the extraction solvent, and for the solubilisation of the analytes at a temperature higher than would be possible at atmospheric pressure. Hereafter, the sample is extracted and collected by the automated filling and voiding of the cell through repeated static cycles. Compared to other solid sample extraction techniques, ASE requires less time, consumes less solvent during extraction and, with the added benefit of automation, has proven effective for several food solid samples.

Evaluation of the performance of ASE for the extraction of natural compounds like curcuminoids, saponins, flavonolignans, terpenes, taxanes, xanthone, flavonoids and artemisinin has already been conducted, as well as the application of ASE for the characterisation of phenolic compounds from fine Alpine plant roots [37]. The advantage of applying pressure is due to the fact that it is able to force the extracting solvent into the matrix and therefore may improve extraction efficiency dramatically. To the best of our knowledge, the present study reports an ASE-based method applied to the extraction of cannabinoids from cannabis row material (inflorescences) for the first time.

Bediol® chemotype was chosen for the optimisation of the ASE working parameters as it encompasses a combination of balanced amounts of THC and CBD, two cannabinoids responsible for most of the clinical effects that medical cannabis can express. In addition, it has been repeatedly suggested that the effect of isolated THC or of any other single cannabinoid is not equivalent to that of whole cannabis preparations, since some of the bioactivity observed could be related also to the presence of acidic cannabinoids. In this context, the use of an analytical method allowing the qualitative and quantitative exhaustive extraction of neutral cannabinoids and its native, acidic forms (THCA and CBDA) from cannabis plant is fundamental to characterise different cannabis varieties, a particularly relevant point when considering medical varieties. That is why the extraction efficacy of ASE was evaluated also for THCA and CBDA.

However, the optimization of effective extraction from cannabis plant is a strategic and very important issue in cannabinoid determination, as it determines the accuracy of the whole analytical method. Therefore, several extraction solvents for ASE extraction of cannabinoids from Bediol® chemotype were evaluated herein.

The best combination in terms of relative area (area analyte/IS) was obtained using methanol as extraction solvent at room temperature and 2 extraction cycles of 5 min each, with a resulting total extraction time of 15 min **(Figure 1)**. These results are in line with a recent study that investigated the use of different extraction methods (dynamic maceration, ultrasound, microwave and supercritical fluid extraction) for the analysis of cannabinoids from fibre-type cannabis varieties [38]. Recoveries calculated by comparing the concentrations of the extracted compounds with those from the MMC calibration curves at two different fortification levels showed an average recovery of 93 and 5.7% as coefficient of variation. Based on obtained MMC calibration curves used for the purpose of validation of ASE procedures the percentage of THC, THCA, CBD and CBDA in Bediol® inflorescence by means of LC-Q-Exactive-Orbitrap-MS analysis was calculated as being: 0.88, 5.7, 0.96 and 7.4%, respectively.

3.1.2. HS-SPME and GC-MS for terpenes fingerprint from Bediol® medical chemotype

In comparison with cannabinoid derivatives, the volatile constituents of *Cannabis sativa* L. have received much less attention. At present, scarce emphasis has been given toward the exhaustive characterisation of the terpenes profile obtained from Cannabis chemotype standardised and certified for medical use [18, 27]. In relation to recent evidence concerning the synergic role of terpenes and cannabinoids (entourage effect) [21], the comprehensive evaluation of terpene compounds especially characterising medical strains is nowadays crucial to correctly managing Cannabis as a complete therapeutic tool. In addition, several medical applications of Cannabis flos involve the vaporisation of inflorescence by using medical vaping equipment to heat the herb thus releasing both cannabinoids and terpenes into the vapour phase. The need

http://dx.doi.org/10.5772/intechopen.79539

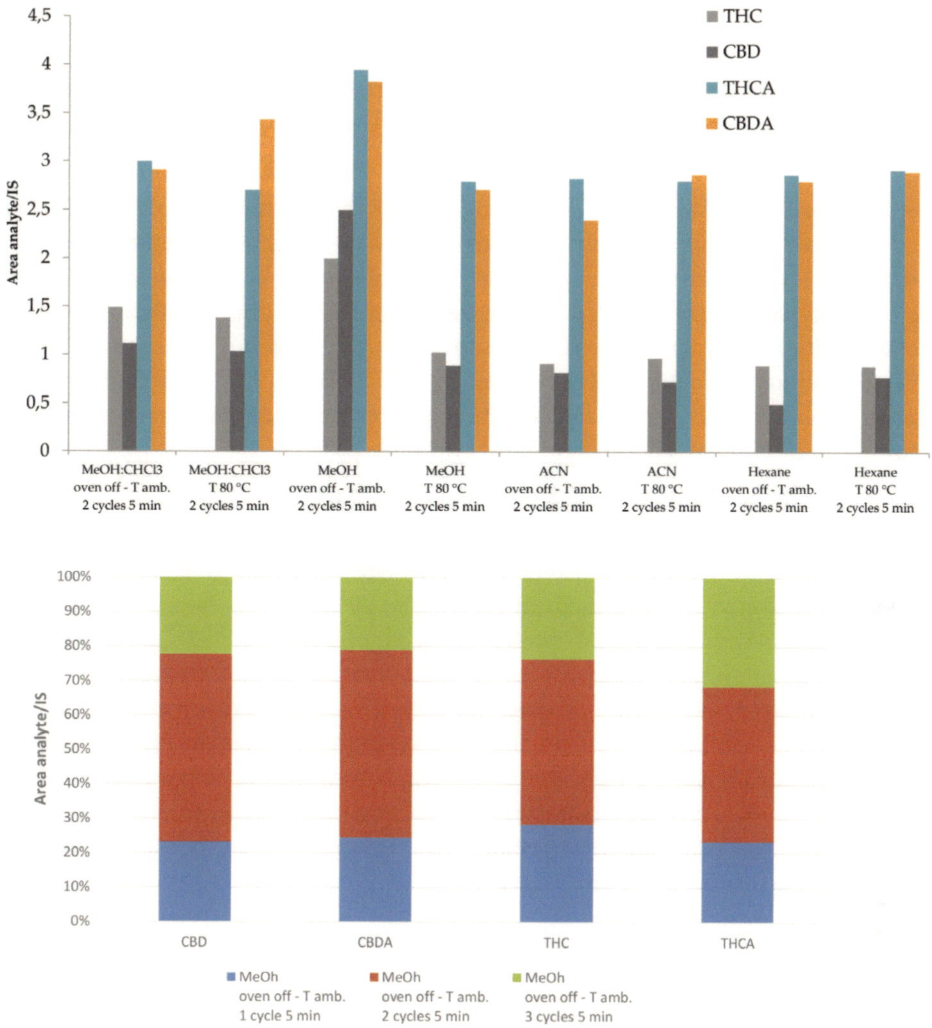

Figure 1. Impact of extraction solvents, temperature and number of extraction cycles on extractability of cannabinoids by using accelerated solvent extraction (ASE) from Bediol® chemotype.

to understand the real terpene profile emitted by medical varieties in order to select the most appropriate varieties for therapeutic use is particularly evident. In the present study, an HS-SPME method was adopted for the preconcentration of the volatile compounds with particular focus on terpenes fraction (mono-di-tri terpenes and sesquiterpenes). HS-SPME is considered a gold analytical technique for the analysis of volatile compounds in general (ref), but scarce data are available about the application of HS-SPME in the analysis of terpenes and in general of the volatile profile from medical cannabis varieties. Nevertheless, a study published recently demonstrates the convenience of HS-SPME in the characterisation of hashish terpene profile [35]. In particular, by the means of HS-SPME, authors were able to isolate and identify a potential volatile marker that might serve as a substance by which the resin and plant material could be discriminated. Volatiles in some Bedrocan® varieties have been previously investigated for their terpene content by GC-FID [29], a technique that provides only a partial volatile profile and is severely limited, as it does not furnish the identification of unknown volatiles, as is feasible with GC-MS facilities accompanied by adequate, up-dated mass spectrum libraries [31, 40].

Furthermore, the terpenes were extracted using ethanol as an extraction solvent [29] and then quantified by using a calibration curve constructed by using generic internal standard. This approach is usually limitative as the polarity of the solvent could dramatically influence the terpene profile obtained and lead to the underestimation of the complex mixture of secondary metabolites emitted by plants as a result [40]. Methods involving headspace sampling appear to be the most opportune option to investigate cannabis volatile profile to obtain a representative profile of their volatile constituents avoiding interference potentially brought by predominant cannabinoids in the resulting chromatogram [41].

It is worth mentioning that the terpenes family includes a great variety of compounds (mono-di-tri and sesquiterpenes) with pronounced chemical differences which consequentially aggravate the dissimilarities in terms of potential clinical effects. It was possible to identify more than 40 monoterpenes in Bediol® medical chemotype by using the optimised HS-SPME and GC-MS. The most representative are presented in **Figure 2.** As a general consideration, β-myrcene was the predominant terpene in Bediol® chemotype as was reported previously [22, 29, 41]. Moreover, this is an extremely important finding as this monoterpene demonstrates a prominent narcotic-like effect that is seemingly responsible for the 'couch lock' phenomenon frequently associated with modern cannabis phenomenology [24]. Furthermore, five other monoterpenes, namely α-terpinolene, β-ocimene, β-phellandrene α-and β-pinene are the major monoterpenes in Bediol® chemotype, as was revealed for other *Cannabis sativa* L. varieties [42]. Interestingly, our analysis revealed the presence of limonene (930 μg/g), which

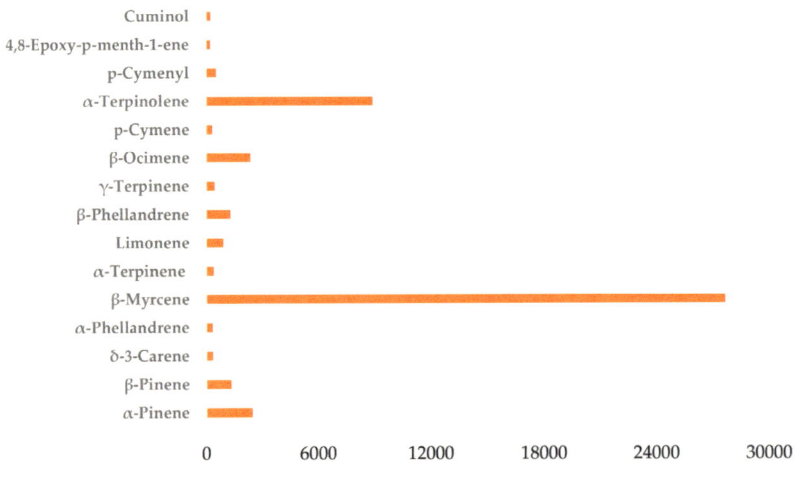

Figure 2. Representative terpenes fraction extracted from Bediol® chemotype by means of HS-SPME and identified using the GC-MS (μg/g).

is in contrast to previously published data for Bediol® inflorescence [29]. This finding is remarkable because the Bediol® chemotype is obtained by hybridising the Bedrocan variety (high THC content) with CBD-predominant varieties. Although the mechanisms underlying the regulation of terpene synthesis in cannabis plants remain to be elucidated, it is possible that selective, individual breeding could influence terpene proportion profiles [22].

Besides the chemical composition of the terpene fraction of Bediol® inflorescence that is comprehensively documented herein, the sesquiterpene fraction was also investigated in detail (**Figure 3**). This flos was particularly rich in trans-caryophyllene which is typical for most of *Cannabis sativa* L. varieties [19, 41, 42], but the significant amount of selina-3,7(11)-dione might be more specific to the Bediol® chemotype. In addition, by the means of mass spectrometry it was possible to identify a compound with a sesquiterpene structure which does not correspond to any known substance from this class. Considering its abundance, a profound examination of this "new", unknown compound is mandatory, as it could be used as a specific Bediol® marker.

Also, this chemotype was principally rich in esters, volatile compounds responsible for, and associated with, "fruity" flavour notes (**Figure 4**). The most abundant ester found is butanoic acid-hexyl ester, which is recognised by its sweet, apple, and apple peel flavour [43]. Its domination in the ester profile of Bediol® candidates this compound as the principal natural flavouring substance for this *Cannabis sativa* L. chemotype.

3.2. Quality analysis of Bediol® oil formulations: cannabinoids and VOC profile

In line with the approval by the Italian Ministry of Health of a decree that regulates the cultivation, processing, and therapeutic uses of Cannabis [16], there has been increasing request for the medicinal oil extracts obtained from the dried flowers [43]. A standardised protocol for oily preparations is therefore also required, but until now has not been formulated. In this

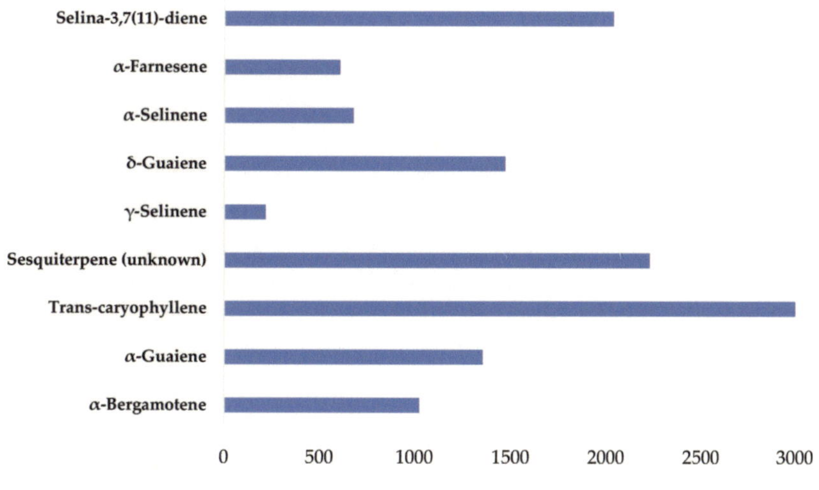

Figure 3. Representative sesquiterpenes fraction extracted from Bediol® chemotype by means of HS-SPME and identified using the GC-MS (μg/g).

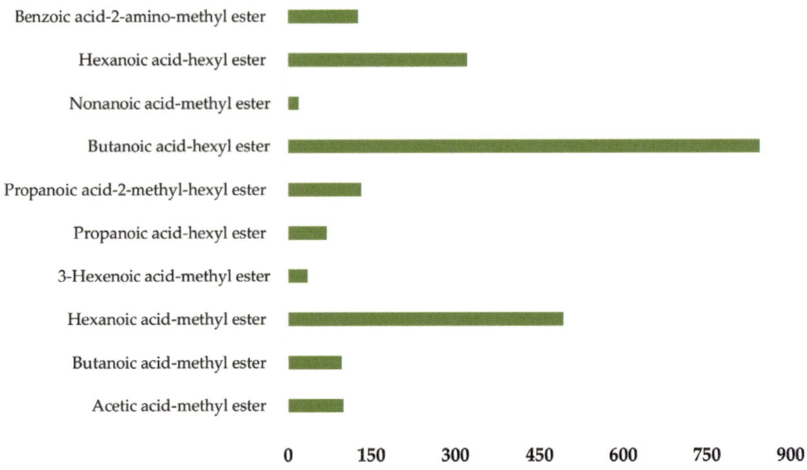

Figure 4. Esters fraction extracted from Bediol® chemotype by means of HS-SPME and identified using the GC-MS (μg/g).

context, cannabis extraction was performed using olive oil and a standardised medicinal cannabis "flos" (according to pharmaceutical standards) [31, 34, 39, 44, 45].

HPLC-MS/MS based analysis has recently been employed for the analysis of cannabinoids in plant materials, extracts and biological matrices [8, 29, 45]. This detection technique has proven to be particularly trustworthy, as there is no risk of native cannabinoids decomposition (decarboxylation of cannabinoid acids during the analysis), which may compromise the accurate assessment of the overall cannabinoids profile. Currently, the most widely used analysers for cannabinoids quantification are the triple quadrupole instruments, which possess excellent sensitivity and selectivity [31, 46]. However, they do not allow structural identification of "*non-target*" compounds.

In this respect, high-resolution accurate mass (HRMS) analyser such as Q-Exactive-Orbitrap-MS, offers the possibility to operate generating an "*in-depth*" qualitative analysis of thousands of compounds in complex biological, environmental or food matrixes providing insights beyond what is currently achievable with classic mass spectrometry instrumentation. Orbitrap mass spectrometer technology is rapidly developing also for cannabinoids profiling in different matrices, because it uniquely provides accurate molecular masses and specific fragmentation patterns for detected species. Moreover, HRMS acquisition mode accumulates all sample data, enabling identification of "unpredicted" compounds with cannabinolic structure and retrospective data analysis without the need to re-run samples.

As an example, a simultaneous identification of 24 synthetic and natural cannabinoids for a wide variety of samples such as herbal cannabis plant material by means of Orbitrap was reported [3]. Moreover, our research group has also recently published results concerning HPLC-Q-Exactive-Orbitrap-MS method for the determination of the seven most important cannabinoids, including four essential cannabinoids (THC, CBD, THCA and CBDA) accompanied with quantification of

CBN, CBG and CBGA [30]. Applying this method, we were able to determine the cannabinoid profile in Bediol® chemotype oils prepared by three different methods, as described in the materials and methods section.

Method 3 (realised by applying a preheating/ultrasounds assisted extraction), showed the highest extraction yields of the neutral cannabinoids CBD and THC. In contrast, method 1 provided the maximal concentrations of THCA, CBDA and CBGA, as a preheating step was not involved. At present, it is important to emphasise that, in the field of the therapeutic uses of cannabinoids related to pharmacological and clinical effects, THC and CBD in their neutral forms are of primary interest, even if there is growing attention toward the acidic forms (**Table 2**) [3].

Furthermore, apart from the targeted compounds revealed, several other untargeted cannabinoids were detected, as well. HRMS analysis has proven to be very useful also in the retrospective evaluation of untargeted isomeric cannabinoids. The structural interpretation of *untargeted* compounds was accomplished from the mass spectra collected in the FS and corresponding dd-MS^2 scan mode, and relied on the information found in the literature [30, 45, 46, 47, 49] and mass spectrum libraries [48]. In this respect, Q-Exactive-Orbitrap-MS analyser is often used in order to obtain structural information of the compounds detected as it provides accurate mass identification for both the precursor and the product ions. Among untargeted molecules, we verified the presence of THCV and CBDV that expressed the same fragmentation behaviour as their C5 equivalents but differed in fragments that contained the C3 side chain [30]. The presence and further quantification of those two compounds seems to be essential as it was revealed that in three models of seizure, cannabis-derived "botanical drug substances" rich in CBDV and CBD exerted significant anticonvulsant effects that were not mediated by the CB1 receptor and were of comparable efficacy with purified CBDV [50]. On the other hand, it is well-known that THCV (also as THC) binds to CB1 and CB2 receptors and acts as a cannabimimetic agonist [50, 51]. Therefore, the pharmacological potency of CBDV and THCV is substantial and, regardless of their relatively small amounts in oil preparations, they may contribute to the physiological efficiency of the overall cannabinoids profile [18], at least as far as Bediol® oil preparation is concerned.

Moreover, in the Bediol® oil extract samples in full scan negative acquisition mode at least four different cannabinoids with the same molecular ions (*m/z* 343.1915) but different retention times were noted (**Figure 5**). Their appearance and intensity varies according to the preparation method used. The fragmentation pattern of peaks at retention time (RT) 9.91 and 12.24 min correspond to tetrahydrocannabinolic acid—C4 (THCA-C4) and cannabidiolic acid—C4 (CBDA-C4). Those two

Preparation method	THC	CBD	CBN	CBG	THC-A	CBD-A	CBG-A
1 [32]	370 ± 23	2010 ± 56	10 ± 0.5	7 ± 0.8	8300 ± 507	14,120 ± 1002	260 ± 23
2 [33]	4520 ± 102	5503 ± 89	56 ± 7	125 ± 21	1808 ± 201	1208 ± 750	114 ± 15
3 [30]	5214 ± 87	7304 ± 108	47 ± 4	102 ± 12	487 ± 42	29 ± 0.75	18 ± 6

Table 2. Quantitative analysis of main cannabinoids from Bediol®'s macerated oil preparations obtained by three different preparation procedures (μg/g, mean ± SD, n = 3).

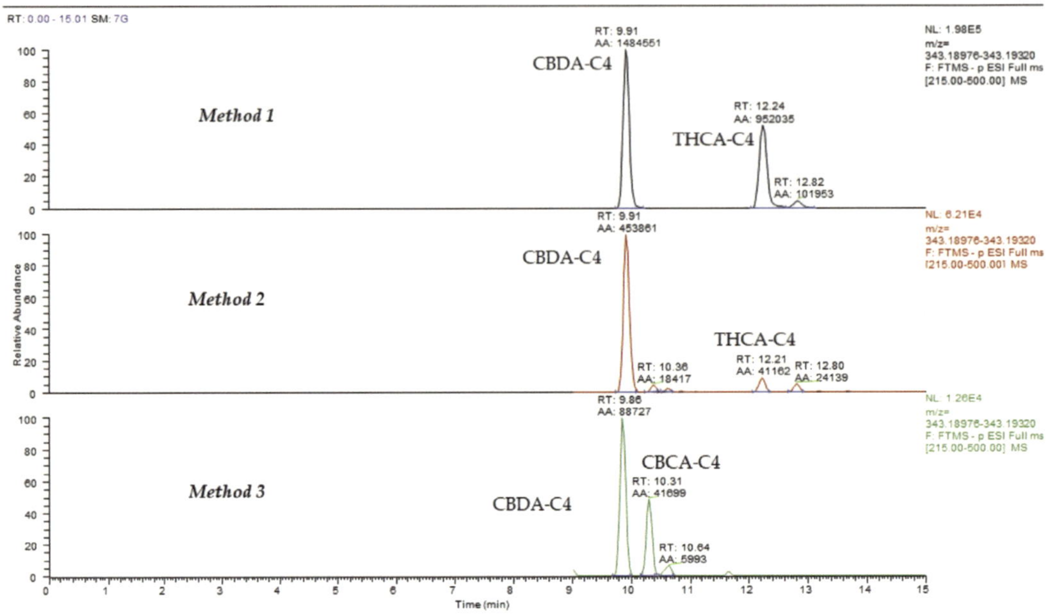

Figure 5. Extracted ion chromatograms from retrospective data analysis which point toward the presence of CBDA-C4; THCA-C4 and CBCA-C4.

acids are respectively homologues of main acids (THCA and CBDA) from which they differ just in the butyl side chain (instead of pentyl). In addition, the presence of the peak 10.31 and its fragmentation profile indicate the presence of cannabichromenic acid C4 (CBCA-C4). In a completely analogous way, the extracted ion chromatograms for *m*/*z* 329.17580 confirm the occurrence of THCVA and CBDVA, the acidic precursors of the above-mentioned THCV and CBDV, just for the oil samples from methods 1 and 2 (**Figure 6**). Additionally, the oil extract obtained by extraction method 3 revealed the presence of cannabichromevarinic acid (CBCVA). This compound, like its neutral counterpart cannabichromevarin CBCV, is not supported by adequate research work to fully understand its eventual distinctive pharmacological and physiological behaviour. However, the fact that extraction method 3 (preheating/ultrasounds) transfers this compound from the inflorescence to the medicinal oil has to be taken into consideration, especially when the signals of THCVA and CBDVA were practically absent in extract 3. This is most likely due to different kinetics of extraction performed by ultrasound that preserves the benzopiranic structure of CBCVA.

All in all, our retrospective analysis of Bediol® medical oil provides clear evidence of the need to develop a standardised procedure for extraction, especially in terms of time and extraction method, since they unambiguously affect the chemical composition of the final product, thus influencing the pharmacological effect of the medicinal preparation that is eventually dispensed to patients.

As far as VOCs profile is concerned, all three preparation methods extracted substantial amounts of terpenes, resembling the profile obtained for the Bediol® inflorescence. Comparing the three different preparation methods, it can be observed that method 1 extracted the highest

http://dx.doi.org/10.5772/intechopen.79539

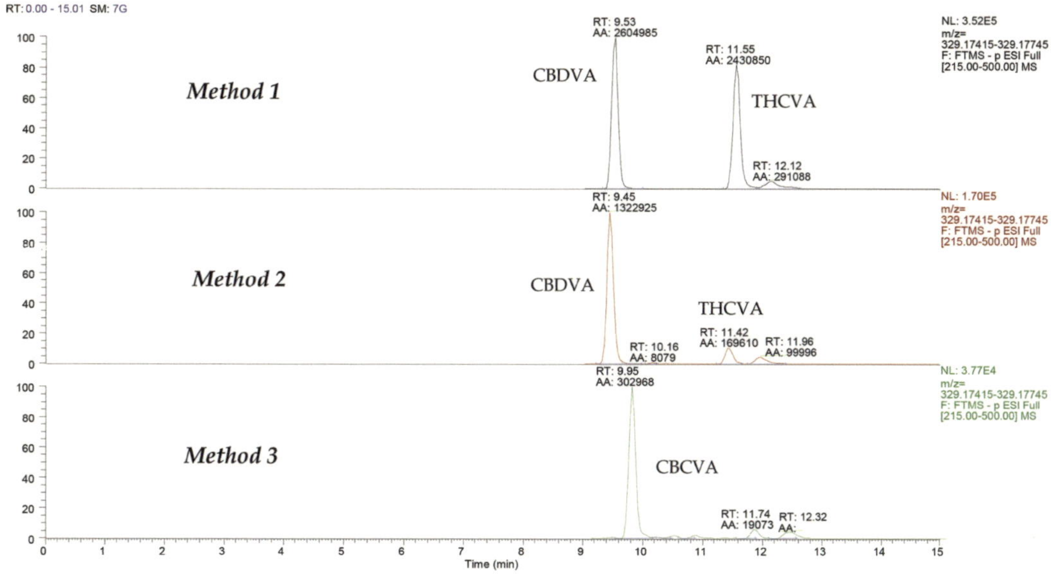

Figure 6. Extracted ion chromatograms from retrospective data analysis which point toward the presence of CBDVA; THCVA and CBCVA.

amount of terpenes, followed by methods 3 and 2 (**Table 3**). This was predictable, as method 1 did not include preheating for decarboxylation, thus the terpene fraction was preserved with evident domination of β-Myrcene. Although preheating the plant material released more of the known active neutral cannabinoids, it simultaneously led to the loss of components such as terpenes by degradation or evaporation.

As regards lipid oxidation products, the opposite trend was shown among the three preparation procedures. In particular, method 3, realised without any heating step, showed minor concentrations of lipid oxidation products. The macerated oil obtained using the method by Romano-Hazekamp (method 1) contained the highest levels of oxidation products, compared with the other two procedures, as expected. This can be related to preparation conditions in which the oil is heated at 98°C for 120 min. The data concerning the formation of lipid oxidation products in cannabis medical oil preparations are extremely limited [30]. The occurrence of aldehydes in the sample obtained by method 1 indicates the initiation of lipid peroxidation of polyunsaturated fatty acids (PUFA) from oils used as a matrix [52, 53]. It is well documented that peroxidation of PUFA leads to the formation of a well-defined series of aldehydes and ketones such as nonenal, hexanal and pentanal, 2-heptenal [54]. The formation rate of lipid oxidation products depends closely on several factors among which the most important are: method preparation temperature, fatty acid composition of oil in which cannabis extract is dissolved and storage conditions [55]. These parameters are crucial to define the ultimate characteristics of the final products to be used for medical treatment. Finally, the presence of 2-furancarboxaldehyde in the oil sample obtained by method 1 confirmed that preheating initiates the series of reactions that leads to the formation of potentially toxic compounds.

Compound class/name	Preparation method		
	1 [32]	2 [33]	3 [30]
Alcohols			
1-Hexanol	31.10 ± 2.8	15 ± 1.3	13.15 ± 2.12
3-Hexen-1-ol	1.10 ± 0.14	0.56 ± 0.12	0.7 ± 0.1
2-Ethyl-1-hexanol	0.22 ± 0.03	n.d.	n.d.
3,3,6-Trimethyl-1,5-heptadien-4-ol	13.1 ± 0.5	7.3 ± 1.93	5.3 ± 0.45
α-Toluenol	0.16 ± 0.03	0.10 ± 0.02	0.08 ± 0.02
Aldehydes			
2-Methyl-butanal	0.42 ± 0.05	n.d.	n.d.
3-Methyl-butanal	0.26 ± 0.03	n.d.	n.d.
Hexanal	1.51 ± 0.13	n.d.	n.d.
Heptanal	1.06 ± 0.29	n.d.	n.d.
2-Hexenal	1.90 ± 0.22	n.d.	n.d.
Octanal	0.54 ± 0.09	0.36 ± 0.01	0.04 ± 0.02
Ketones			
6-Methyl-5 hepten-2 one	1.8 ± 0.15	0.98 ± 0.14	0.28 ± 0.08
3-Methyl-3-cyclohexen-1-one	3.01 ± 0.67	0.58 ± 0.14	0.19 ± 0.05
Esters			
Acetic acid-methyl ester	0.41 ± 0.09	n.d.	n.d.
3-Hexen-1-ol-acetate	0.51 ± 0.02	0.22 ± 0.03	0.18 ± 0.01
Propanoic acid-hexyl ester	1.84 ± 0.01	0.99 ± 0.17	0.90 ± 0.1
Propanoic acid-2-methyl-hexyl ester	2.47 ± 0.01	1.55 ± 0.25	1.70 ± 0.09
Butanoic acid-hexyl ester	21.01 ± 0.21	10.80 ± 2.72	16 ± 0.82
Hexanoic acid-hexyl ester	1.78 ± 0.54	1.23 ± 0.28	1.43 ± 0.22
Benzoic acid-2-amino-methyl ester	0.55 ± 0.04	0.53 ± 0.16	0.53 ± 0.04
Mono/di/triterpenes			
α-Pinene	109 ± 1.4	12.37 ± 2.54	29.0 ± 0.39
α-Thujene	5.41 ± 0.45	2.12 ± 0.34	2.71 ± 0.11
Camphene	2.27 ± 0.15	0.67 ± 0.09	0.30 ± 0.01
β-Pinene	55.04 ± 7.0	14.57 ± 1.54	17.20 ± 0.67
Sabinene	1.82 ± 0.14	0.2 ± 0.07	n.d.
δ-3-Carene	18.4 ± 1.93	6.62 ± 0.90	7.44 ± 0.13
α-Phellandrene	19.00 ± 2.21	10.67 ± 1.93	5.57 ± 0.51
β-Myrcene	1074.2 ± 30	227.77 ± 35.1	458.0 ± 2.74
α-Terpinene	13.90 ± 1.27	10.20 ± 1045	16.56 ± 1.14
Limonene	32.4 ± 4.13	14.39 ± 1.75	18.17 ± 1.38

Compound class/name	Preparation method		
	1 [32]	2 [33]	3 [30]
Eucalyptol	5.2 ± 0.58	3.14 ± 0.76	4.84 ± 0.46
β-Phellandrene	52.00 ± 7.57	27.25 ± 4.37	35.83 ± 1.57
Cis-ocimene	2.70 ± 0.20	1.47 ± 0.24	0.72 ± 0.11
γ-Terpinene	13.87 ± 1.13	14 ± 2.36	8.50 ± 0.48
β-Ocimene	107.22 ± 6	49.0 ± 6.7	64.88 ± 1.15
p-Cymene	11.86 ± 1.11	6.7 ± 0.63	4.7 ± 0.49
α-Terpinolene	253.3 ± 20.9	157.78 ± 19.46	197.14 ± 1.08
1,3,8-p-Menthatriene	0.63 ± 0.01	0.37 ± 0.03	0.27 ± 0.04
p-Cymenyl	6.3 ± 0.18	6.84 ± 1.46	8.07 ± 0.33
Isomenthone	n.d.	0.16 ± 0.02	0.57 ± 0.08
4,8-Epoxy-p-menth-1-ene	12.11 ± 0.12	4.57 ± 1.01	2.80 ± 0.27
β-Linalool	0.89 ± 0.05	0.83 ± 0.19	0.66 ± 0.05
p-Menth-2-en-1-ol	0.42 ± 0.05	n.d.	n.d.
4-Terpineol	2.60 ± 0.01	2.65 ± 0.78	2.61 ± 0.18
Verbenol	2.41 ± 0.13	1.56 ± 0.63	2.21 ± 0.08
1,8-Menthadien-4-ol	7.00 ± 0.32	5.34 ± 1.55	6.15 ± 0.25
α-Terpineol	4.66 ± 0.15	3.63 ± 1.15	3.45 ± 0.20
Borneol	1.07 ± 0.16	0.89 ± 0.26	0.77 ± 0.02
p-Menth-1-en-3-ol	0.85 ± 0.03	0.39 ± 0.06	0.25 ± 0.03
Trans-3-caren-2-ol	1.00 ± 0.05	0.64 ± 0.11	0.52 ± 0.04
Cuminol	4.60 ± 0.36	3.42 ± 0.66	4.29 ± 0.23
Sesquiterpenes			
α-Santalene	0.94 ± 0.16	0.61 ± 0.08	0.57 ± 0.06
α-Bergamotene	4.66 ± 1.03	3.17 ± 0.63	4.28 ± 0.83
α-Guaiene	8.94 ± 2.17	6.97 ± 1.14	7.05 ± 1.93
Trans-caryophyllene	27.64 ± 4.78	20.60 ± 3.11	21.07 ± 3.13
α-Humulene	10.62 ± 2.35	7.11 ± 1.39	8.00 ± 1.73
δ-Guaiene	7.50 ± 2.11	5.84 ± 0.94	5.90 ± 1.41
β-Selinene	1.15 ± 0.26	0.83 ± 0.11	0.90 ± 0.29
α-Selinene	1.78 ± 0.07	1.07 ± 0.11	1.90 ± 0.45
α-Farnesene	0.63 ± 0.20	0.42 ± 0.06	0.54 ± 0.16
Selina-3,7(11)-diene	7.40 ± 2.30	5.60 ± 0.78	6.65 ± 1.93
Nerolidol	0.37 ± 0.08	0.35 ± 0.11	0.46 ± 0.18
Furans			
2-Furancarboxaldehyde	0.32 ± 0.05	n.d.	n.d.

Compound class/name	Preparation method		
	1 [32]	2 [33]	3 [30]
Dihydro-2(3H)-furanone	0.24 ± 0.06	0.16	n.d.
5-Ethyl-2(5H)-furanone	0.32 ± 0.04	0.27 ± 0.03	n.d.
Miscellaneous			
Dimethyl sulfide	0.63 ± 0.12	n.d.	n.d.
Methyl-pyrazine	n.d.	n.d.	n.d.
2,5-Dimethyl-pyrazine	n.d.	0.22 ± 0.07	0.16 ± 0.09
Dibutylformamide	n.d.	n.d.	n.d.
Acetylpyrrole	0.32 ± 0.07	0.41 ± 0.05	0.38 ± 0.06

Data are expressed in μg/g (mean value ± SD, n = 3).

Table 3. Volatile compounds extracted and identified by HS-SPME-GC/MS in Bediol® oil obtained from different preparation methods.

4. Conclusions

In this study, an analytical protocol involving the combination of HS-SPME coupled to GC–MS and ASE coupled to HPLC-HRMS (Orbitrap®) was applied for the in-depth profiling and fingerprinting of cannabinoids and terpenes in an authorised medical grade variety of *Cannabis sativa* L. (Bediol®). HS-SPME was shown to be an excellent technique to investigate both the cannabis inflorescence and derived macerated oil volatile composition. In particular, HS-SPME extraction provides an accurate profile concerning plausible terpenes fingerprint of different cannabis chemotypes, as presented in this study.

LC-HRMS-Orbitrap, used to investigate cannabinoids extracted from inflorescences and macerated oils, showed high-throughput performances, as it can be used both for quantification of *target* analytes and to investigate *untargeted* fraction to obtain a very complex prolife as an expression of plant phytocomplex at the same time.

These approaches are nowadays essential and pivotal in order to understand the composition of *Cannabis sativa* chemotypes currently used for their role in therapeutic management, as they are able to provide comprehensive information essential to then correlate the phytochemical characteristics of cannabis and the clinical results obtained when managed and administered to patients as well.

Acknowledgements

The present study was conducted according to the authorization released to Dr. Lorenzo Calvi by Ministero della Salute (SP/065, protocol number) for the supply and detention of narcotic

http://dx.doi.org/10.5772/intechopen.79539

drugs and/or psychotropic substances for scientific purposes. The present paper is partially funded and realised within the project ITALIAN MOUNTAIN LAB, Ricerca e Innovazione per l'ambiente ed. i Territori di Montagna—Progetto FISR Fondo integrativo speciale per la ricerca.

Author details

Lorenzo Calvi[1], Radmila Pavlovic[1,2], Sara Panseri[3]*, Luca Giupponi[1,2], Valeria Leoni[1,2] and Annamaria Giorgi[1,2]

*Address all correspondence to: sara.panseri@unimi.it

1 Department of Agricultural and Environmental Sciences—Production, Landscape, Agroenergy, Università degli Studi di Milano, Milan, Italy

2 CRC-Ge.S.Di.Mont.—Centre for Applied Studies in the Sustainable Management and Protection of the Mountain Environment, CRC-Ge.S.Di.Mont—Università degli Studi di Milano, Brescia, Italy

3 Department of Health, Animal Science and Food Safety, Università degli Studi di Milano, Milan, Italy

References

[1] Leung L. Cannabis and its derivatives: Review of medical use. Journal of the American Board of Family Medicine. 2011;**24**:452-462

[2] Borgelt LM, Franson KL, Nussbaum AM, Wang GS. The pharmacologic and clinical effects of medical cannabis. Pharmacotherapy. 2013;**33**:195-209

[3] Whiting PF, Wolff RF, Deshpande S, Di Nisio M, Duffy S, Hernandez AV et al. Cannabinoids for medical use: A systematic review and meta-analysis. JAMA. 2015;**313**:2456-2473

[4] Mead A. The legal status of cannabis (marijuana) and cannabidiol (CBD) under U.S. law. Epilepsy & Behavior. 2017;**70**:288-291

[5] Brenneisen R. Chemistry and analysis of phytocannabinoids and other Cannabis constituents. In: ElSohly MA, editor. Marijuana and the Cannabinoids. 1st ed. Totowa, New Jersey: Humana Press Inc.; 2007. pp. 17-49

[6] Alexander SPH, Mathie A, Peters JA. Guide to receptors and channels (GRAC), 4th ed. British Journal of Pharmacology. 2009;**158**(Suppl. 1):S1-S254

[7] Flores-Sanchez IJ, Verpoorte R. Secondary metabolism in Cannabis. Phytochemistry Reviews. 2008;**7**:615-639

[8] Pavlovic R, Nenna G, Calvi L, Panseri P, Borgonovo G, Giupponi L, Cannazza G, Giorgi A. Quality traits of "Cannabidiol oils": Cannabinoids content, terpene fingerprint and oxidation

stability of European commercially available preparations. Molecules. May 20 2018;**23**(5): pii:E1230. DOI:10.3390/molecules23051230

[9] Radwan MM, ElSohly MA, Slade D, Ahmed SA, Khan JA, Ross SA. Biologically active cannabinoids from high-potency Cannabis sativa. Journal of Natural Products. 2009;**72**: 906-911

[10] Russo EB. Cannabinoids in the management of difficult to treat pain. Therapeutics and Clinical Risk Management. 2008;**4**:245-259

[11] Rong C, Lee Y, Carmona NE, Cha DS, Ragguett RM, Rosenblat JD, Mansur RB, Ho RC, McIntyre RS. Cannabidiol in medical marijuana: Research vistas and potential opportunities. Pharmacological Research. 2017;**121**:213-218

[12] www.ema.europa.eu/sativex/

[13] FDA Briefing Document: **P**eripheral and Central Nervous System Drugs Advisory Committee Meeting; April 19, 2018, NDA 210365

[14] www.emcdda.europa.eu/topics/cannabis

[15] Regulation (EU) No. 1307/2013 of the European Parliament and of the Council of 17 December 2013 establishing rules for direct payments to farmers under support schemes within the framework of the common agricultural policy and repealing Council Regulation (EC) No. 637/2008 and Council Regulation (EC) No. 73/2009

[16] Decreto 9 novembre 2015: Funzioni di Organismo statale per la cannabis previsto dagli articoli 23 e 28 della convenzione unica sugli stupefacenti del 1961, come modificata nel 1972. Available: http://www.gazzettaufficiale.it/eli/id/2015/11/30/15A08888/sg;jsessionid=p1rnwNujUKlqQ5azhA%20Q95A__.ntc-as3-guri2a

[17] http://www.emcdda.europa.eu/html.cfm/index146601EN.html

[18] Citti C, Ciccarella G, Braghiroli D, Parenti C, Vandelli MA, Cannazza G. Medicinal cannabis: Principal cannabinoids concentration and their stability evaluated by a high-performance liquid chromatography coupled to diode array and quadrupole time of flight mass pectrometry method. Journal of Pharmaceutical and Biomedical Analysis. 2016;**128**:201-209

[19] Hazekamp A. The medicinal power of cannabis [Cannabinoïden werken - Bewezen - pijnstillend: De medicinale kracht v an cannabis]. Pharmaceutisch Weekblad. 2007;**142**(44): 38-41

[20] ElSohly MA, editor. Marijuana and the Cannabinoids. 1st ed. Totowa, New Jersey: Humana Press Inc.; 2007

[21] Elzinga S, Fischedick R, Podkolinski J, Raber C. Cannabinoids and terpenes as chemotaxonomic markers in cannabis. Natural Products Chemistry and Research. 2015;**3**:81

[22] Aizpurua-Olaizola O, Soydaner U, Öztürk E, Schibano D, Simsir Y, Navarro P, Etxebarria N, Usobiaga A. Evolution of the cannabinoid and terpene content during the growth of

Cannabis sativa plants from different chemotypes. Journal of Natural Products. 2016;**79**: 324-331

[23] Lewis MA, Russo EB, Smith KM. Pharmacological foundations of Cannabis chemovars. Planta Medica. 2018;**84**(4):225-233

[24] Russo EB. Taming THC: Potential cannabis synergy and phytocannabinoid-terpenoid entourage effects. British Journal of Pharmacology. 2011;**163**:1344-1364

[25] Gertsch J, Leonti M, Raduner S, Racz I, Chen JZ, Xie XQ, et al. Beta-caryophyllene is a dietary cannabinoid. Proceedings of the National Academy of Sciences of the United States of America. 2008;**105**:S9099-S9104

[26] Gertsch J, Raduner S, Altmann KH. New natural noncannabinoid ligands for cannabinoid type-2 (CB2) receptors. Journal of Receptor and Signal Transduction Research. 2006;**26**: S709-S730

[27] Russo EB, Jiang HE, Li X, Sutton A, Carboni A, del Bianco F, et al. Phytochemical and genetic analyses of ancient Cannabis from Central Asia. Journal of Experimental Botany. 2008;**59**:4171-4182

[28] Fischedick JT, Hazekamp A, Erkelens T, Choi YH, Verpoorte R. Metabolic fingerprinting of *Cannabis sativa* L., cannabinoids and terpenoids for chemotaxonomic and drug standardization purposes. Phytochemistry. 2010;**71**:2058-2073

[29] Citti C, Braghiroli DM, Vandelli A, Cannazza G. Pharmaceutical and biomedical analysis of cannabinoids: A critical review. Journal of Pharmaceutical and Biomedical Analysis. 2018;**147**:566-579

[30] Calvi L, Pentimalli D, Panseri S, Giupponi L, Gelmini F, Beretta G, et al. Comprehensive quality evaluation of medical *Cannabis sativa L.* inflorescence and macerated oils based on HS-SPME coupled to GC–MS and LC-HRMS (q-exactive orbitrap®) approach. Journal of Pharmaceutical and Biomedical Analysis. 2018;**150**:208-219

[31] Chiesa L, Labella GF, Giorgi A, Panseri S, Pavlovic R, Bonacci S, Arioli F. The occurrence of pesticides and persistent organic pollutants in Italian organic honeys from different productive areas in relation to potential environmental pollution. Chemosphere. 2016;**59**:482-490

[32] Romano L, Hazekamp A. Cannabis oil: Chemical evaluation of an upcoming cannabis based medicine. Cannabinoids. 2013;**1**:1-11

[33] Pacifici R, Marchei E, Salvatore F, Guandalini L, Busardò FP, Pichini S. Evaluation of cannabinoids concentration and stability in standardized preparations of cannabis tea and cannabis oil by ultra-high performance liquid chromatography tandem mass spectrometry. Clinical Chemistry and Laboratory Medicine. 2017;**0**:1-9

[34] Azmir J, Zaidul ISM, Rahman MM, Sharif KM, Mohamed A, Sahena F, Jahurul MHA, Ghafoor K, Norulaini NAN, Omar AKM. Techniques for extraction of bioactive compounds from plant materials: A review. Journal of Food Engineering. 2013;**117**(4):426-436

[35] http://aevnmont.free.fr/SACH-BOOKS/Petrochemistry/Oil%20Extraction%20and%20Analysis/1893997782_CH03.PDF

[36] Hossain M, Barry-Ryan C, Martin-Diana AB, Brunton N. Optimisation of accelerated solvent extraction of antioxidant compounds from rosemary (*Rosmarinus officinalis* L.), marjoram (*Origanum majorana* L.) and oregano (*Origanum vulgare* L.) using response surface methodology. Food Chemistry. 2011;**126**:339-346

[37] Giupponi L, Pentimalli D, Manzo A, Panseri S, Giorgi A. Effectiveness of fine root fingerprinting as a tool to identify plants of the Alps: Results of preliminary study. Plant Biosystems. 2017; in press

[38] Brighenti V, Pellati F, Steinbach M, Maran D, Benvenuti S. Development of a new extraction technique and HPLC method for theanalysis of non-psychoactive cannabinoids in fibre-type *Cannabis sativa* L. (hemp). Journal of Pharmaceutical and Biomedical Analysis. 2018;**143**:228-236

[39] Marchini LM, Charvoz C, Dujourdy L, Baldovini N, Filippi JJ. Multidimensional analysis of cannabis volatile constituents: Identification of 5,5-dimethyl-1-vinylbicyclo[2.1.1] hexane as a volatile marker of hashish, the resin of *Cannabis sativa*. Journal of Chromatography A. 2014;**1370**:200-215

[40] Wiebelhaus N, Hamblin D, Kreitals NM, Almirall JR. Differentiation of marijuana headspace volatiles from other plants and hemp products using capillary microextraction of volatiles (CMV) coupled to gas-chromatography-mass spectrometry (GC-MS). Forensic Chemistry. 2016;**2**:1-8

[41] Sexton M, Shelton K, Haley P, West M. Evaluation of cannabinoid and terpenoid content: Cannabis flower compared to supercritical CO_2 concentrate. Planta Medica. 2018;**84**(4): 234-241

[42] Wang S, Saito T, Ohkawa K, Ohara H, Suktawee S, Ikeura H, Kondo S. Abscisic acid is involved in aromatic ester biosynthesis related with ethylene in green apples. Journal of Plant Physiology. 2018. DOI: 10.1016/j.jplph.2017.12.007. Epub 2017 Dec 16

[43] Carcieri C, Tomasello C, Simiele M, De Nicolò A, Avataneo V, Canzoneri L, Cusato J, Di Perri G, D'Avolio A. Cannabinoids concentration variability in cannabis olive oil galenic preparations. The Journal of Pharmacy and Pharmacology. 2017. DOI: 10.1111/jphp.12845

[44] Casiraghi A, Roda G, Casagni E, Cristina C, Musazzi UM, Franzè S, et al. Extraction method and analysis of cannabinoids in Cannabis olive oil preparations. Planta Medica. 2018;**84**:242-249

[45] Aizpurua-Olaizola O, Omar J, Navarro P, Olivares M, Etxebarria N, Usobiaga A. Identification and quantification of cannabinoids in *Cannabis sativa* L. plants by high performance liquid chromatography-mass spectrometry. Analytical and Bioanalytical Chemistry. 2014; **406**:7549-7560

[46] Citti C, Pacchetti B, Vandelli MA, Forni F, Cannazza G. Analysis of cannabinoids in commercial hemp seed oil and decarboxylation kinetics studies of cannabidiolic acid (CBDA). Journal of Pharmaceutical and Biomedical Analysis. 2018;**149**:532-540

[47] Lebel P, Waldron KC, Furtos A. Rapid determination of 24 synthetic and natural cannabinoids for LC-MS-MS screening in natural products and drug inspection applications. Current Trends in Mass Spectrometry. 2015;**13**:8-15

[48] Lewis MM, Yang Y, Wasilewski E, Clarke HA, Kotra LP. Chemical profiling of medical Cannabis extracts. ACS Omega. 2017;**2**(9):6091-6103

[49] https://www.mzcloud.org/

[50] Iannotti FA, Hill CL, Leo A, Alhusaini A, Soubrane C, Mazzarella E, Russo E, Whalley BJ, Di Marzo V, Stephens GJ. Nonpsychotropic plant cannabinoids, cannabidivarin (CBDV) and cannabidiol (CBD), activate and desensitize transient receptor potential vanilloid 1 (TRPV1) channels in vitro: Potential for the treatment of neuronal hyperexcitability. ACS Chemical Neuroscience. 2014;**5**:1131-1141

[51] Thomas A, Stevenson LA, Wease KN. Evidence that the plant cannabinoid Delta 9-tetrahydrocannabivarin is a cannabinoid CB1 and CB2 receptor antagonist. British Journal of Pharmacology. 2005;**146**(7):917-926

[52] Pisanti S, Malfitano AM, Ciaglia E, Lamberti A, Ranieri R, Cuomo G, et al. Cannabidiol: State of the art and new challenges for therapeutic applications. Pharmacology & Therapeutics. 2017;**175**:133-150

[53] Guillén MD, Goicoechea E. Toxic oxygenated alpha, beta-unsaturated aldehydes and their study in foods: A review. Critical Reviews in Food Science and Nutrition. 2008;**48**(2):119-136

[54] Panseri S, Soncin S, Chiesa LM, Biondi PA. A headspace solid-phase microextraction gas-chromatographic mass-spectrometric method (HS-SPME-GC/MS) to quantify hexanal in butter during storage as marker of lipid oxidation. Food Chemistry. 2011;**127**:886-889

[55] Sapino S, Carlotti ME, Peira E, Gallarate M. Hemp-seed and olive oils: Their stability against oxidation and use in O/W emulsions. Journal of Cosmetic Science. 2005;**56**(4):227-251

Section 3

Clinical Research

Chapter 5

The United Chemicals of Cannabis: Beneficial Effects of Cannabis Phytochemicals on the Brain and Cognition

Katrina Weston-Green

Additional information is available at the end of the chapter

http://dx.doi.org/10.5772/intechopen.79266

Abstract

'Medicinal cannabis' can be defined as pharmaceutical grade cannabis-based products used for the treatment of illness. Beneficial treatment effects of cannabidiol (CBD), a major non-intoxicating compound isolated from the cannabis plant, have been shown in multiple states of cognitive impairment, including neurodegenerative (Alzheimer's, Huntington's and Parkinson's disease), neuroinflammatory (sepsis-induced encephalopathy) and neurological disorders (ischemic brain injury). CBD can also treat some of the symptoms of schizophrenia, including cognitive deficits (impairments in learning and memory), which is a major symptom domain of the illness that is largely resistant to existing antipsychotic medications. However, empirical evidence suggests the presence of an 'entourage effect' in cannabis; that is, observations that medicinal cannabis seems to work better in some instances when administered as a whole-plant extract. While scientific evidence highlights isolated CBD as a strong candidate for treating cognitive impairment, the entourage effect suggests that the co-operation of other plant molecules could provide further benefits. This chapter explores the scientific evidence surrounding the benefits of CBD and other specific key phytochemicals in cannabis: linalool, α-pinene, β-caryophyllene, flavonoids and anthocyanin, on brain health and cognition.

Keywords: medicinal cannabis, entourage effect, synergy, cannabidiol, CBD, terpenes, linalool, alpha-pinene, beta-caryophyllene, phenol, flavonoid, anthocyanins, purple cannabis, marijuana, cognition, learning, memory, brain, therapeutics, neuroprotection, inflammation

1. Introduction

Research shows that certain molecules identified in the cannabis plant are able to improve aspects of cognition. Cognition encompasses multiple aspects of thought processing including decision-making, processing speed, attention span, learning and memory. Cognitive dysfunction can occur in a range of illnesses and disease states, for example Alzheimer's disease, dementia, Parkinson's disease, schizophrenia, hypoxic ischemia, stroke and meningitis. There is particularly strong evidence in the existing literature to support the pro-cognitive effects of the cannabinoid, cannabidiol (CBD) in disease states. There is also evidence that other phytochemicals in cannabis provide benefits for brain health and cognitive function. Furthermore, the suggested presence of an 'entourage effect' may mean that the therapeutic potential of CBD could be boosted through synergistic interactions with other phytochemicals. Therefore, certain cannabis strains may confer greater benefits for particular clinical indications, presenting unique opportunities for the discovery of novel personalised therapeutics. Identifying specific beneficial compounds could underpin selective breeding of plant cultivars with phytochemical profiles optimised towards restoring brain function in diseases associated with cognitive dysfunction.

2. Cannabidiol (CBD) and the brain

CBD is a major cannabinoid of *C. sativa*, considered a metabolic by-product rather than a biosynthetic product of the plant [1]. There has been a recent burst of studies showing beneficial effects of CBD in the brain, with evidence pointing to CBD as a promising novel therapy for a range of disorders. Based on its ability to change brain function and behaviour, it is, by definition 'psychoactive', but CBD is non-intoxicating and there is currently no evidence that it causes the deleterious hallucinogenic, paranoia and anxiety-inducing effects of the delta-tetrahydrocannabinol (Δ-THC) type chemicals, particularly Δ9-THC that is primarily responsible for the 'high' induced by recreational cannabis [2]. Instead, CBD has a broad spectrum of therapeutic properties, including antipsychotic, anxiolytic, immunomodulatory, anti-inflammatory, neuroprotective and pro-cognitive benefits in humans and preclinical disease models. Although its mechanisms of action are currently unclear, studies show that CBD is a cannabinoid 1 receptor (CB1) negative allosteric modulator [3], is a partial agonist of the dopamine D2 high receptor sub-type [4] and increases anandamide (AEA) signalling [5], possibly through inhibition of the AEA catabolic enzyme, fatty acid amide hydrolase (FAAH) [6].

2.1. Cannabidiol protects against cognitive harms of high-THC Cannabis

In terms of cognition, our recent systematic review by Osborne et al. [7] revealed a body of clinical and pre-clinical evidence supporting the pro-cognitive effects of CBD. We identified reports demonstrating that CBD can protect against cognitive harms of cannabis. For example, recreational users of cannabis containing higher (>0.75%) CBD performed better in verbal memory testing during acute intoxication compared to users of cannabis with the same Δ9-THC levels but low (<0.14%) CBD [reviewed in 7]. CBD pre-treatment (600 mg oral) also protected against deficits in verbal learning and memory, and aspects of working memory during a Δ9-THC (1.5 mg/kg intravenous (i.v.)) challenge in healthy participants ($n = 22$) [reviewed in 7].

http://dx.doi.org/10.5772/intechopen.79266

Imaging studies over the past decade have revealed altered brain morphology in key regions of the brain implicated in cognition in cannabis users. For example, chronic heavy cannabis users (n = 15) exhibit reduced brain volume in the hippocampus and amygdala compared to matched non-using controls (n = 16) [8], and hippocampal shape aberrations were detected in cannabis users (n = 15 male chronic heavy users) that were exacerbated in people with co-morbid schizophrenia (n = 8 males) compared to healthy controls [9]. Interestingly, regular users of low CBD cannabis had reduced hippocampal volumes compared to non-users; a reduction that was not observed in the participants either using cannabis containing CBD or in former users [10]. The authors of that study concluded that CBD could reduce harm to brain health caused by cannabis use, while periods of abstinence could recover damage in the parameters examined [10]. Recently, it was reported that 10-weeks of oral CBD treatment (200 mg) increased the volume of discrete hippocampal regions in cannabis users (n = 18), with higher growth observed in heavy compared to light cannabis users [11]. Overall, these studies point to a protective effect of CBD on cognitive regions of the brain during cannabis use in humans; however, larger scale placebo-controlled trials are required. A potential mechanism for these benefits may relate to the neuroprotective characteristics of CBD, particularly its ability to stimulate neurogenesis, synaptic formation and neurite outgrowth (reveiwed in [12]).

Similar results supporting a protective role of CBD have been reported in pre-clinical studies. For example, CBD (0.5 mg/kg) increased visual learning and memory, and procedural learning in Rhesus monkeys co-administered Δ9-THC (0.2 or 0.5 mg/kg) compared to those administered Δ9-THC alone; however, spatial working memory was further impaired by combined treatment (reviewed in [7]). Chronic Δ9-THC exposure in adolescent mice (3 mg/kg daily) reduced recognition memory that persisted into adulthood, but this was not apparent in the group receiving CBD (3 mg/kg CBD) co-treatment during Δ9-THC exposure [13]. On the other hand, research shows that there are no beneficial effects of CBD on cognition, including verbal learning and memory, social recognition, executive function, spatial memory or conditioned learning, when administered to healthy subjects (humans or rodents) (reviewed in [7, 13]).

2.2. Cannabidiol treatment for neurological disorders and inflammatory disease states

2.2.1. Alzheimer's disease

Alzheimer's disease is the most common form of dementia. It is a progressive neurological disorder characterised by the presence of plaques and neurofibrillary tangles in the brain. Amyloid β peptides form densely packed extracellular filaments (plaques) that block cell signalling and trigger neuroinflammation. Neurofibrillary tangles are caused by transport-associated proteins called tau that form twisted structures during oxidative stress and block transport of nutrients and other essentials for neuronal function [14]. The progressive disruption and destruction of synapses results in memory loss and cognitive dysfunction. A role for cannabinoids as a therapy for Alzheimer's disease has been proposed, in part due to the neuroprotective, anti-inflammatory and anti-oxidant properties of cannabinoids, as well as the role of the endocannabinoid system in memory and Alzheimer's disease pathology (reviewed in [15]). One study found that Sativex®, containing Δ9-THC and CBD, reduced tau and amyloid deposition in the hippocampus and cortex in a mouse model of tauopathy [16]. In addition, Δ9-THC and CBD administration improved memory deficits in AβPP/PS1 transgenic mice with an Alzheimer-like phenotype, but not in mice with cognitive decline associated with healthy ageing [17]. Another study attributed CBD treatment (20 mg/kg oral, daily for 8 months) of social recognition deficits in AβPP/PS1 mice with the prevention of neuroinflammation and cholesterol homeostasis rather than a reduction in amyloid load [18]. Clinical studies are required to confirm whether CBD/Δ9-THC therapies can improve brain health and function in people with Alzheimer's disease or dementia.

2.2.2. Huntington's disease

Huntington's disease is a progressive neurodegenerative disease of genetic origins, manifesting in motor impairment, cognitive decline and behavioural symptoms. In a double-blinded, placebo-controlled, cross-over clinical trial, Sativex® (orally administered in 12 sprays/day) was unable to improve cognitive, motor or behavioural scores in a cohort of patients with Huntington's disease (n = 24) compared to placebo-treated controls after 12-weeks of treatment [19]. In a smaller double-blinded, randomised cross-over study, CBD alone (10 mg/kg/day, oral) also yielded no symptom efficacy, including recall memory, in 15 patients Huntington's disease after 6-weeks of treatment [20]. However, large cohort studies of CBD administration in people with Huntington's disease are required.

2.2.3. Parkinson's disease

Parkinson's disease occurs through the progressive degeneration of dopaminergic neurons in the midbrain, resulting in severe motor impairment and loss of motor control. CBD is a prime novel therapeutic candidate for the treatment of Parkinson's disease due to its neuroprotective properties. However, one clinical study reported no improvement in motor or general symptoms scores in patients treated with CBD (75 or 300 mg/day) compared to placebo-treated controls (n = 7/group), although, overall quality of life was significantly improved in the 300 mg CBD treatment group compared to placebo-treated controls [21]. Another clinical study (open-label pilot study, n = 6) of Parkinson's disease patients with psychosis revealed significant improvements to psychiatric scores, but not motor function following CBD (>150 mg/day oral CBD) administration for 4-weeks in combination with existing L-dopa medication [22]. On the other hand, CBD (0.5 or 5 mg/kg CBD administered in four injections) prevented cognition and motor dysfunction when administered prior to reserpine treatment in a rodent model of Parkinson's disease [23].

2.2.4. Ischemic brain injury

Brain injury due to blood flow impediment and hypoxic damage can result in immediate and progressive cognitive decline. Ischemic brain injury can occur following events such as a stroke, cardiac arrest, near drowning or birth complications resulting in perinatal asphyxia.

Rats exposed to hypoxic ischemia at birth exhibited recognition memory deficits that were attenuated by CBD (1 mg/kg) administered subcutaneously 10 min post-ischemia, while CBD treatment (3, 10 or 30 mg/kg 30 min pre- and 3, 24 and 48 h post-ischemic insult) increased spatial memory compared to placebo-treated ischemic rats (reviewed in [7]). In a subsequent study, acute CBD treatment (5 mg/kg, intraperitoneal (i.p.)) reduced apoptosis, neuronal loss and neuroinflammation in ischemic in neonatal rats [24], providing mechanistic clues about the behavioural restorative effects of CBD during hypoxic brain damage. A clinical trial investigating THC:CBD efficacy on spasticity following a stroke has been registered [25]; however, cognitive testing has not been proposed as a treatment outcome.

2.2.5. *Sepsis-induced encephalopathy*

Sepsis is a potentially life-threatening systemic inflammatory state that occurs as the body attempts to eliminate a pathogen. It can cause rapid cognitive impairment, particularly memory decline that was initially considered a transient state restored through the destruction of the pathogen and attenuation of the inflammatory response. However, sepsis is also associated with encephalopathy, a disease state of the brain that can manifest symptoms ranging from mild personality changes to cognitive and motor impairment, lethargy and coma. Sepsis-induced encephalopathy can be caused by increased permeability of the blood brain barrier and neuroinflammation that can lead to permanent functional impairment and enhance susceptibility to subsequent neurodegenerative disorders post-recovery [26]. Sub-chronic CBD treatment improved associative learning in a rodent model of sepsis (CBD administered either 2.5, 5 or 10 mg/kg daily for 9 days) compared to vehicle-treated controls (reviewed in [7]). CBD (single acute dose 3 mg/kg, i.v.) treatment also preserved blood–brain barrier integrity, restored normal vascular endothelial function and reduced inflammation in the mouse brain during endotoxic shock induced by administration of lipopolysaccharide (LPS) [27], a cell wall component of Gram-negative bacteria that can be used to model an excessive pro-inflammatory response in the host.

2.2.6. *Schizophrenia*

Schizophrenia is a chronic neurodevelopmental disorder characterised by three main symptom domains: positive (e.g., hallucinations, delusions and paranoia), negative (e.g., social withdrawal, flattened emotional expression, lack of motivation) and cognitive deficits. Existing antipsychotic medications confer minimal to no cognitive benefits (in some instances can further impair cognition) [28], and can cause serious weight gain and diabetes side-effects [29, 30]. We recently discovered that chronic CBD (10 mg/kg CBD, i.p., twice daily (b.i.d.)) treated cognitive impairment (learning, working and recognition memory) and social interaction deficits in a rat prenatal infection (poly I:C) model of schizophrenia-like phenotypes [31]. No behavioural changes were observed in healthy rats administered CBD and CBD did not cause weight gain side-effects [31]. An earlier clinical study (phase II, single-centred, double-blinded, randomised parallel-group controlled clinical trial of CBD vs. amisulpride) had reported improved positive and negative symptoms in people with schizophrenia following 4 weeks of CBD treatment, with therapeutic efficacy similar to the commercial antipsychotic, amisulpride; however, cognitive function was not examined [5]. More recently, a multi-centre double-blinded parallel-group clinical trial examined the efficacy of CBD co-treatment with the patient's existing antipsychotic medication on a range of endpoints, including positive, negative and cognitive scores and Clinical Global Impression scales (CGI, measuring illness severity, improvement and response to treatment) [32]. Results showed significant improvements in positive (not negative) symptoms and CGI scores, as well as some improvement in cognitive performance (did not reach statistical significance, $p = 0.068$ CBD vs. placebo) when CBD was combined with the patient's existing antipsychotic medications [32].

2.3. Conclusions on the use of CBD in neurological disease

There is substantial scientific evidence to show the beneficial effects of CBD in the brain, with protection and treatment efficacy for various cognitive behaviours conferred in multiple disease states. Overall, there seems to be a general requirement for further placebo-controlled clinical trials, as well as investigation of long-term efficacy and safety in different populations of people. Evidence for illness-specific optimal dosing regimens (dose, route of administration, timing and number of daily doses, effect of concurrent medications, etc.) is also required. In addition, similar to our rodent study of CBD effects on cognition in schizophrenia [31], most studies use either isolated CBD or combined THC and CBD. While this methodology enables investigators to attribute results to a specific compound, it may not be the optimal therapeutic approach as cannabis-derived plant molecules are thought to interact and produce a synergy that enhances therapeutic effects—termed the 'entourage effect'.

3. The entourage effect

The entourage effect is defined as the act by which compounds (both cannabis phytochemicals and compounds from the endogenous cannabinoid system) augment or support the effects of major cannabinoids, for example, Δ9-THC, CBD, 2-arachidonoyl-glycerol (2-AG) [33, 34]. This phenomenon has been likened to an orchestra where 'many musicians support and harmonise the melody provided by the soloists' [34]. Compounds can exert synergistic effects through several mechanisms, for example by interacting with each other to improve bioavailability of beneficial compounds, or through combined actions on different therapeutic targets [35].

The concept of a cannabis entourage effect is largely based on anecdotal evidence from medicinal and recreational users attesting to the notion that cannabis 'works better' as a whole plant extract and its existence has been argued back and forth over time. However, there is evidence to suggest that the cannabis plant contains active ingredients as well as 'synergists' that boost drug effects above that of the isolated compound. Indeed, early description of a potential synergy between molecules in the cannabis plant came from a study in the 1970s that reported a 2–4 times greater deficits in parameters such as processing tasks and motor function in subjects administered Brazilian cannabis samples compared to Δ9-THC [36]. The phrase 'entourage effect' was first described in 1998 in response to the finding that certain endogenous molecules (2-linoleoyl-glycerol (2-LG) and 2-palmitoyl-glycerol (2-PG)) potentiated the effects of the endocannabinoid, 2-AG [33]. Interestingly, cultured hippocampal neurons exposed to CBD-rich plant extracts exhibit a significantly greater intracellular signalling response compared to CBD alone [37]. This provides preliminary (*in-vitro*) evidence that CBD-rich plant extracts exert greater effects on cells of the hippocampus (a region of the brain highly implicated in learning and memory) than isolated CBD. Overall, it may be possible to boost the pro-cognitive therapeutic efficacy of CBD through a synergistic approach. Studies show that cannabinoids other than CBD could confer beneficial effects on the brain through synergistic mechanisms, for example, the parent phytocannabinoid cannabigerol (CBG) exerted greater analgesic effects on mice than Δ9-THC alone, while CBG and cannabichromene (CBC) both have anti-depressant effects in rodents (reviewed in [38]) and CBG is neuroprotective in a mouse model of Huntington's Disease [39]. However, section 4 will focus on several key non-cannabinoid cannabis phytochemicals with promising evidence of positive effects on brain function.

4. Non-cannabinoid phytochemicals of Cannabis: terpenes, flavonoids and anthocyanins

The cannabis plant contains hundreds of phytochemicals, with new compounds and metabolites frequently identified. The concentration of chemicals in a cannabis plant can be influenced by multiple factors including nutrition, humidity, temperature, age of plant, strain, harvest time, plant stress, organ and storage conditions [1, 40]. Therefore, plant phytochemical composition is highly variable. Variability identified even within the same strain has led some authors to conclude that the name of a plant strain does not necessarily indicate potency or chemical composition [41]. However, others found that when grown under standardised conditions, certain cannabis strains can provide reproducible terpene and phytocannabinoid profiles that have been considered chemotaxonomic markers [42]. Furthermore, cannabinoid content can be used to classify plants into chemovars (plants with distinct photochemical profiles): Type I Δ9-THC-dominant, Type II Δ9-THC and CBD, Type III CBD-dominant and distinctions can be made outside these classes based on specific terpene profiles [43]. Therefore, it is possible to optimise plants to reproduce a distinct chemical composition and, potentially, specific medicinal characteristics.

4.1. Terpenes: linalool, alpha-pinene and beta-caryophyllene

Terpenes have been described as the most abundant class of small natural molecules by mass on Earth, undertaking innumerable structural and functional roles in most life forms on the planet (e.g., cholesterols for structural and signalling components of cell membranes, retinal in the eye for vision, carotenoids in photosynthesis) [44]. In cannabis, they create fragrances and flavours, but are also found in other plants and commonly used as safe food additives [38]. Terpenes can cross the blood brain barrier due to their lipophilic nature and studies have demonstrated a range of health benefits for some terpenes found in cannabis.

4.1.1. Linalool

Linalool is a monoterpene abundant in aromatic plants, such as lavender and purple basil [45]. Evidence shows that chronic administration of linalool reverses deficits in spatial memory and learning, with reduced amyloid plaque deposition and tau dysfunction in the hippocampus in rodent models of Alzheimer's disease [46, 47], using 25 mg/kg and 100 mg/kg linalool, respectively. Linalool also prevented deficits in spatial memory, motor function, neuroinflammation and post-ischemic neurodegeneration in a rat model of global cerebral ischemia, following oral daily administration (25 mg/kg) for 1 month [48]. However, reduced short and long-term recognition memory (50 and 100 mg/kg linalool, i.p.) [49] and memory acquisition (3% preparation for inhalation) [50] were found when linalool was administered as a single dose to healthy rats. This apparent contradiction in findings could be attributed to the administration of linalool to healthy vs. cognitively impaired rats, suggesting that the compound exerts benefits in a disease state but is detrimental when not patho physiologically required; however, further investigation is necessary to confirm.

4.1.2. Alpha-pinene

Alpha-pinene (α-pinene) is a highly abundant monoterpene found in coniferous trees (e.g., pine and fir) and cannabis [51] that, according to cannabis culture, provides pine-needle fragrances and tastes to cannabis. In mice with cognitive deficits caused by scopolamine-induced blockade of acetylcholine neurotransmission (apparent in advanced stages of Alzheimer's disease [52]), α-pinene (10 mg/kg, i.p.) improved working and spatial memory, and increased markers of acetylcholine synthesis in the cortex [53]. Inhalation of α-pinene can also influence major neurotransmitter signalling in the brain, for example it improved quality and duration of sleep in mice by modulating the major inhibitory neurotransmitter signalling system, gamma-aminobutyric acid (γ-aminobutyric acid, GABA)) [54], and decreased anxiety-like behaviour that was associated with increased tyrosine hydroxylase (the rate limiting enzyme for dopamine synthesis) in the midbrain [55]. Another study reported significant improvements in avoidance memory of cognitively impaired mice following administration of an essential oil obtained from a Korean fir tree containing α-pinene [56]; however, the results cannot be entirely attributed to this terpene due to the use of whole-plant extract containing other constituents.

4.1.3. Beta-caryophyllene

Beta-caryophyllene (β-caryophyllene) is a sesquiterpene that has a weak woody-spicy characteristic, abundant in cloves, black pepper, cinnamon and thyme [57, 58]. In a mouse model of Alzheimer's disease, β-caryophyllene reversed spatial memory deficits, reduced β-amyloid deposition in the hippocampus and cortex, and reduced neuroinflammation when administered for 10 weeks (48 mg/kg, oral) [59]. In rats with chronic cerebral ischemia resembling vascular dementia, β-caryophyllene (administered in a hydroxypropyl-β-cyclodextrin inclusion complex delivery system to enhance its bioavailability) attenuated cognitive deficits and increased cerebral blood flow [60]. β-caryophyllene also prevented oxidative stress in the cortex of rats following transient global cerebral hypoperfusion/reperfusion [61].

Neurological scores were improved in mice administered β-caryophyllene (24 and 72 mg/kg, i.p.) following an induced stroke [62] and anti-depressant-like behaviour was reported in healthy mice following β-caryophyllene, through mechanisms involving catecholamine (adrenergic) neurotransmission [63]. Overall, the studies provide some evidence to support the role of β-caryophyllene as pro-cognitive, with anti-inflammatory, neuroprotective and anti-depressant effects.

4.2. Phenolic acids: flavonoids and anthocyanins

In addition to terpenes, cannabis plants contain phenolic compounds, including flavonoids and anthocyanins [40, 64–66]. Flavonoids are commonly consumed by humans through dietary fruit, vegetable, tea and wine intake. Anthocyanins are a group of flavonoids responsible for the blue-violet and red-orange colours of plant organs. Certain strains of cannabis plants exhibit a purple phenotype (**Figure 1**), which is widely attributed to anthocyanin content in recreational cannabis culture; however, experimental data showing anthocyanin levels of purple compared to non-purple strains appear to be lacking.

Flavonoids and anthocyanins are extensively researched due to their neuroprotective, anti-inflammatory and pro-cognitive characteristics and can pass the blood brain barrier [67]. For example, one study found that anthocyanin pre-treatment (200 mg/kg orally for 7 days) prevented cognitive deficits in a rat model of dementia [68]. Flavonoids improve working memory, processing speed, executive function and episodic memory in humans (reviewed in [69, 70]) and stimulate neurogenesis, synaptic plasticity and reduced neuroinflammation in the hippocampus (reviewed in [71]). Anthocyanin-rich cherry juice improved verbal fluency and short- and long-term memory performance in people with mild-to-moderate dementia during a 12 week randomised, controlled clinical trial of older people (+70 years) with mild to moderate dementia (200 ml/day cherry juice vs. control juice lacking anthocyanin) [72]. Interestingly, both cherries and cannabis plants contain phenolic acids related to flavonoid and anthocyanin biosynthesis pathways [65, 73]. Indeed, hemp seed extract can contain phenolic compound levels that are comparable to Japanese plums [74, 75]. Japanese plums are an important source of

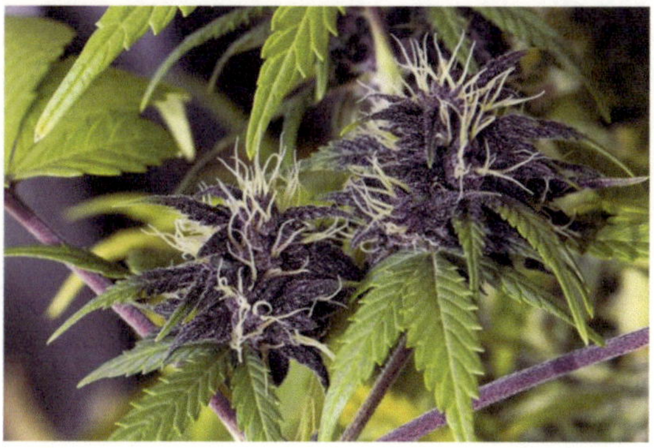

Figure 1. Inflorescence of purple cannabidiol (CBD)-rich, low Δ9-tetrahydrocannabinol (Δ9-THC) medicinal cannabis cultivar, GHM Genetic Development, Amsterdam, The Netherlands (2018).

anthocyanins, with particularly high levels in darker purple, blue and black coloured fruits [75]. Similar to cannabis plants, the phytochemical profile of Japanese plum varieties is influenced by horticultural practices, processing and storage conditions [75]. Other commercial plants, such as violet cauliflower and Thai purple basil, gain their unusual purple colouring through modifications to anthocyanin regulatory genes [76, 77]. Therefore, it is possible that plants can be manipulated naturally and artificially (i.e., genetically) to maximise anthocyanin content.

4.3. Conclusions on the effects of terpenes and flavonoids on the brain

The terpenes linalool, α-pinene and β-caryophyllene, as well as flavonoids and anthocyanins confer pro-cognitive, neuroprotective and anti-inflammatory effects in models of cerebral ischemia and Alzheimer's disease, as well as some anxiolytic effects. Most studies have been conducted in pre-clinical (rodent) models; however, pro-cognitive effects of flavonoids and anthocyanins have been shown in human clinical studies of dementia. Overall, combinations of CBD with other key phytochemicals found in cannabis could confer benefits on brain health through a multi-target synergy (entourage effect); however, further research is required.

5. Overall conclusion

This chapter has identified a consensus in the scientific literature that specific phytochemicals (CBD, linalool, α-pinene, β-caryophyllene, flavonoids and anthocyanins) found in cannabis plants are beneficial for cognition and brain health in a number of disease states. These compounds are psychoactive as they alter the brain to effect behaviour, and there is some evidence that they can differentially affect healthy individuals (e.g., CBD has no cognitive benefits and linalool has detrimental effects on cognition in healthy subjects). Therefore, societal consideration of 'medicinal cannabis' as a true medicine is necessary, that is, prescribed for patients who require treatment of a clinically diagnosed illness. Further research is needed to inform optimal prescription for treating specific illnesses, including dose, route of administration, long-term clinical efficacy, safety and side effects. There is some evidence to support the existence of an 'entourage effect'—such synergism could arise from a multi-target approach. The united benefits of specific terpenes and flavonoids could boost the therapeutic potential of CBD to improve cognition in disease states that manifest impairment; we are currently investigating these synergies in my laboratory. An other exciting future area of investigation is the identification of select cannabis phytochemical profiles that will treat specific illnesses with optimal efficacy. Following this, efforts towards standardising horticultural and cannabis plant processing practices to ensure optimal and reproducible medicines can be directed towards a proven goal—a translational interface between medical science and horticulture.

Acknowledgements

I wish to acknowledge the work of Ashleigh L. Osborne, Professor Nadia Solowij and Distinguished Professor Xu-Feng Huang as co-investigators on our project examining the pro-cognitive effects of CBD in a rodent model of schizophrenia. Thanks to Mr. Heiko Hampsink, GHM Genetic Development, The Netherlands, for supplying the purple cannabis photo. I extend gratitude to Mr. Thomas Forrest (Indicated Technology, Australia) and Mr. Heiko Hampsink for generously sharing their knowledge of cannabis horticulture.

Conflict of interest

There are no conflicts of interest to declare.

Notes/Thanks/Other declarations

I dedicate this book chapter to my husband, M. Green, for his tireless support.

Author details

Katrina Weston-Green[1,2,3,4*]

*Address all correspondence to: katrina_green@uow.edu.au

1 Neuropharmacology and Molecular Psychiatry Research Laboratory, School of Medicine, Faculty of Science, Medicine and Health, University of Wollongong, NSW, Australia

2 Molecular Horizons, Faculty of Science, Medicine and Health, University of Wollongong, NSW, Australia

3 Illawarra Health and Medical Research Institute, Wollongong, NSW, Australia

4 Australian Centre for Cannabinoid Clinical and Research Excellence, New Lambton Heights, NSW, Australia

References

[1] Citti C, Pacchetti B, Vandelli MA, Forni F, Cannazza G. Analysis of cannabinoids in commercial hemp seed oil and decarboxylation kinetics studies of cannabidiolic acid (CBDA). Journal of Pharmaceutical and Biomedical Analysis. 2018;**149**:532-540. DOI: 10.1016/j.jpba.2017.11.044

[2] ElSohly MA, Gul W. Constituents of Cannabis. In: Pertwee R, editor. Handbook of Cannabis. Oxford, UK: Oxford University Press; 2014. DOI: 10.1093/acprof:oso/9780199662685.001.0001

[3] Laprairie RB, Bagher AM, Kelly ME, Denovan-Wright EM. Cannabidiol is a negative allosteric modulator of the cannabinoid CB1 receptor. British Journal of Pharmacology. 2015;**172**(20):4790-4805. DOI: 10.1111/bph.13250

[4] Seeman P. Cannabidiol is a partial agonist at dopamine D2 high receptors, predicting its antipsychotic clinical dose. Translational Psychiatry. 2016;**6**(10):e920. DOI: 10.1038/tp.2016.195

[5] Leweke FM, Piomelli D, Pahlisch F, Muhl D, Gerth CW, Hoyer C, Klosterkötter J, Hellmich M, Koethe D. Cannabidiol enhances anandamide signaling and alleviates psychotic symptoms of schizophrenia. Translational Psychiatry. 2012;**2**:e94. DOI: 10.1038/tp.2012.15

[6] Elmes MW, Kaczocha M, Berger WT, Leung K, Ralph BP, Wang L, Sweeney JM, Miyauchi JT, Tsirka SE, Ojima I, Deutsch DG. Fatty acid-binding proteins (FABPs) are intracellular carriers for Delta9-tetrahydrocannabinol (THC) and cannabidiol (CBD). Journal of Biological Chemistry. 2015;**290**(14):8711-8721. DOI: 10.1074/jbc.M114.618447

[7] Osborne AL, Solowij N, Weston-Green K. A systematic review of the effect of cannabidiol on cognitive function: Relevance to schizophrenia. Neuroscience and Biobehavioral Reviews. 2017;**72**:310-324. DOI: 10.1016/j.neubiorev.2016.11.012

[8] Yucel M, Solowij N, Respondek C, Whittle S, Fornito A, Pantelis C, Lubman DI. Regional brain abnormalities associated with long-term heavy cannabis use. Archives of General Psychiatry. 2008;**65**(6):694-701. DOI: 10.1001/archpsyc.65.6.694

[9] Solowij N, Walterfang M, Lubman DI, Whittle S, Lorenzetti V, Styner M, Velakoulis D, Pantelis C, Yucel M. Alteration to hippocampal shape in cannabis users with and without schizophrenia. Schizophrenia Research. 2013;**143**(1):179-184. DOI: 10.1016/j.schres.2012.10.040

[10] Yucel M, Lorenzetti V, Suo C, Zalesky A, Fornito A, Takagi MJ, Lubman DI, Solowij N. Hippocampal harms, protection and recovery following regular cannabis use. Translational Psychiatry. 2016;**6**:e710. DOI: 10.1038/tp.2015.201

[11] Beale C, Broyd SJ, Chye Y, Suo C, Schira M, Galettis P, Martin JH, Yucel M, Solowij N. Prolonged Cannabidiol treatment effects on hippocampal subfield volumes in current Cannabis users. Cannabis and Cannabinoid Research. 2018;**3**(1):94-107. DOI: 10.1089/can.2017.0047

[12] Campos AC, Fogaça MV, Sonego AB, Guimarães FS. Cannabidiol, neuroprotection and neuropsychiatric disorders. Pharmacological Research. 2016;**112**:119-127. DOI: 10.1016/j.phrs.2016.01.033

[13] Murphy M, Mills S, Winstone J, Leishman E, Wager-Miller J, Bradshaw H, Mackie K. Chronic adolescent Delta(9)-tetrahydrocannabinol treatment of male mice leads to long-term cognitive and behavioral dysfunction, which are prevented by concurrent Cannabidiol treatment. Cannabis and Cannabinoid Research. 2017;**2**(1):235-246. DOI: 10.1089/can.2017.0034

[14] Bloom GS. Amyloid-beta and tau: The trigger and bullet in Alzheimer disease pathogenesis. JAMA Neurology. 2014;**71**(4):505-508. DOI: 10.1001/jamaneurol.2013.5847

[15] Karl T, Cheng D, Garner B, Arnold JC. The therapeutic potential of the endocannabinoid system for Alzheimer's disease. Expert Opinion on Therapeutic Targets. 2012;**16**(4): 407-420. DOI: 10.1517/14728222.2012.671812

[16] Casarejos MJ, Perucho J, Gomez A, Munoz MP, Fernandez-Estevez M, Sagredo O, Fernandez Ruiz J, Guzman M, de Yebenes JG, Mena MA. Natural cannabinoids improve dopamine neurotransmission and tau and amyloid pathology in a mouse model of tauopathy. Journal of Alzheimer's Disease. 2013;**35**(3):525-539. DOI: 10.3233/jad-130050

[17] Aso E, Andres-Benito P, Ferrer I. Delineating the efficacy of a Cannabis-based medicine at advanced stages of dementia in a murine model. Journal of Alzheimer's Disease. 2016;**54**(3):903-912. DOI: 10.3233/jad-160533

[18] Cheng D, Spiro AS, Jenner AM, Garner B, Karl T. Long-term cannabidiol treatment prevents the development of social recognition memory deficits in Alzheimer's disease transgenic mice. Journal of Alzheimer's Disease. 2014;**42**(4):1383-1396. DOI: 10.3233/jad-140921

[19] Lopez-Sendon Moreno JL, Garcia Caldentey J, Trigo Cubillo P, Ruiz Romero C, Garcia Ribas G, Alonso Arias MA, Garcia de Yebenes MJ, Tolon RM, Galve-Roperh I, Sagredo O, Valdeolivas S, Resel E, Ortega-Gutierrez S, Garcia-Bermejo ML, Fernandez Ruiz J, Guzman M, Garcia de Yebenes Prous J. A double-blind, randomized, cross-over, placebo-controlled, pilot trial with Sativex in Huntington's disease. Journal of Neurology. 2016;**263**(7):1390-1400. DOI: 10.1007/s00415-016-8145-9

[20] Consroe P, Laguna J, Allender J, Snider S, Stern L, Sandyk R, Kennedy K, Schram K. Controlled clinical trial of cannabidiol in Huntington's disease. Pharmacology Biochemistry and Behavior. 1991;**40**(3):701-708. DOI: 10.1016/0091-3057(91)90386-G

[21] Chagas MH, Zuardi AW, Tumas V, Pena-Pereira MA, Sobreira ET, Bergamaschi MM, dos Santos AC, Teixeira AL, Hallak JE, Crippa JA. Effects of cannabidiol in the treatment of patients with Parkinson's disease: An exploratory double-blind trial. Journal of Psychopharmacology. 2014;**28**(11):1088-1098. DOI: 10.1177/0269881114550355

[22] Zuardi AW, Crippa JA, Hallak JE, Pinto JP, Chagas MH, Rodrigues GG, Dursun SM, Tumas V. Cannabidiol for the treatment of psychosis in Parkinson's disease. Journal of Psychopharmacology. 2009;**23**(8):979-983. DOI: 10.1177/0269881108096519

[23] Peres FF, Levin R, Suiama MA, Diana MC, Gouvêa DA, Almeida V, Santos CM, Lungato L, Zuardi AW, Hallak JEC, Crippa JA, Vânia DA, Silva RH, Abílio VC. Cannabidiol prevents motor and cognitive impairments induced by reserpine in rats. Frontiers in Pharmacology. 2016;**7**:343. DOI: 10.3389/fphar.2016.00343

[24] Ceprian M, Jimenez-Sanchez L, Vargas C, Barata L, Hind W, Martinez-Orgado J. Cannabidiol reduces brain damage and improves functional recovery in a neonatal rat model of arterial ischemic stroke. Neuropharmacology. 2017;**116**:151-159. DOI: 10.1016/j.neuropharm.2016.12.017

[25] Marinelli L, Balestrino M, Mori L, Puce L, Rosa GM, Giorello L, Curra A, Fattapposta F, Serrati C, Gandolfo C, Abbruzzese G, Trompetto C. A randomised controlled cross-over double-blind pilot study protocol on THC:CBD oromucosal spray efficacy as an add-on therapy for post-stroke spasticity. BMJ Open. 2017;**7**(9):e016843. DOI: 10.1136/bmjopen-2017-016843

[26] Widmann CN, Heneka MT. Long-term cerebral consequences of sepsis. The Lancet Neurology. 2014;**13**(6):630-636. DOI: 10.1016/S1474-4422(14)70017-1

[27] Ruiz-Valdepeñas L, Martínez-Orgado JA, Benito C, Millán Á, Tolón RM, Romero J. Cannabidiol reduces lipopolysaccharide-induced vascular changes and inflammation in the mouse brain: An intravital microscopy study. Journal of Neuroinflammation. 2011;**8**(1):5. DOI: 10.1186/1742-2094-8-5

[28] Nielsen RE, Levander S, Kjaersdam Telléus G, Jensen SOW, Østergaard Christensen T, Leucht S. Second-generation antipsychotic effect on cognition in patients with schizophrenia—A meta-analysis of randomized clinical trials. Acta Psychiatrica Scandinavica. 2015;**131**(3):185-196. DOI: 10.1111/acps.12374

[29] Weston-Green K, Huang XF, Deng C. Alterations to melanocortinergic, GABAergic and cannabinoid neurotransmission associated with olanzapine-induced weight gain. PLoS One. 2012;**7**(3):e33548. DOI: 10.1371/journal.pone.0033548

[30] Weston-Green K, Huang XF, Deng C. Second generation antipsychotic-induced type 2 diabetes: A role for the muscarinic M3 receptor. CNS Drugs. 2013;**27**(12):1069-1080. DOI: 10.1007/s40263-013-0115-5

[31] Osborne AL, Solowij N, Babic I, Huang XF, Weston-Green K. Improved social interaction, recognition and working memory with Cannabidiol treatment in a prenatal infection (poly I:C) rat model. Neuropsychopharmacology. 2017;**42**(7):1447-1457. DOI: 10.1038/npp.2017.40

[32] McGuire P, Robson P, Cubala WJ, Vasile D, Morrison PD, Barron R, Taylor A, Wright S. Cannabidiol (CBD) as an adjunctive therapy in schizophrenia: A multicenter randomized controlled trial. American Journal of Psychiatry. 2017;**175**(3):225-231. DOI: 10.1176/appi.ajp.2017.17030325

[33] Ben-Shabat S, Fride E, Sheskin T, Tamiri T, Rhee M-H, Vogel Z, Bisogno T, De Petrocellis L, Di Marzo V, Mechoulam R. An entourage effect: Inactive endogenous fatty acid glycerol esters enhance 2-arachidonoyl-glycerol cannabinoid activity. European Journal of Pharmacology. 1998;**353**(1):23-31. DOI: 10.1016/S0014-2999(98)00392-6

[34] Piomelli D, Russo EB. The Cannabis sativa versus *Cannabis indica* debate: An interview with Ethan Russo, MD. Cannabis and Cannabinoid Research. 2016;**1**(1):44-46. DOI: 10.1089/can.2015.29003.ebr

[35] Wagner H, Ulrich-Merzenich G. Synergy research: Approaching a new generation of phytopharmaceuticals. Phytomedicine. 2009;**16**(2-3):97-110. DOI: 10.1016/j.phymed.2008.12.018

[36] Carlini EA, Karniol IG, Renault PF, Schuster CR. Effects of marihuana in laboratory animals and in man. British Journal of Pharmacology. 1974;**50**(2):299-309

[37] Ryan D, Drysdale AJ, Pertwee RG, Platt B. Differential effects of cannabis extracts and pure plant cannabinoids on hippocampal neurones and glia. Neuroscience Letters. 2006;**408**(3):236-241. DOI: 10.1016/j.neulet.2006.09.008

[38] Russo EB. Taming THC: Potential cannabis synergy and phytocannabinoid-terpenoid entourage effects. British Journal of Pharmacology. 2011;**163**(7):1344-1364. DOI: 10.1111/j.1476-5381.2011.01238.x

[39] Valdeolivas S, Navarrete C, Cantarero I, Bellido ML, Munoz E, Sagredo O. Neuro protective properties of cannabigerol in Huntington's disease: Studies in R6/2 mice and 3-nitropropionate-lesioned mice. Neurotherapeutics. 2015;**12**(1):185-199. DOI: 10.1007/s13311-014-0304-z

[40] Andre CM, Hausman J-F, Guerriero G. *Cannabis sativa*: The plant of the thousand and one molecules. Frontiers in Plant Science. 2016;**7**(19). DOI: 10.3389/fpls.2016.00019

[41] Elzinga S, Fischedick J, Podkolinski R, Raber J. Cannabinoids and terpenes as chemotaxonomic markers in Cannabis. Natural Products Chemistry & Research. 2015;**3**(181). DOI: 10.4172/2329-6836.1000181

[42] Fischedick JT, Hazekamp A, Erkelens T, Choi YH, Verpoorte R. Metabolic fingerprinting of *Cannabis sativa* L, cannabinoids and terpenoids for chemotaxonomic and drug standardization purposes. Phytochemistry. 2010;**71**(17-18):2058-2073. DOI: 10.1016/j.phytochem.2010.10.001

[43] Lewis MA, Russo EB, Smith KM. Pharmacological foundations of Cannabis chemovars. Planta Medica. 2018;**84**(4):225-233. DOI: 10.1055/s-0043-122240

[44] Oldfield E, Lin F-Y. Terpene biosynthesis: Modularity rules. Angewandte Chemie (International Ed. in English). 2012;**51**(5):1124-1137. DOI: 10.1002/anie.201103110

[45] Yavari M, Mirdamadi S, Masoudi S, Tabatabaei-Anaraki M, Larijani K, Rustaiyan A. Composition and antibacterial activity of the essential oil of a green type and a purple type of *Ocimum basilicum* L. from Iran. Journal of Essential Oil Research. 2011;**23**(1):1-4. DOI: 10.1080/10412905.2011.9700421

[46] Sabogal-Guáqueta AM, Osorio E, Cardona-Gómez GP. Linalool reverses neuropathological and behavioral impairments in old triple transgenic Alzheimer's mice. Neuropharmacology. 2016;**102**:111-120. DOI: 10.1016/j.neuropharm.2015.11.002

[47] Xu P, Wang K, Lu C, Dong L, Gao L, Yan M, Aibai S, Yang Y, Liu X. The protective effect of lavender essential oil and its main component linalool against the cognitive deficits induced by D-galactose and aluminum trichloride in mice. Evidence-based Complementary and Alternative Medicine. 2017;**2017**:7426538. DOI: 10.1155/2017/7426538

[48] Sabogal-Guaqueta AM, Posada-Duque R, Cortes NC, Arias-Londono JD, Cardona-Gomez GP. Changes in the hippocampal and peripheral phospholipid profiles are

associated with neurodegeneration hallmarks in a long-term global cerebral ischemia model: Attenuation by linalool. Neuropharmacology. 2018;**135**:555-571. DOI: 10.1016/j.neuropharm.2018.04.015

[49] Coelho VR, Gianesini J, Von Borowski R, Mazzardo-Martins L, Martins DF, Picada JN, Santos ARS, Brum LFS, Pereira P. (−)-linalool, a naturally occurring monoterpene compound, impairs memory acquisition in the object recognition task, inhibitory avoidance test and habituation to a novel environment in rats. Phytomedicine. 2011;**18**(10):896-901. DOI: 10.1016/j.phymed.2011.02.010

[50] Linck VM, da Silva AL, Figueiró M, Caramão EB, Moreno PRH, Elisabetsky E. Effects of inhaled linalool in anxiety, social interaction and aggressive behavior in mice. Phytomedicine. 2010;**17**(8):679-683. DOI: 10.1016/j.phymed.2009.10.002

[51] Booth JK, Page JE, Bohlmann J. Terpene synthases from *Cannabis sativa*. PLoS One. 2017;**12**(3):e0173911. DOI: 10.1371/journal.pone.0173911

[52] Schliebs R, Arendt T. The cholinergic system in aging and neuronal degeneration. Behavioural Brain Research. 2011;**221**(2):555-563. DOI: 10.1016/j.bbr.2010.11.058

[53] Lee GY, Lee C, Park GH, Jang JH. Amelioration of scopolamine-induced learning and memory impairment by alpha-Pinene in C57BL/6 mice. Evidence-based Complementary and Alternative Medicine. 2017;**2017**:4926815. DOI: 10.1155/2017/4926815

[54] Yang H, Woo J, Pae AN, Um MY, Cho NC, Park KD, Yoon M, Kim J, Lee CJ, Cho S. Alpha-Pinene, a major constituent of pine tree oils, enhances non-rapid eye movement sleep in mice through GABAA-benzodiazepine receptors. Molecular Pharmacology. 2016;**90**(5):530-539. DOI: 10.1124/mol.116.105080

[55] Kasuya H, Okada N, Kubohara M, Satou T, Masuo Y, Koike K. Expression of BDNF and TH mRNA in the brain following inhaled administration of alpha-pinene. Phytotherapy Research. 2015;**29**(1):43-47. DOI: 10.1002/ptr.5224

[56] Kim K, Bu Y, Jeong S, Lim J, Kwon Y, Cha DS, Kim J, Jeon S, Eun J, Jeon H. Memory-enhancing effect of a supercritical carbon dioxide fluid extract of the needles of *Abies koreana* on scopolamine-induced amnesia in mice. Bioscience, Biotechnology, and Biochemistry. 2006;**70**(8):1821-1826. DOI: 10.1271/bbb.50608

[57] Gertsch J, Leonti M, Raduner S, Racz I, Chen J-Z, Xie X-Q, Altmann K-H, Karsak M, Zimmer A. Beta-caryophyllene is a dietary cannabinoid. Proceedings of the National Academy of Sciences of the United States of America. 2008;**105**(26):9099-9104. DOI: 10.1073/pnas.0803601105

[58] Nurdjannah N, Bermawie N, 11 - Cloves A2. In: Peter KV, editor. Handbook of Herbs and Spices. 2 ed. Cambridge, UK: Woodhead Publishing; 2012. pp. 197-215. DOI: 10.1533/9780857095671.197

[59] Cheng Y, Dong Z, Liu S. Beta-Caryophyllene ameliorates the Alzheimer-like phenotype in APP/PS1 mice through CB2 receptor activation and the PPARgamma pathway. Pharmacology. 2014;**94**(1-2):1-12. DOI: 10.1159/000362689

[60] Lou J, Teng Z, Zhang L, Yang J, Ma L, Wang F, Tian X, An R, Yang M, Zhang Q, Xu L, Dong Z. beta-Caryophyllene/hydroxypropyl-beta-cyclodextrin inclusion complex improves cognitive deficits in rats with vascular dementia through the cannabinoid receptor type 2-mediated pathway. Frontiers in Pharmacology. 2017;**8**:2. DOI: 10.3389/fphar.2017.00002

[61] Poddighe L, Carta G, Serra MP, Melis T, Boi M, Lisai S, Murru E, Muredda L, Collu M, Banni S, Quartu M. Acute administration of beta-caryophyllene prevents endocannabinoid system activation during transient common carotid artery occlusion and reperfusion. Lipids in Health and Disease. 2018;**17**(1):23. DOI: 10.1186/s12944-018-0661-4

[62] Yang M, Lv Y, Tian X, Lou J, An R, Zhang Q, Li M, Xu L, Dong Z. Neuroprotective effect of beta-caryophyllene on cerebral ischemia-reperfusion injury via regulation of necroptotic neuronal death and inflammation: In vivo and in vitro. Frontiers in Neuroscience. 2017;**11**:583. DOI: 10.3389/fnins.2017.00583

[63] Oliveira DR, Silva DM, Florentino IF, de Brito A, Fajemiroye JO, Silva DPB, da Rocha F, Costa EA, De Carvalho PG. Monoamine involvement in the antidepressant-like effect of beta-caryophyllene. CNS & Neurological Disorders Drug Targets. 2018. DOI: 10.2174/1871527317666180420150249

[64] Flores-Sanchez IJ, Verpoorte R. Secondary metabolism in Cannabis. Phytochemistry Reviews. 2008;**7**(3):615-639. DOI: 10.1007/s11101-008-9094-4

[65] Docimo T, Consonni R, Coraggio I, Mattana M. Early Phenylpropanoid biosynthetic steps in *Cannabis sativa*: Link between genes and metabolites. International Journal of Molecular Sciences. 2013;**14**(7):13626-13644. DOI: 10.3390/ijms140713626

[66] Lesma G, Consonni R, Gambaro V, Remuzzi C, Roda G, Silvani A, Vece V, Visconti GL. Cannabinoid-free *Cannabis sativa* L. grown in the Po valley: Evaluation of fatty acid profile, antioxidant capacity and metabolic content. Natural Product Research. 2014;**28**(21):1801-1807. DOI: 10.1080/14786419.2014.926354

[67] Youdim KA, Dobbie MS, Kuhnle G, Proteggente AR, Abbott NJ, Rice-Evans C. Interaction between flavonoids and the blood-brain barrier: In vitro studies. Journal of Neurochemistry. 2003;**85**(1):180-192

[68] Gutierres JM, Carvalho FB, Schetinger MRC, Marisco P, Agostinho P, Rodrigues M, Rubin MA, Schmatz R, da Silva CR, de Cognato PG, Farias JG, Signor C, Morsch VM, Mazzanti CM, Bogo M, Bonan CD, Spanevello R. Anthocyanins restore behavioral and biochemical changes caused by streptozotocin-induced sporadic dementia of Alzheimer's type. Life Sciences. 2014;**96**(1):7-17. DOI: 10.1016/j.lfs.2013.11.014

[69] Bell L, Lamport JD, Butler TL, Williams MC. A review of the cognitive effects observed in humans following acute supplementation with flavonoids, and their associated mechanisms of action. Nutrients. 2015;**7**(12):10290-10306. DOI: 10.3390/nu7125538

[70] Spencer JP. The impact of fruit flavonoids on memory and cognition. The British Journal of Nutrition. 2010;**104**(Suppl 3):S40-S47. DOI: 10.1017/s0007114510003934

[71] Vauzour D. Effect of flavonoids on learning, memory and neurocognitive performance: Relevance and potential implications for Alzheimer's disease pathophysiology. Journal of the Science of Food and Agriculture. 2014;**94**(6):1042-1056. DOI: 10.1002/jsfa.6473

[72] Kent K, Charlton K, Roodenrys S, Batterham M, Potter J, Traynor V, Gilbert H, Morgan O, Richards R. Consumption of anthocyanin-rich cherry juice for 12 weeks improves memory and cognition in older adults with mild-to-moderate dementia. European Journal of Nutrition. 2017;**56**(1):333-341. DOI: 10.1007/s00394-015-1083-y

[73] Kent K, Charlton KE, Jenner A, Roodenrys S. Acute reduction in blood pressure following consumption of anthocyanin-rich cherry juice may be dose-interval dependant: A pilot cross-over study. International Journal of Food Sciences and Nutrition. 2016;**67**(1):47-52. DOI: 10.3109/09637486.2015.1121472

[74] Smeriglio A, Galati EM, Monforte MT, Lanuzza F, D'Angelo V, Circosta C. Polyphenolic compounds and antioxidant activity of cold-pressed seed oil from Finola cultivar of *Cannabis sativa* L. Phytotherapy Research. 2016;**30**(8):1298-1307. DOI: 10.1002/ptr.5623

[75] Fanning KJ, Topp B, Russell D, Stanley R, Netzel M. Japanese plums (*Prunus salicina* Lindl.) and phytochemicals—Breeding, horticultural practice, postharvest storage, processing and bioactivity. Journal of the Science of Food and Agriculture. 2014;**94**(11): 2137-2147. DOI: 10.1002/jsfa.6591

[76] Chiu L-W, Zhou X, Burke S, Wu X, Prior RL, Li L. The purple cauliflower arises from activation of a MYB transcription factor. Plant Physiology. 2010;**154**(3):1470-1480. DOI: 10.1104/pp.110.164160

[77] Phippen WB, Simon JE. Anthocyanin inheritance and instability in purple basil (*Ocimum basilicum* L.). Journal of Heredity. 2000;**91**(4):289-296

Chapter 6

Modulation of Pain by Endocannabinoids in the Periphery

Megan L. Uhelski, Iryna Khasabova and
Donald A. Simone

Additional information is available at the end of the chapter

http://dx.doi.org/10.5772/intechopen.79673

Abstract

Activation of cannabinoid receptors using systemic treatments produces analgesia in a variety of experimental pain models, but these effects are hindered by sedation and motor impairment mediated by receptors in the central nervous system. Targeting the endocannabinoid system in the periphery can bypass these unwanted side effects while still producing analgesia in both acute and chronic pain states. This chapter discusses the different approaches to increasing peripheral endocannabinoid activity in experimental models of acute and chronic pain, including inflammatory pain, neuropathic pain, and sickle cell disease. We also explore how these treatments alter nociceptive activity in the peripheral nervous system.

Keywords: pain, hyperalgesia, nociceptors, primary afferent nerve fibers, cannabinoids

1. Introduction

Although the cannabis plant (*Cannabis sativa*) has been used as a folk remedy to treat various ailments for thousands of years, it is only within the last century that its active components have been isolated and identified. While some of its effects are well documented, its impact on pain had been less clear due to confounding effects on mood, motor impairment, and sedation. Isolation of the psychoactive components of the cannabis plant and the development of synthetic cannabinoid compounds enabled more rigorous testing. Identification of a cannabinoid receptor (CB1) in 1988 gave insight into the mechanisms of the cannabis effect, as did the discovery of endogenous ligands, referred to as endocannabinoids [1–4]. Studies in rats showed that when applied intravenously or directly to the spinal cord, cannabinoid agonists attenuated responses to noxious mechanical and thermal stimulation in nociceptive spinal neurons [5–7]. These early studies provided the first evidence of a direct effect of cannabinoids in pain inhibition and led to further investigations to identify the mechanisms underlying cannabinoid effects on neuronal activity.

The endogenous cannabinoid system consists of two well-characterized receptor subtypes, CB1 and CB2, and their endogenous ligands, from which anandamide (AEA) and 2-arachidonoyl glycerol (2-AG) are the most studied [8–10]. Cannabinoid receptors are G-protein coupled, mainly to $G_{i/o}$, which inhibits adenylyl cyclase [3, 11], and voltage-dependent Ca^{2+} channels [12]. CB1 receptors are expressed primarily in the nervous system, but are also present in non-neuronal tissues. CB2 receptors are mainly located peripherally, and are associated with modulation of immune cells [4, 13, 14]. Since CB receptors are widely distributed, their activation produces a wide variety of behavioral and physiological responses.

1.1. Role of the endocannabinoid system in anti-nociception and neuroprotection

Activation of cannabinoid receptors has been shown to produce anti-nociception in experimental models of inflammatory pain, including formalin [15, 16], carrageenan [17–19], CFA, complete Freund's adjuvant [20], and capsaicin [19, 21–24]. In addition, the administration of cannabinoid antagonists has been shown to enhance pain behavior in formalin and carrageenan models [15, 18], suggesting that tonic activation of cannabinoid receptors contributes to anti-nociception in response to inflammation. Systemic administration of cannabinoid agonists has also been shown to attenuate neuropathic pain following peripheral nerve injury (CCI model [25], partial sciatic nerve ligation [26], spinal nerve injury [27], L5/L6 ligation [28, 29]), diabetic neuropathy (type 1 [30–32] and type 2 [32]), and chemotherapy induced peripheral neuropathy [33–36]. In humans, cannabinoid agonists attenuated post-operative pain [37] and also enhanced the analgesic efficacy of opioids [38]. Two small clinical evaluations of the efficacy of (−)Δ9-tetrohydrocannabinol (THC), the main psychoactive compound of the cannabis plant, reported pain relief comparable to codeine [39, 40]. Unfortunately, higher doses tended to produce significant side effects including sedation, dizziness, ataxia and blurred vision.

In addition to anti-nociception, the endocannabinoid system has a neuroprotective function. In a model of cerebral ischemia, cannabinoid agonists, cannabidiol and THC attenuated toxicity related to the activity of excitatory neurotransmitters in the rat cerebral cortex independent from CB1 and CB2 receptors [41]. Cannabidiol is known to have low affinity for cannabinoid receptors, and has also been shown to act as a negative allosteric modulator at the CB1 receptor and a reverse agonist at the CB2 receptor [42, 43]. Another study reported the involvement of CB1 receptors in the reduction of neuronal loss [44]. Further, an *in vitro* study of hypoxic ischemia demonstrated a possible role for CB2 receptors [45]. The endogenous cannabinoid ligand, 2-AG, was shown to be neuroprotective in a model of traumatic brain injury, resulting in reduced edema and neuronal loss in the hippocampus [46]. Endocannabinoids have also been shown to protect against neurodegenerative diseases, including Alzheimer's disease, where the inhibition of microglial activation may prevent pathological changes associated with beta amyloid [47]. There is also evidence that cannabinoids possess antioxidant properties through the activity of cannabinoid receptors located on microglia, astrocytes, and other immune cells, where activation inhibits the release of pro-inflammatory substances [48–54]. Increased expression of CB2 on microglia and astrocytes has been observed in the area of lesion [54]. The administration of a CB2 agonist slowed the progression of amyotrophic lateral sclerosis in mice, and the activation of the endocannabinoid system protected against myelin degeneration in multiple sclerosis through a combination of immunosuppression and neuroprotection [55–57]. In studies of peripheral neuropathy produced by chemotherapy, WIN 55,212-2 prevented the development of neuropathy induced by cisplatin treatment [33], and when WIN 55,212-2 treatment was initiated after sciatic nerve ligation (CCI model of neuropathic pain), mechanical hyperalgesia failed to develop by 14 days post-injury [58].

2. Targeting the peripheral endocannabinoid system in chronic pain

A major limitation to the systemic use of cannabinoid agonists as treatment for chronic pain is that activation of cannabinoid receptors in the central nervous system is associated with undesirable side effects, including sedation and catalepsy [59]. Targeting endocannabinoid activity in the peripheral nervous system bypasses these unwanted side effects while still producing analgesia in animal models of inflammatory pain, bone cancer pain, neuropathic pain and sickle cell disease. Continued research into the specific mechanisms of analgesia produced by activation of the endocannabinoid system in the periphery could identify new targets for pain which could serve as stand-alone therapies or be integrated into a multifaceted treatment approach. This chapter will review studies that have investigated the analgesic effects of treatments that target the peripheral endocannabinoid system, whether through direct activation of cannabinoid receptors or through modulation of endocannabinoid metabolism.

2.1. Synthetic cannabinoids in rodent models of pain: inflammation, bone cancer pain, neuropathic pain and sickle cell disease

Local administration of cannabinoid receptor agonists, as opposed to systemic treatment, can produce analgesia without centrally-mediated side effects. Intraplantar administration of the non-selective cannabinoid receptor agonist WIN 55,212–2 attenuated heat and mechanical hyperalgesia in an acute cutaneous heat injury model in rats. This was blocked by a CB1 receptor antagonist, and partially blocked by a CB2 receptor antagonist, suggesting that while both receptor subtypes play a role in anti-nociception during acute pain, the effect was primarily mediated through activation of CB1 receptors [60]. WIN 55,212–2 also decreased mechanical hyperalgesia in the tumor-bearing hind paw in a mouse model of bone cancer pain [61]. The anti-hyperalgesic effect was mediated by both CB1 and CB2 receptors. Importantly, intraplantar administration did not induce catalepsy, which normally occurs when cannabinoid agonists are injected systemically and can confound behavioral measures of nociception [62]. Recordings from the tibial nerve of tumor-bearing mice showed that intraplantar WIN 55,212-2 attenuated sensitization of C-fiber nociceptors as evidenced by a decrease in spontaneous discharge and reduced responses evoked by mechanical stimuli responses evoked by mechanical stimulation, effects which were blocked by both CB1 and CB2 antagonists [63] (**Figure 1**).

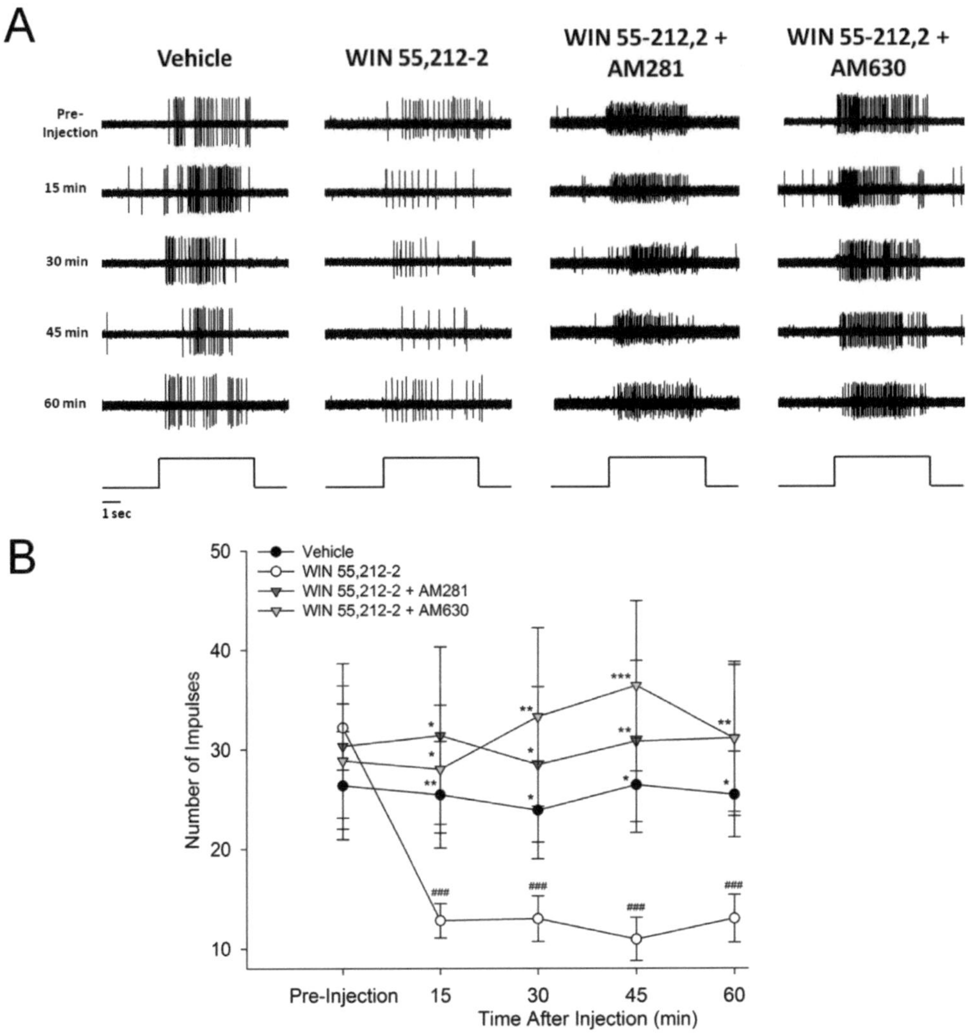

Figure 1. Effect of non-selective cannabinoid receptor agonist WIN 55,212-2 on responses of C-fiber nociceptors evoked by suprathreshold mechanical stimulation. (A) Representative examples of nociceptor responses evoked by 147 mN before injection and at 15, 30, 45 and 60 min after intraplantar administration of vehicle or WIN 55,212-2 alone or preceded by the CB1 receptor antagonist AM281 or CB2 antagonist AM630. The time of application of the stimulus is shown at the bottom of each column. (B) Mean (±SEM) number of evoked impulses before and at 15, 30, 45 and 60 min after intraplantar administration of vehicle, WIN 55,212–2, WIN 55,212–2 + AM281, and WIN 55,212–2 + AM630. Evoked responses were not changed following injection of vehicle but decreased following WIN 55,212-2. This was blocked by pretreatment with AM281 or AM630. * $p < .05$, ** $p \leq .01$, *** $p < .001$ vs. WIN 55,212–2; ### $p < .001$ vs. pre-injection value (from Uhelski et al. [63]).

In a model of inflammatory pain, intraplantar administration of the non-selective cannabinoid receptor agonist CP 55,940 attenuated CFA-induced hyperalgesia in mice expressing human sickle hemoglobin (BERK and hBERK1) as well as controls expressing normal human hemoglobin (HbA-BERK) [64].

The analgesic effect of intraplantar WIN 55,212-2 showed more variability in models of neuropathic pain. In a sciatic nerve ligation model, only the highest dose tested (250 μg) produced an anti-hyperalgesic effect, but the injection altered withdrawal latencies to heat and mechanical response thresholds in both the treated and non-treated hind paw, suggesting that the drug effect was not limited to the periphery [65]. This effect was also seen in rats with partial sciatic nerve ligation (Seltzer model of neuropathic pain); however, the effect was blocked by the intraplantar administration of a CB1 antagonist but not when that same antagonist was administered by the intrathecal route [26], indicating that the ability of WIN 55,212-2 to produce anti-nociception in the contralateral paw is not necessarily mediated by activation of CB1 receptors in the central nervous system. In a rat model of chemotherapy-induced peripheral neuropathy produced by paclitaxel treatment, intraplantar administration of WIN 55,212-2 had no effect on mechanical or heat hyperalgesia, whereas systemic treatment produced anti-nociception [65]. In contrast, intraplantar administration of WIN 55,212-2 attenuated mechanical allodynia associated with streptozotocin-induced diabetic neuropathy [31]. A non-selective cannabinoid receptor agonist naphthalen-1-yl-(4-pentyloxynaphthalen-1-yl)methanone, a novel compound which does not appear to cross the blood–brain barrier, reduced mechanical hyperalgesia in a rats with partial sciatic nerve ligation when administered orally [66], indicating that peripherally-restricted activation of cannabinoid receptors can produce adequate analgesia with an oral dosing regimen.

Receptor-selective synthetic cannabinoids also produce analgesic effects. In rats given an intraplantar injection of CFA, arachidonyl-2′-chloroethylamide (ACEA) and (R)-(+)-methanandamide (methAEA), stable mimics of AEA that preferentially bind CB1 receptors, reduced mechanical hyperalgesia and decreased evoked responses in Aδ-fiber nociceptors. The reduction in mechanical hyperalgesia was blocked by a CB1 receptor antagonist, but not by a CB2 antagonist. Notably, neither drug had any effect on mechanical withdrawal thresholds or paw withdrawal frequency in naïve rats, and no changes were seen in evoked responses of Aδ-fiber nociceptors isolated from nerves innervating normal, non-inflamed paws [67]. The CB1 receptor agonist arachidonylcyclopropylamide (ACPA) attenuated hyperalgesia in a mouse model of bone cancer pain [68].

Intraplantar administration of AM1241, which preferentially binds to the CB2 receptor, reduced withdrawal responses to noxious heat in naïve rats, and no central side effects were observed when this compound was administered systemically [69]. Intraplantar administration of AM1241 reduced capsaicin-evoked nocifensive behaviors and hyperalgesia [70], reduced hyperalgesia and edema in carrageenan-induced inflammation [71], and reduced hyperalgesia in a mouse model of bone cancer pain [68].

The endocannabinoids AEA and 2-AG have also been assessed for their peripheral anti-nociceptive properties. Intraplantar administration of AEA prevented the development of CFA-induced hyperalgesia and inflammation, while systemic administration of AEA had no effect [19]. This indicates that in order for AEA to inhibit the inflammatory pain that follows CFA injection, high levels of the drug must be present at the site of injury, which is difficult to achieve under normal conditions given that AEA has a short half-life due to rapid degradation by enzymes. Intraplantar AEA also inhibited capsaicin-induced edema and reduced formalin-induced nociceptive behaviors via CB1 receptor activation [15, 19, 72]. Intraplantar AEA was far more effective at inhibiting formalin-induced behaviors than intravenous AEA [15]. Formalin-evoked behaviors were also inhibited by intraplantar administration of 2-AG, an effect blocked by a CB2 receptor antagonist but not a CB1 antagonist [73]. In rats with inflammation produced by carrageenan administration to the hind paw, evoked responses of nociceptive spinal dorsal horn neurons were reduced following intraplantar administration of AEA [74]. The reduction in evoked activity was blocked by a CB2 antagonist, but not a CB1 antagonist. Intraplantar administration of AEA did not produce any changes in evoked responses of spinal neurons in control rats. Intraplantar AEA decreased hyperalgesia in the tumor-bearing paw in a mouse model of bone cancer pain, and this was blocked by a CB1 receptor antagonist [75]. Intraplantar 2-AG also decreased hyperalgesia in the tumor-bearing paw and the anti-hyperalgesia was mediated by CB2 receptors [76]. Intraplantar AEA has also been shown to decrease hyperalgesia following cisplatin treatment [77]. The mechanism of anti-nociception produced by AEA is complex, and the subtype of cannabinoid receptors involved in its effect seems to differ under acute and chronic pain states. AEA has strong analgesic effects when applied to the site of inflammation or neuropathic pain; however, it should be noted that elevated levels of AEA can also increase excitability of nociceptors through activation of TRPV1 receptors that induces Ca^{2+} influx. This effect was shown in cultured dorsal root ganglion (DRG) neurons sensitive to heat stimulation [78]. It should also be noted that endocannabinoid interactions with ion channels and other binding sites separate from cannabinoid receptors can also produce changes in neuronal function.

In addition to direct cannabinoid receptor agonists, there are drugs which modify endocannabinoid metabolism and thereby alter levels of endocannabinoids. For example, compounds that inhibit enzymes that break down endocannabinoids increase the amount of endocannabinoids available for binding to cannabinoid receptors. URB597 ((3′-(aminocarbonyl)[1,1′-biphenyl]-3-yl)-cyclohexylcarbamate) targets fatty acid amide hydrolase (FAAH), an enzyme which breaks down AEA. Intraplantar administration of URB597 decreased hyperalgesia and C-fiber nociceptor sensitization in chemotherapy-induced peripheral neuropathy following cisplatin treatment, effects which were blocked by a CB1 receptor antagonist but not a CB2 antagonist. Biochemical analysis of skin showed that URB597 increased local levels of AEA without altering the levels of other endocannabinoids [79], indicating that increased activation of CB1 receptors by AEA was the source of decreased nociceptor excitability and analgesia. Intraplantar URB597 also decreased hyperalgesia and C-fiber nociceptor sensitization in a transgenic mouse model of sickle cell disease (SCD, HbSS-BERK). These effects were also blocked by a CB1 receptor antagonist but not by a CB2 receptor antagonist (**Figure 2**). Importantly, intraplantar administration of URB597 still had an anti-hyperalgesic effect in sickle mice with CB2 receptors knocked out (HbSS-BERK-CBR2$^{-/-}$, [80], confirming mediation by CB1 receptors.

Systemic application of URB937 (N-cyclohexyl-carbamic acid, 3′-(aminocarbonyl)-6-hydroxy [1,1′-biphenyl]-3-yl ester), a FAAH inhibitor that is restricted to the periphery and cannot cross the blood-brain barrier, produced analgesic effects in sciatic nerve ligation (Bennett model of

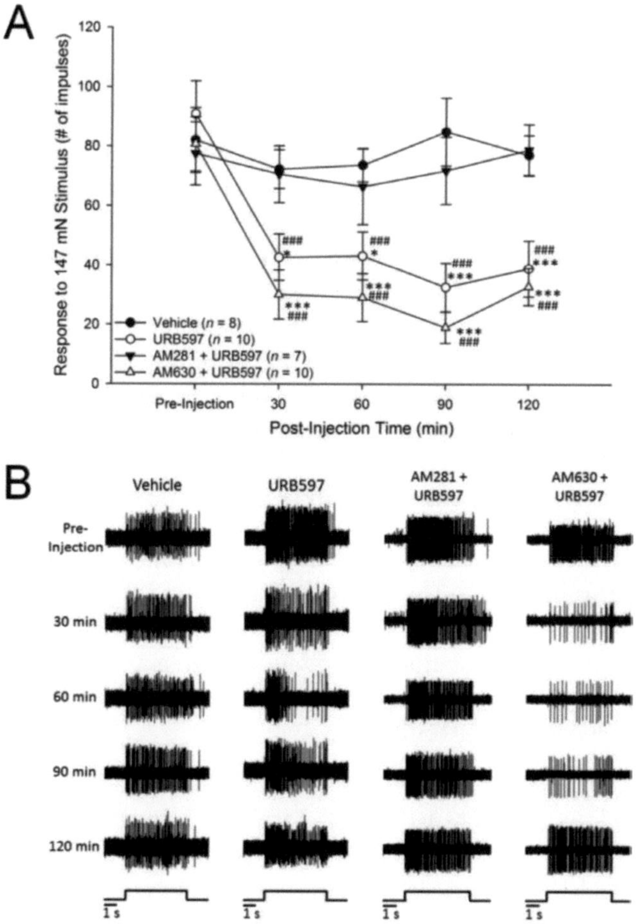

Figure 2. (A) Intraplantar administration of the FAAH inhibitor URB597 decreased evoked responses in C-fiber nociceptors isolated from HbSS-BERK sickle mice. Data show the mean (±SEM) number of impulses evoked by 147 mN before and at 30, 60, 90 and 120 min after various drug treatments. The number of evoked impulses was reduced following intraplantar administration of URB597 at 30, 60, 90, and 120 min post-injection, and this effect was blocked by the CB1 receptor antagonist AM281, but not CB2 receptor antagonist AM630. *$p < .05$, **$p < .005$, ***$p \leq .001$ vs. the vehicle-treated group. ###$p < .001$ indicates significant differences from pre-injection value. (B) Representative examples of responses of individual C-fibers evoked by 147 mN for 5 s before (pre-injection) and at 30, 60, 90 and 120 min after intraplantar injection of vehicle, URB597, URB597 + AM281, and URB597 + AM630. The time of mechanical stimulation is illustrated at the bottom of each column. Reproduced from Uhelski et al. [80].

neuropathic pain) and carrageenan-induced inflammation in the affected hind paw, but did not alter responses on the non-affected hind paw [81, 82]. In cisplatin-treated mice, URB597 delayed and decreased the hyperalgesic effect of cisplatin [77]. Unfortunately, sustained pharmacological inhibition of FAAH results in endocannabinoid catabolism by alternative pathways, which are not dependent upon FAAH [83], thus limiting their clinical effectiveness. FAAH knockout mice have elevated levels of N-acylethanolamines and N-acyl taurines, show reduced responses to noxious stimuli, and are hypersensitive to AEA [84].

Monoacylglycerol lipase (MAGL) is an enzyme that breaks down 2-AG. Inhibition of MAGL produces analgesia under inflammatory conditions. Intraplantar administration of MAGL-inhibitor URB602 (N-[1,1′-Biphenyl]-3-yl-carbamic acid, cyclohexyl ester) attenuated formalin-evoked nociceptive behaviors [73]. Combining URB602 with 2-AG enhanced the anti-nociceptive effects of each [73]. The effect of URB602 was blocked by both CB1 and CB2 antagonists, whereas the effects of 2-AG were only blocked by a CB2 antagonist, suggesting that the URB602 does not behave as selective and/or potent inhibitor of MAGL [85] and that its effects are not dependent on only 2-AG, but may involve the inhibition of FAAH as well. In a mouse model of bone cancer pain, JZL184, a selective MAGL inhibitor, attenuated hyperalgesia in the tumor-bearing hind paw [76]. JZL184 elevates levels of 2-AG but not AEA following acute systemic administration, and the anti-hyperalgesic effect was shown to be dependent on CB2 (but not CB1) receptors. In contrast, intraplantar injection of JZL184 in cisplatin-treated mice decreased hyperalgesia by inhibiting both MAGL and FAAH and normalizing 2-AG and AEA levels in the plantar skin and DRG [86].

2.2. Mechanisms underlying peripheral effects of endocannabinoids

There is a large body of evidence demonstrating that activation of cannabinoid receptors in the periphery produces analgesia. This effect appears to be the result of decreased nociceptor excitability, and there are several mechanisms that could contribute to this effect. These include direct activation of cannabinoid receptors that are expressed by nociceptors as well as activation of cannabinoid receptors expressed in the surrounding non-neuronal tissue that indirectly modulate neuronal excitability.

Studies of mRNA and protein expression have identified CB1 receptors on nociceptive neurons, and selectively knocking out CB1 receptors in $Na_v1.8$-expressing neurons increased sensitivity to noxious heat, enhanced CFA-induced inflammation, and decreased the analgesic effect of WIN 55,212-2 [87–89]. Further, blocking either CB1 or CB2 receptors in the periphery inhibited the anti-nociceptive effect of systemic WIN 55,212-2 to the same degree, suggesting that peripheral cannabinoid receptors are a major site of action for cannabinoid receptor-mediated analgesia [90]. The application of cannabinoid agonist WIN 55, 212–2 and CP 55,940 to cultured primary afferent neurons reduced evoked Ca^{2+} influx in intermediate-diameter neurons, but not small-diameter neurons, though immunoreactivity for CB1 was detected in both cell populations [12, 91]. This indicates that reduction of calcium influx is just one of the inhibitory actions that can result from CB1 activation. Activation of CB1 receptors has also been shown to inhibit the release of calcitonin gene-related peptide (CGRP) from the nerve terminals of nociceptive primary afferent fibers in isolated skin from the rat hind paw [19], which could lead to reduced nociceptor excitability.

Expression of cannabinoid receptors can be modified in chronic pain states, which can enhance the effects of cannabinoid agonists. In a mouse model of bone cancer pain, the DRG ipsilateral to the tumor-bearing hind paw showed increased expression of CB1 receptors. Enhanced CB1 receptor expression in the DRG may explain why small-diameter neurons co-cultured with cancer cells were responsive to CB1 receptor agonists (which attenuated evoked calcium influx), while small-diameter DRG neurons in naïve mice were not [75] (**Figure 3**).

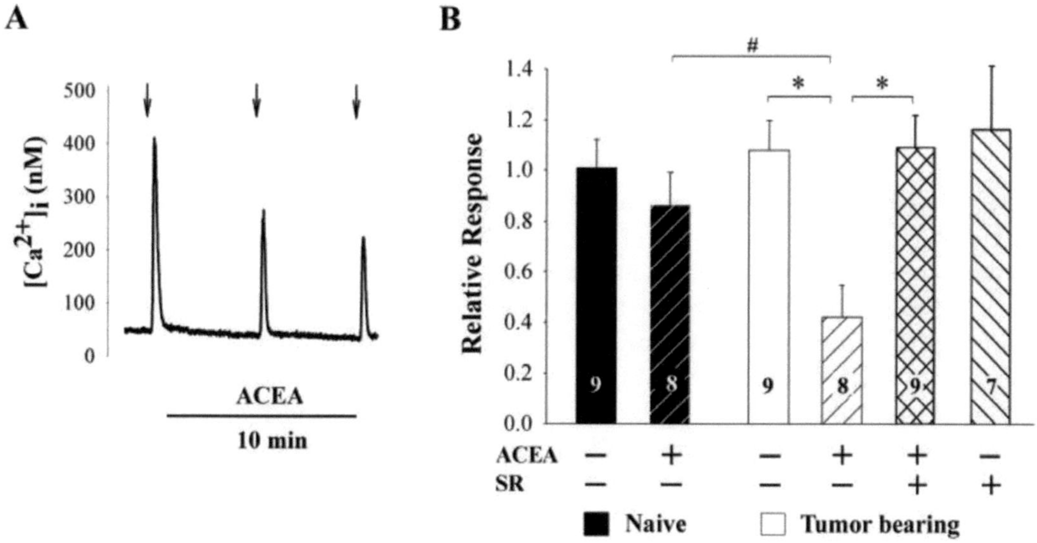

Figure 3. Small DRG neurons (<500 μm²) isolated from DRG L3-L5 of tumor-bearing mice and maintained *in vitro* in control medium for 20–28 h exhibited a change in sensitivity to the CB1 agonist ACEA. (A) The trace represents cannabinoid agonist inhibition of the Ca^{2+} transient evoked by brief superfusion with KCl (50 mM, 10 s, arrows). ACEA (1 μM) was included in the superfusate following the first test with KCl. (B) ACEA attenuated the Ca^{2+} transient evoked by KCl (50 mM) in neurons isolated from L3-L5 DRGs of tumor-bearing mice, but not in those from naïve mice. Involvement of CB1 receptors in the response to ACEA was confirmed by blocking the inhibitory effect by co-application of the CB1 receptor antagonist SR141716A (SR, 1 μM). Relative response was defined as the amplitude of the response of a neuron to KCl in the presence of ACEA divided by the amplitude of the response in the absence of ACEA. *Significantly different at $p < 0.001$; #significantly different at $p < 0.01$ (one-way ANOVA with Tukey's multiple comparisons test). Reproduced from Khasabova et al. [75].

CB2 receptor mRNA and protein are increased in the lumbar DRG after spinal nerve ligation (SNL) or CCI (Bennett model of neuropathic pain), but not CFA-induced inflammation [92]. The effect appears to be localized to microglia [92, 93], though there is some evidence of enhanced neuronal expression after SNL, including increased expression in the nerve proximal to the ligation [94]. In a mouse model of bone cancer pain, tumors showed high levels of CB2 receptor protein levels, and CB2 receptor proteins were also elevated in plantar skin of the tumor-bearing hind paw [76]. Taken together, these results support to the notion that endocannabinoid-mediated inhibition of peripheral nociceptor activity is necessary to prevent exaggerated responses to noxious stimuli and that tonic activation of endocannabinoids aids in suppressing pain, inflammation, and nociceptor sensitization after injury. Further evidence is shown by differences in levels of endocannabinoids in naïve, acute inflammation, and chronic pain conditions. In models of chronic pain from bone cancer and chemotherapy-induced peripheral neuropathy, the level of AEA was decreased in the skin of the plantar hind paw due to increased FAAH mRNA expression and AEA uptake in DRG neurons ipsilateral to a tumor-bearing hind paw [75, 95]. In cisplatin-treated mice, expression of 2-AG and AEA are both decreased in the plantar skin and DRG [86].

3. Conclusions

Concerns about the safety of commonly used analgesic drugs have hindered the treatment of patients with chronic pain. Continued exploration of mechanisms underlying nociceptive processing under naïve, acute and chronic pain states has helped identify specific targets for the development of new treatment approaches that could solve some of the problems associated with chronic use of opiates and NSAIDs. This includes the use of drugs which target the endocannabinoid system. Early investigations identified problems with the systemic use of compounds derived from the cannabis plant, including sedation, mood alterations, and motor effects, a direct consequence of binding to cannabinoid receptors in the brain. By targeting the peripheral endocannabinoid system, the negative side effects of cannabinoids can be bypassed, providing analgesia without impairment of normal function. Work with animal models has shown that activation of cannabinoid receptors in the periphery can be useful for a wide variety of pain conditions, including inflammation, bone cancer pain, chemotherapy-induced peripheral neuropathy, and sickle cell disease. Analgesia can be achieved through direct receptor activation or through the restoration of endocannabinoid levels, both of which decrease signs of sensitization in peripheral nociceptors. Thus, specific treatments could target known alterations in endocannabinoid levels associated with different chronic pain conditions. Drugs targeting the peripheral endocannabinoid system could be used as effective analgesics or in combination with currently available therapies to maximize pain relief while minimizing harmful side effects.

Acknowledgements

This work was supported by NIH grants HL135895 and HL117664.

Conflict of interest

The authors have no conflicts of interest to declare.

Author details

Megan L. Uhelski*, Iryna Khasabova and Donald A. Simone

*Address all correspondence to: muhelski@umn.edu

Department of Diagnostic and Biological Sciences, School of Dentistry,
University of Minnesota, Minneapolis, MN USA

References

[1] Devane WA, Dysarz F3, Johnson MR, Melvin LS, Howlett AC. Determination and characterization of a cannabinoid receptor in rat brain. Molecular Pharmacology. 1988 Nov 1;**34**(5):605-613

[2] Devane WA, Hanus L, Breuer A, Pertwee RG, Stevenson LA, Griffin G, Gibson D, Mandelbaum A, Etinger A, Mechoulam R. Isolation and structure of a brain constituent that binds to the cannabinoid receptor. Science. 1992 Dec 18;**258**(5090):1946-1949. DOI: 10.1126/science.1470919

[3] Matsuda LA, Lolait SJ, Brownstein MJ, Young AC, Bonner TI. Structure of a cannabinoid receptor and functional expression of the cloned cDNA. Nature. 1990 Aug;**346**(6284):561

[4] Munro S, Thomas KL, Abu-Shaar M. Molecular characterization of a peripheral receptor for cannabinoids. Nature. 1993 Sep;**365**(6441):61

[5] Hohmann AG, Martin WJ, Tsou K, Walker JM. Inhibition of noxious stimulus-evoked activity of spinal cord dorsal horn neurons by the cannabinoid WIN 55,212-212. Life Sciences. 1995 May 5;**56**(23-24):2111-2118. DOI: 10.1016/0024-3205(95)00196-D

[6] Hohmann AG, Tsou K, Walker JM. Cannabinoid modulation of wide dynamic range neurons in the lumbar dorsal horn of the rat by spinally administered WIN55,212-2. Neuroscience Letters. 1998 Dec 4;**257**(3):119-122. DOI: 10.1016/S0304-3940(98)00802-7

[7] Hohmann AG, Tsou K, Walker JM. Cannabinoid suppression of noxious heat-evoked activity in wide dynamic range neurons in the lumbar dorsal horn of the rat. Journal of Neurophysiology. 1999 Feb 1;**81**(2):575-583. DOI: 10.1152/jn.1999.81.2.575

[8] Griffin G, Tao Q, Abood ME. Cloning and pharmacological characterization of the rat CB2 cannabinoid receptor. Journal of Pharmacology and Experimental Therapeutics. 2000 Mar 1;**292**(3):886-894

[9] Fride E, Mechoulam R. Pharmacological activity of the cannabinoid receptor agonist, anandamide, a brain constituent. European Journal of Pharmacology. 1993 Feb 9;**231**(2): 313-314. DOI: 10.1016/0014-2999(93)90468-W

[10] Di Marzo V, Bifulco M, De Petrocellis L. The endocannabinoid system and its therapeutic exploitation. Nature Reviews Drug discovery. 2004 Sep;**3**(9):771. DOI: 10.1038/nrd1495

[11] Pacher P, Bátkai S, Kunos G. The endocannabinoid system as an emerging target of pharmacotherapy. Pharmacological Reviews. 2006 Sep 1;**58**(3):389-462. DOI: 10.1124/pr.58.3.2

[12] Khasabova IA, Simone DA, Seybold VS. Cannabinoids attenuate depolarization-dependent Ca^{2+} influx in intermediate-size primary afferent neurons of adult rats. Neuroscience. 2002 Dec 2;**115**(2):613-625

[13] Facci L, Dal Toso R, Romanello S, Buriani A, Skaper SD, Leon A. Mast cells express a peripheral cannabinoid receptor with differential sensitivity to anandamide and palmitoylethanolamide. Proceedings of the National Academy of Sciences. 1995 Apr 11;**92**(8): 3376-3380. DOI: 10.1073/pnas.92.8.3376

[14] Galiègue S, Mary S, Marchand J, Dussossoy D, Carrière D, Carayon P, Bouaboula M, Shire D, Fur G, Casellas P. Expression of central and peripheral cannabinoid receptors in human immune tissues and leukocyte subpopulations. The FEBS Journal. 1995 Aug 1;**232**(1):54-61. DOI: 10.1111/j.1432-1033.1995.tb20780.x

[15] Calignano A, La Rana G, Giuffrida A, Piomelli D. Control of pain initiation by endogenous cannabinoids. Nature. 1998 Jul;**394**(6690):277. DOI: 10.1038/28393

[16] Moss DE, Johnson RL. Tonic analgesic effects of Δ9-tetrahydrocannabinol as measured with the formalin test. European Journal of Pharmacology. 1980 Feb 8;**61**(3):313-315

[17] Elmes SJ, Winyard LA, Medhurst SJ, Clayton NM, Wilson AW, Kendall DA, Chapman V. Activation of CB1 and CB2 receptors attenuates the induction and maintenance of inflammatory pain in the rat. Pain. 2005 Dec 5;**118**(3):327-335. DOI: 10.1016/j.pain.2005.09.005

[18] Clayton N, Marshall FH, Bountra C, O'shaughnessy CT. CB1 and CB2 cannabinoid receptors are implicated in inflammatory pain. Pain. 2002 Apr 1;**96**(3):253-260. DOI: 10.1016/S0304-3959(01)00454-7

[19] Richardson JD, Kilo S, Hargreaves KM. Cannabinoids reduce hyperalgesia and inflammation via interaction with peripheral CB1 receptors. Pain. 1998 Mar 1;**75**(1):111-119

[20] Martin WJ, Loo CM, Basbaum AI. Spinal cannabinoids are anti-allodynic in rats with persistent inflammation. Pain. 1999 Aug 1;**82**(2):199-205

[21] Ko MC, Woods JH. Local administration of Δ9-tetrahydrocannabinol attenuates capsaicin-induced thermal nociception in rhesus monkeys: A peripheral cannabinoid action. Psychopharmacology. 1999 Apr 1;**143**(3):322-326

[22] Li J, Daughters RS, Bullis C, Bengiamin R, Stucky MW, Brennan J, Simone DA. The cannabinoid receptor agonist WIN 55,212-2 mesylate blocks the development of hyperalgesia produced by capsaicin in rats. Pain. 1999 May 1;**81**(1-2):25-33

[23] Johanek LM, Heitmiller DR, Turner M, Nader N, Hodges J, Simone DA. Cannabinoids attenuate capsaicin-evoked hyperalgesia through spinal and peripheral mechanisms. Pain. 2001 Sep 1;**93**(3):303-315. DOI: 10.1016/S0304-3959(01)00336-0

[24] Rukwied R, Watkinson A, McGlone F, Dvorak M. Cannabinoid agonists attenuate capsaicin-induced responses in human skin. Pain. 2003 Apr 1;**102**(3):283-288

[25] Herzberg U, Eliav E, Bennett GJ, Kopin IJ. The analgesic effects of R (+)-WIN 55,212-2 mesylate, a high affinity cannabinoid agonist, in a rat model of neuropathic pain. Neuroscience Letters. 1997 Jan 17;**221**(2-3):157-160. DOI: 10.1016/S0304-3940(96)13308-5

[26] Fox A, Kesingland A, Gentry C, McNair K, Patel S, Urban L, James I. The role of central and peripheral Cannabinoid1 receptors in the antihyperalgesic activity of cannabinoids in a model of neuropathic pain. Pain. 2001 May 1;**92**(1-2):91-100. DOI: 10.1016/S0304-3959(00)00474-7

[27] Bridges D, Ahmad K, Rice AS. The synthetic cannabinoid WIN55, 212-2 attenuates hyperalgesia and allodynia in a rat model of neuropathic pain. British Journal of Pharmacology. 2001;**133**:586-594. DOI: 10.1038/sj.bjp.0704110

[28] Scott DA, Wright CE, Angus JA. Evidence that CB-1 and CB-2 cannabinoid receptors mediate antinociception in neuropathic pain in the rat. Pain. 2004 May 1;**109**(1-2):124-131. DOI: 10.1016/j.pain.2004.01.020

[29] Ibrahim MM, Deng H, Zvonok A, Cockayne DA, Kwan J, Mata HP, Vanderah TW, Lai J, Porreca F, Makriyannis A, Malan TP. Activation of CB2 cannabinoid receptors by AM1241 inhibits experimental neuropathic pain: Pain inhibition by receptors not present in the CNS. Proceedings of the National Academy of Sciences. 2003 Sep 2;**100**(18):10529-10533. DOI: 10.1073/pnas.1834309100

[30] Doğrul A, Gül H, Yıldız O, Bilgin F, Güzeldemir ME. Cannabinoids blocks tactile allodynia in diabetic mice without attenuation of its antinociceptive effect. Neuroscience Letters. 2004 Sep 16;**368**(1):82-86. DOI: 10.1016/j.neulet.2004.06.060

[31] Ulugol A, Karadag HC, Ipci Y, Tamer M, Dokmeci I. The effect of WIN 55,212-2, a cannabinoid agonist, on tactile allodynia in diabetic rats. Neuroscience Letters. 2004 Nov 23; **371**(2-3):167-170

[32] Vera G, López-Miranda V, Herradón E, Martín MI, Abalo R. Characterization of cannabinoid-induced relief of neuropathic pain in rat models of type 1 and type 2 diabetes. Pharmacology Biochemistry and Behavior. 2012 Aug 1;**102**(2):335-343. DOI: 10.1016/j.pbb.2012.05.008

[33] Vera G, Chiarlone A, Cabezos PA, Pascual D, Martín MI, Abalo R. WIN 55,212-2 prevents mechanical allodynia but not alterations in feeding behaviour induced by chronic cisplatin in the rat. Life Sciences. 2007 Jul 19;**81**(6):468-479. DOI: 10.1016/j.lfs.2007.06.012

[34] Vera G, Cabezos PA, Martín MI, Abalo R. Characterization of cannabinoid-induced relief of neuropathic pain in a rat model of cisplatin-induced neuropathy. Pharmacology Biochemistry and Behavior. 2013 Apr 1;**105**:205-212. DOI: 10.1016/j.pbb.2013.02.008

[35] Burgos E, Gómez-Nicola D, Pascual D, Martín MI, Nieto-Sampedro M, Goicoechea C. Cannabinoid agonist WIN 55,212-2 prevents the development of paclitaxel-induced peripheral neuropathy in rats. Possible involvement of spinal glial cells. European Journal of Pharmacology. 2012;**682**:62-72. DOI: 10.1016/j.ejphar.2012.02.008

[36] Deng L, Guindon J, Vemuri VK, Thakur GA, White FA, Makriyannis A, Hohmann AG. The maintenance of cisplatin-and paclitaxel-induced mechanical and cold allodynia is suppressed by cannabinoid CB 2 receptor activation and independent of CXCR4 signaling in models of chemotherapy-induced peripheral neuropathy. Molecular Pain. 2012 Dec;**8**(1):71. DOI: 10.1186/1744-8069-8-71

[37] Raft D, Gregg J, Ghia J, Harris L. Effects of intravenous tetrahydrocannabinol on experimental and surgical pain; psychological correlates of the analgesic response. Clinical Pharmacology & Therapeutics. 1977 Jan 1;**21**(1):26-33

[38] Yesilyurt O, Dogrul A, Gul H, Seyrek M, Kusmez O, Ozkan Y, Yildiz O. Topical cannabinoid enhances topical morphine antinociception. Pain. 2003 Sep 1;**105**(1-2):303-308. DOI: 10.1016/S0304-3959(03)00245-8

[39] Noyes R, Brunk SF, Avery DH, Canter A. The analgesic properties of delta-9-tetrahydrocannabinol and codeine. Clinical Pharmacology & Therapeutics. 1975 Jul 1;**18**(1):84-89

[40] Noyes R, Brunk SF, Baram DA, Canter A. Analgesic effect of delta-9-tetrahydrocannabinol. The Journal of Clinical Pharmacology. 1975 Feb 3;**15**(2-3):139-143

[41] Hampson AJ, Grimaldi M, Axelrod J, Wink D. Cannabidiol and (−)Δ9-tetrahydrocannabinol are neuroprotective antioxidants. Proceedings of the National Academy of Sciences. 1998 Jul 7;**95**(14):8268-8273. DOI: 10.1073/pnas.95.14.8268

[42] Thomas A, Baillie GL, Phillips AM, Razdan RK, Ross RA, Pertwee RG. Cannabidiol displays unexpectedly high potency as an antagonist of CB1 and CB2 receptor agonists in vitro. British journal of pharmacology. 2007 Mar 1;**150**(5):613-623

[43] Laprairie RB, Bagher AM, Kelly ME, Denovan-Wright EM. Cannabidiol is a negative allosteric modulator of the cannabinoid CB1 receptor. British Journal of Pharmacology. 2015 Oct 1;**172**(20):4790-4805

[44] Nagayama T, Sinor AD, Simon RP, Chen J, Graham SH, Jin K, Greenberg DA. Cannabinoids and neuroprotection in global and focal cerebral ischemia and in neuronal cultures. Journal of Neuroscience. 1999 Apr 15;**19**(8):2987-2995

[45] Fernández-López D, Martínez-Orgado J, Nuñez E, Romero J, Lorenzo P, Moro MÁ, Lizasoain I. Characterization of the neuroprotective effect of the cannabinoid agonist WIN-55212 in an in vitro model of hypoxic-ischemic brain damage in newborn rats. Pediatric Research. 2006 Aug;**60**(2):169. DOI: 10.1203/01.pdr.0000228839.00122.6c

[46] Panikashvili D, Simeonidou C, Ben-Shabat S, Hanuš L, Breuer A, Mechoulam R, Shohami E. An endogenous cannabinoid (2-AG) is neuroprotective after brain injury. Nature. 2001 Oct;**413**(6855):527. DOI: 10.1038/35097089

[47] Ramírez BG, Blázquez C, del Pulgar TG, Guzmán M, de Ceballos ML. Prevention of Alzheimer's disease pathology by cannabinoids: Neuroprotection mediated by blockade of microglial activation. Journal of Neuroscience. 2005 Feb 23;**25**(8):1904-1913. DOI: 10.1523/JNEUROSCI.4540-04.2005

[48] Molina-Holgado F, Lledó A, Guaza C. Anandamide suppresses nitric oxide and TNF-α responses to Theiler's virus or endotoxin in astrocytes. Neuroreport. 1997 May 26;**8**(8): 1929-1933

[49] Molina-Holgado F, Molina-Holgado E, Guaza C, Rothwell NJ. Role of CB1 and CB2 receptors in the inhibitory effects of cannabinoids on lipopolysaccharide-induced nitric oxide release in astrocyte cultures. Journal of Neuroscience Research. 2002 Mar 15;**67**(6):829-836. DOI: 10.1002/jnr.10165

[50] Puffenbarger RA, Boothe AC, Cabral GA. Cannabinoids inhibit LPS-inducible cytokine mRNA expression in rat microglial cells. Glia. 2000 Jan 1;**29**(1):58-69

[51] Marsicano G, Moosmann B, Hermann H, Lutz B, Behl C. Neuroprotective properties of cannabinoids against oxidative stress: Role of the cannabinoid receptor CB1. Journal of Neurochemistry. 2002 Feb 1;**80**(3):448-456

[52] Facchinetti F, Del Giudice E, Furegato S, Passarotto M, Leon A. Cannabinoids ablate release of TNFα in rat microglial cells stimulated with lipopolysaccharide. Glia 2003 Jan 15; **41**(2):161-168. DOI: 10.1002/glia.10177

[53] Sheng WS, Hu S, Min X, Cabral GA, Lokensgard JR, Peterson PK. Synthetic cannabinoid WIN55, 212-2 inhibits generation of inflammatory mediators by IL-1β-stimulated human astrocytes. Glia. 2005 Jan 15;**49**(2):211-219. DOI: 10.1002/glia.20108

[54] Fernández-Ruiz J, Romero J, Velasco G, Tolón RM, Ramos JA, Guzmán M. Cannabinoid CB2 receptor: A new target for controlling neural cell survival? Trends in Pharmacological Sciences. 2007 Jan 1;**28**(1):39-45. DOI: 10.1016/j.tips.2006.11.001

[55] Pryce G, Ahmed Z, Hankey DJ, Jackson SJ, Croxford JL, Pocock JM, Ledent C, Petzold A, Thompson AJ, Giovannoni G, Cuzner ML, Baker D. Cannabinoids inhibit neurodegeneration in models of multiple sclerosis. Brain. 2003 Oct 1;**126**(10):2191-2202. DOI: 10.1093/brain/awg224

[56] Maresz K, Pryce G, Ponomarev ED, Marsicano G, Croxford JL, Shriver LP, Ledent C, Cheng X, Carrier EJ, Mann MK, Giovannoni G. Direct suppression of CNS autoimmune inflammation via the cannabinoid receptor CB 1 on neurons and CB 2 on autoreactive T cells. Nature Medicine. 2007 Apr;**13**(4):492. DOI: 10.1038/nm1561

[57] Croxford JL, Pryce G, Jackson SJ, Ledent C, Giovannoni G, Pertwee RG, Yamamura T, Baker D. Cannabinoid-mediated neuroprotection, not immunosuppression, may be more relevant to multiple sclerosis. Journal of Neuroimmunology. 2008 Jan 1;**193**(1): 120-129. DOI: 10.1016/j.jneuroim.2007.10.024

[58] Costa B, Colleoni M, Conti S, Trovato AE, Bianchi M, Sotgiu ML, Giagnoni G. Repeated treatment with the synthetic cannabinoid WIN 55,212-2 reduces both hyperalgesia and production of pronociceptive mediators in a rat model of neuropathic pain. British Journal of Pharmacology. 2004 Jan 1;**141**(1):4-8. DOI: 10.1038/sj.bjp.0705587

[59] Castaneto MS, Gorelick DA, Desrosiers NA, Hartman RL, Pirard S, Huestis MA. Synthetic cannabinoids: Epidemiology, pharmacodynamics, and clinical implications. Drug & Alcohol Dependence. 2014 Nov 1;**144**:12-41. DOI: 10.1016/j.drugalcdep.2014.08.005

[60] Johanek LM, Simone DA. Activation of peripheral cannabinoid receptors attenuates cutaneous hyperalgesia produced by a heat injury. Pain. 2004 Jun 1;**109**(3):432-442. DOI: 10.1016/j.pain.2004.02.020

[61] Potenzieri C, Harding-Rose C, Simone DA. The cannabinoid receptor agonist, WIN 55, 212-2, attenuates tumor-evoked hyperalgesia through peripheral mechanisms. Brain Research. 2008 Jun 18;**1215**:69-75. DOI: 10.1016/j.brainres.2008.03.063

[62] Martin BR, Compton DR, Thomas BF, Prescott WR, Little PJ, Razdan RK, Johnson MR, Melvin LS, Mechoulam R. Behavioral, biochemical, and molecular modeling evaluations of cannabinoid analogs. Pharmacology Biochemistry and Behavior. 1991 Nov 1;**40**(3):471-478

[63] Uhelski ML, Cain DM, Harding-Rose C, Simone DA. The non-selective cannabinoid receptor agonist WIN 55,212-2 attenuates responses of C-fiber nociceptors in a murine model of cancer pain. Neuroscience. 2013 Sep 5;**247**:84-94. DOI: 10.1016/j.neuroscience.2013.05.003

[64] Kohli DR, Li Y, Khasabov SG, Gupta P, Kehl LJ, Ericson ME, Nguyen J, Gupta V, Hebbel RP, Simone DA, Gupta K. Pain-related behaviors and neurochemical alterations in mice expressing sickle hemoglobin: Modulation by cannabinoids. Blood. 2010 Jul 22;**116**(3):456-465. DOI: 10.1182/blood-2010-01-260372

[65] Pascual D, Goicoechea C, Suardíaz M, Martín MI. A cannabinoid agonist, WIN 55,212-2, reduces neuropathic nociception induced by paclitaxel in rats. Pain. 2005 Nov 1;**118**(1-2): 23-34. DOI: 10.1016/j.pain.2005.07.008

[66] Dziadulewicz EK, Bevan SJ, Brain CT, Coote PR, Culshaw AJ, Davis AJ, Edwards LJ, Fisher AJ, Fox AJ, Gentry C, Groarke A. Naphthalen-1-yl-(4-pentyloxynaphthalen-1-yl) methanone: A potent, orally bioavailable human CB1/CB2 dual agonist with antihyperalgesic properties and restricted central nervous system penetration. Journal of Medicinal Chemistry. 2007 Aug 9;**50**(16):3851-3856. DOI: 10.1021/jm070317a

[67] Potenzieri C, Brink TS, Pacharinsak C, Simone DA. Cannabinoid modulation of cutaneous Aδ nociceptors during inflammation. Journal of Neurophysiology. 2008 Nov;**100**(5): 2794-2806. DOI: 10.1152/jn.90809.2008

[68] Khasabova IA, Gielissen J, Chandiramani A, Harding-Rose C, Odeh DA, Simone DA, Seybold VS. CB1 and CB2 receptor agonists promote analgesia through synergy in a murine model of tumor pain. Behavioural Pharmacology. 2011 Sep;**22**(5-6):607-616. DOI: 10.1097/FBP.0b013e3283474a6d

[69] Malan TP Jr, Ibrahim MM, Deng H, Liu Q, Mata HP, Vanderah T, Porreca F, Makriyannis A. CB2 cannabinoid receptor-mediated peripheral antinociception. Pain. 2001 Sep 1;**93**(3): 239-245

[70] Hohmann AG, Farthing JN, Zvonok AM, Makriyannis A. Selective activation of cannabinoid CB2 receptors suppresses hyperalgesia evoked by intradermal capsaicin. Journal of Pharmacology and Experimental Therapeutics. 2004 Feb 1;**308**(2):446-453. DOI: 10.1124/jpet.103.060079

[71] Quartilho A, Mata HP, Ibrahim MM, Vanderah TW, Porreca F, Makriyannis A, Malan TP. Inhibition of inflammatory Hyperalgesia by activation of peripheral CB2 cannabinoid receptors. Anesthesiology. 2003 Oct 1;**99**(4):955-960

[72] Guindon J, De Léan A, Beaulieu P. Local interactions between anandamide, an endocannabinoid, and ibuprofen, a nonsteroidal anti-inflammatory drug, in acute and inflammatory pain. Pain. 2006 Mar 1;**121**(1-2):85-93. DOI: 10.1016/j.pain.2005.12.007

[73] Guindon J, Desroches J, Beaulieu P. The antinociceptive effects of intraplantar injections of 2-arachidonoyl glycerol are mediated by cannabinoid CB2 receptors. British Journal of Pharmacology. 2007 Mar 1;**150**(6):693-701. DOI: 10.1038/sj.bjp.0706990

[74] Sokal DM, Elmes SJ, Kendall DA, Chapman V. Intraplantar injection of anandamide inhibits mechanically-evoked responses of spinal neurones via activation of CB2 receptors in anaesthetised rats. Neuropharmacology. 2003 Sep 1;**45**(3):404-411

[75] Khasabova IA, Khasabov SG, Harding-Rose C, Coicou LG, Seybold BA, Lindberg AE, Steevens CD, Simone DA, Seybold VS. A decrease in anandamide signaling contributes to the maintenance of cutaneous mechanical hyperalgesia in a model of bone cancer pain. Journal of Neuroscience. 2008 Oct 29;**28**(44):11141-11152

[76] Khasabova IA, Chandiramani A, Harding-Rose C, Simone DA, Seybold VS. Increasing 2-arachidonoyl glycerol signaling in the periphery attenuates mechanical hyperalgesia in a model of bone cancer pain. Pharmacological Research. 2011 Jul 1;**64**(1):60-67. DOI: 10.1016/j.phrs.2011.03.007

[77] Khasabova IA, Khasabov S, Paz J, Harding-Rose C, Simone DA, Seybold VS. Cannabinoid type-1 receptor reduces pain and neurotoxicity produced by chemotherapy. Journal of Neuroscience. 2012 May 16;**32**(20):7091-7101. DOI: 10.1523/JNEUROSCI.2847-08.2008

[78] Fischbach T, Greffrath W, Nawrath H, Treede RD. Effects of anandamide and noxious heat on intracellular calcium concentration in nociceptive DRG neurons of rats. Journal of Neurophysiology. 2007 Aug;**98**(2):929-938. DOI: 10.1152/jn.01096.2006

[79] Uhelski ML, Khasabova IA, Simone DA. Inhibition of anandamide hydrolysis attenuates nociceptor sensitization in a murine model of chemotherapy-induced peripheral neuropathy. Journal of Neurophysiology. 2014 Dec 10;**113**(5):1501-1510. DOI: 10.1152/jn.00692.2014

[80] Uhelski ML, Gupta K, Simone DA. Sensitization of C-fiber nociceptors in mice with sickle cell disease is decreased by local inhibition of anandamide hydrolysis. Pain. 2017 Sep 1;**158**(9):1711-1722. DOI: 10.1097/j.pain.0000000000000966

[81] Clapper JR, Moreno-Sanz G, Russo R, Guijarro A, Vacondio F, Duranti A, Tontini A, Sanchini S, Sciolino NR, Spradley JM, Hohmann AG. Anandamide suppresses pain initiation through a peripheral endocannabinoid mechanism. Nature Neuroscience. 2010 Oct;**13**(10):1265. DOI: 10.1038/nn.2632

[82] Moreno-Sanz G, Sasso O, Guijarro A, Oluyemi O, Bertorelli R, Reggiani A, Piomelli D. Pharmacological characterization of the peripheral FAAH inhibitor URB937 in female rodents: Interaction with the Abcg2 transporter in the blood-placenta barrier. British Journal of Pharmacology. 2012 Dec 1;**167**(8):1620-1628. DOI: 10.1111/j.1476-5381.2012.02098.x

[83] Yu M, Ives D, Ramesha CS. Synthesis of prostaglandin E2 ethanolamide from anandamide by cyclooxygenase-2. Journal of Biological Chemistry. 1997 Aug 22;**272**(34):21181-21186. DOI: 10.1074/jbc.272.34.21181

[84] Cravatt BF, Demarest K, Patricelli MP, Bracey MH, Giang DK, Martin BR, Lichtman AH. Supersensitivity to anandamide and enhanced endogenous cannabinoid signaling in mice lacking fatty acid amide hydrolase. Proceedings of the National Academy of Sciences. 2001 Jul 31;**98**(16):9371-9376. DOI: 10.1073/pnas.161191698

[85] Vandevoorde S, Jonsson KO, Labar G, Persson E, Lambert DM, Fowler CJ. Lack of selectivity of URB602 for 2-oleoylglycerol compared to anandamide hydrolysis in vitro. British Journal of Pharmacology. 2007 Jan 1;**150**(2):186-191. DOI: 10.1038/sj.bjp.0706971

[86] Khasabova IA, Yao X, Paz J, Lewandowski CT, Lindberg AE, Coicou L, Burlakova N, Simone DA, Seybold VS. JZL184 is anti-hyperalgesic in a murine model of cisplatin-induced peripheral neuropathy. Pharmacological Research. 2014 Dec 1;**90**:67-75. DOI: 10.1016/j.phrs.2014.09.008

[87] Hohmann AG, Herkenham M. Localization of central cannabinoid CB1 receptor messenger RNA in neuronal subpopulations of rat dorsal root ganglia: A double-label in situ hybridization study. Neuroscience. 1999 May 1;**90**(3):923-931. DOI: 10.1016/S0306-4522(98)00524-7

[88] Bridges D, Rice ASC, Egertova M, Elphick MR, Winter J, Michael GJ. Localisation of cannabinoid receptor 1 in rat dorsal root ganglion using in situ hybridisation and immunohistochemistry. Neuroscience. 2003;**119**:803-812. DOI: 10.1016/S0306-4522(03)00200-8

[89] Agarwal N, Pacher P, Tegeder I, Amaya F, Constantin CE, Brenner GJ, Rubino T, Michalski CW, Marsicano G, Monory K, Mackie K. Cannabinoids mediate analgesia largely via peripheral type 1 cannabinoid receptors in nociceptors. Nature Neuroscience. 2007;**10**:870. DOI: 10.1038/nn1916

[90] Zhu CZ, Mikusa JP, Fan Y, Hollingsworth PR, Pai M, Chandran P, Daza AV, Yao BB, Dart MJ, Meyer MD, Decker MW. Peripheral and central sites of action for the non-selective cannabinoid agonist WIN 55,212-2 in a rat model of post-operative pain. British Journal of Pharmacology. 2009 Jun 1;**157**(4):645-655. DOI: 10.1111/j.1476-5381.2009.00184.x

[91] Khasabova IA, Harding-Rose C, Simone DA, Seybold VS. Differential effects of CB1 and opioid agonists on two populations of adult rat dorsal root ganglion neurons. Journal of Neuroscience. 2004 Feb 18;**24**(7):1744-1753. DOI: 10.1523/JNEUROSCI.4298-03.2004

[92] Zhang J, Hoffert C, Vu HK, Groblewski T, Ahmad S, O'donnell D. Induction of CB2 receptor expression in the rat spinal cord of neuropathic but not inflammatory chronic pain models. European Journal of Neuroscience. 2003 Jun 1;**17**(12):2750-2754. DOI: 10.1046/j.1460-9568.2003.02704.x

[93] Beltramo M, Bernardini N, Bertorelli R, Campanella M, Nicolussi E, Fredduzzi S, Reggiani A. CB2 receptor-mediated antihyperalgesia: Possible direct involvement of neural mechanisms. European Journal of Neuroscience. 2006;**23**:1530-1538. DOI: 10.1111/j.1460-9568.2006.04684.x

[94] Wotherspoon G, Fox A, McIntyre P, Colley S, Bevan S, Winter J. Peripheral nerve injury induces cannabinoid receptor 2 protein expression in rat sensory neurons. Neuroscience. 2005 Jan 1;**135**(1):235-245. DOI: 10.1016/j.neuroscience.2005.06.009

[95] Khasabova IA, Holman M, Morse T, Burlakova N, Coicou L, Harding-Rose C, Simone DA, Seybold VS. Increased anandamide uptake by sensory neurons contributes to hyperalgesia in a model of cancer pain. Neurobiology of Disease. 2013 Oct 1;**58**:19-28. DOI: 10.1016/j.nbd.2013.04.018

Chapter 7

Possible Role of the Endocannabinoid System in Tourette Syndrome

Natalia Szejko, Ewgeni Jakubovski and
Kirsten Müller-Vahl

Additional information is available at the end of the chapter

http://dx.doi.org/10.5772/intechopen.79895

Abstract

Tourette syndrome (TS) is a neuropsychiatric disorder with childhood onset. The core symptoms are motor and vocal tics. The majority of patients also suffer from psychiatric comorbidities. The pathophysiology of TS is not clear, but changes in different neurotransmitter systems—in particular the dopaminergic system—have been confirmed. Since there is increasing evidence that cannabis-based medicine (CBM) is effective in the treatment of TS, an involvement of the endocannabinoid system in the pathophysiology of TS has been suggested. The purpose of this chapter is to present existing evidence suggesting a pathophysiological role of the endocannabinoid system in TS and to summarize available data on beneficial treatment effects of CBM in patients with TS.

Keywords: Tourette syndrome, cannabis-based medicine, tics, THC, cannabinoids, cannabis

1. Introduction

1.1. Symptoms of Tourette syndrome

Tourette syndrome (TS) is a childhood onset neuropsychiatric disorder that is present in approximately 1% of the population [1]. For unknown reasons, it occurs 3–4 times more often in men than in women. To fulfill the diagnostic criteria for TS, multiple motor and at least one vocal tic must be present for a minimal period of 1 year before 18 years of age.

Tics are sudden, repetitive involuntary movements or vocalizations. Both vocal and motor tics can be further differentiated into a simple or complex presentation. Simple motor tics involve only one group of muscles in a brief jerk-like movement, with examples such as eye blinking, head jerking or shoulder shrugging. Complex motor tics, on the contrary, involve multiple groups of muscles or resemble purposeful movements. Examples of complex motor tics are as follows: touching people or objects, echopraxia (mirroring another person's actions) or copropraxia (involuntary performing of obscene gestures). Simple vocal tics are short vocalizations, for example throat clearing, sniffing or grunting. Complex vocal tics involve the involuntary production of words or entire sentences, for example echolalia (repeating another person's words), palilalia (repeating one's own words) and coprolalia (involuntary pronunciation of obscene words). Although coprolalia is often associated with TS, it is only present in approximately 10% of patients [2]. The majority of patients report a premonitory urge that proceeds the tics. This is often described as an "uncomfortable" physical sensation located in a particular body part or as a more generalized feeling [3]. Most (adult) patients are able to control their tics for a short period of time.

In almost 90% of TS patients, tics are accompanied by other co-occurring psychiatric disorders such as attention deficit/hyperactivity disorder (ADHD), obsessive–compulsive disorder (OCD), self-injurious behaviors (SIB), anxiety disorders and depression [4].

1.2. Course and causes of Tourette syndrome

Tics typically first emerge between 5 and 7 years of age and increase in severity until they reach a peak in early adolescence (most often at the age of 10–12 years). After this worst-ever period, tics—in most cases—decrease until a mild to minimal degree of severity is reached in early adulthood [5]. At the same time, TS is characterized by spontaneous fluctuations and waxing and waning over time. The occurrence of tics is influenced by various environmental factors. While the majority of patients experience fewer tics when relaxing or concentrating (e.g. when practicing sports, playing musical instruments or computer games), tics often increase with stress, tiredness and infections.

To date, no single cause of TS was identified; instead, several lines of evidence suggested that TS is caused by an interplay between genetic [6] and environmental factors [7]. For example, there is clear evidence that prenatal and perinatal complications including low birth weight and maternal smoking during pregnancy [8, 9] may represent such epigenetic factors. In contrast, the influence of infections [7] and immunological factors [10] is still unclear. As for the pathophysiology of TS, most studies suggest a major involvement of the dopaminergic system [11–17]; however, several other neurotransmitter systems might play a role including the serotonergic [12, 18], histaminergic [19], glutamatergic [20], GABAergic [21], cholinergic [22], and noradrenergic systems [23]. Furthermore, it is believed that disturbances of cortico-striato-thalamo-cortical (CSTC) pathways play a role in the generation of tics [24].

1.3. Treatment of Tourette syndrome

Both European [25–27] as well as Canadian [28] treatment guidelines for TS recommend application of behavioral psychotherapy techniques (either habit reversal training or exposure and response prevention training), pharmacotherapy and, in otherwise treatment resistant very severely affected patients, surgical intervention using deep brain stimulation. Like in the case of many psychiatric disorders, treatment is only available on a symptomatic level. Available treatments for TS alleviate symptoms to more tolerable degree quite successfully, but cannot eradicate tics completely. However, treatment for tics is not necessary in all cases, but should be taken into consideration, when tics interfere with daily life functions or cause significant emotional distress. The drugs most often used in the treatment of tics are atypical antipsychotics including aripiprazole, risperidone, sulpiride, and (in Germany) tiapride. If these drugs are not effective or not well tolerated, only few alternative options remain, including alpha-2-agonists (in case of comorbid ADHD), topiramate, tetrabenazine and, rarely, botulinum toxin. While the antipsychotics are by far the most widely used drugs for the treatment of TS, they bring along considerable side effects load such as sedation, weight gain, metabolic changes, and acute dyskinesia [25].

In summary, a large number of patients with TS are unsatisfied with available treatments—either due to insufficient efficacy or because of clinically relevant side effects—and therefore, further treatment alternatives need to be developed.

2. Possible role of the endocannabinoid system in Tourette syndrome

The main function of the central endocannabinoid system (ECS) is inhibitory modulation of other neurotransmitter systems. Among other brain regions, cannabinoid type 1 receptors (CB1) are expressed with high density in the basal ganglia [29] indicating a paramount role of the ECS in the control of movements. In TS, there is substantial evidence for an involvement of the dopaminergic system. However, until today it is unclear, whether these alterations represent the primary cause of the disease or are related to secondary or compensatory changes. In addition to the dopaminergic hypothesis in TS, changes in several other transmitter systems have been suggested including the glutamatergic, GABAergic, serotonergic, noradrenergic and histaminergic systems. Since the ECS is a highly important modulatory system in the brain that influences and controls all important neurotransmitter systems, it can be speculated that TS might be caused by a dysfunction in the ECS system. This hypothesis is in line with studies reporting about an involvement of several different neurotransmitter systems in TS. In addition, alterations within the ECS would explain the complex clinical presentation of TS including both hyperkinetic movements with tics and a large variety of psychiatric manifestations.

Noteworthy, there is a strong interaction between the dopaminergic and the ECS [29, 30], particularly in basal ganglia regions including the striatum [31] and the globus pallidus [32]. Since there is substantial evidence for an involvement of the dopaminergic system in the pathobiology of TS, it, therefore, can also be speculated that CBM may inhibit dopaminergic activity in brain areas associated with motor control resulting in a reduction of hyperkinetic movements such as tics [33]. However, one might also speculate that the modulation of other neurotransmitter systems including glutamate and GABA might result in a reduction of tics.

Until today, only one neuroimaging study has been performed using single photon emission computed tomography (SPECT) and [123I]AM281 to investigate the ECS in patients with TS [34].

In this study, it could be demonstrated that CB1 receptor binding is reduced after treatment with THC. Since in this study, no control group has been included, no statement is possible, whether CB1 receptor binding is changed in patients with TS. So far, genetic analyses failed to demonstrate any genetic variations in the cannabinoid receptor gene (CNR1) in TS [35].

3. Cannabis-based medicine in patients with Tourette syndrome

3.1. Retrospective reports on self-medication

A substantial number of patients with TS report using cannabis illegally in order to improve their tics or comorbid psychiatric disorders. While doing so, most of these patients rely on their own judgment and self-medicate without a proper consultation with their treating physician. Such an observation was first described in two small case series published in 1988 and 1993 [36]. Sandyk et al. [37] described three male patients, who benefitted both in terms of tics and comorbid psychiatric symptoms after smoking 0.5–2 marijuana cigarettes per day. Hemming et al. [36] reported a case of a 36-year-old man, who smoked a marijuana cigarette every day and claimed to be symptom-free for 1 year. More recently, Müller-Vahl et al. [38] conducted a retrospective survey about self-medication with cannabis in 64 patients with TS seen at a specialized Tourette outpatient clinic in Germany. Seventeen patients indicated to use marijuana illegally as self-treatment for their symptoms, and 14 of them reported beneficial effects not only on tics, but also on different comorbidities. Interestingly, none of the patients reported clinically relevant adverse events (AEs) or a deterioration of tics after the use of marijuana. This effect was not influenced by concomitant use of antipsychotics or selective serotonin reuptake inhibitors (SSRIs).

Finally, Abi-Jaoude et al. [39] in Canada reported results from a retrospective analysis investigating efficacy and safety of smoked cannabis in 19 adults with TS. Patients experienced an average improvement of their tic severity measured with the Total Tic Score (TTS) of the Yale Global Tic Severity Scale (YGTSS) of approximately 60%. Altogether, 18 out of 19 patients experienced an improvement of their TS symptoms. All patients included in this study had used cannabis for self-medication for more than 1 year. Most often reported AEs were a feeling of "being high", decreased concentration, increased anxiety, increased appetite, sedation, irritability, dry mouth, and dry eyes. However, no serious adverse events (SAEs) were reported.

3.2. Prospective case studies using different cannabis-based medicines

To date, there is a small number of prospective case studies available providing increasing evidence that CBM might be effective and well tolerated in adults with TS. Interestingly, in these case reports, different CBMs have been used. While most of these studies report about beneficial effects in adults, only very recently, first promising case reports in minors have been published.

3.2.1. *Case studies using tetrahydrocannabinol*

In 1999, Müller-Vahl et al. [40] published the first case of a 25-year old patient with TS treated with oral tetrahydrocannabinol (THC). This patient suffered from a complex TS and a number of additional psychiatric disorders such as ADHD, obsessive–compulsive behavior (OCB), SIB, anxiety disorder, and impulsivity. According to the patient's report, self-medication with smoked cannabis (2–3 g/day) caused a clinically relevant improvement of all these symptoms. Therefore, the patient was prospectively treated once with a single dose of 10 mg THC. This resulted in a significant reduction of tics of about 80% as well as an improvement in attention, impulse control, OCB, and premonitory urges. In addition, neuropsychological tests showed improvements in signal detection, sustained attention, and reaction time in the absence of AEs.

The same group described another case of a 24-year old female, who had an improvement of tics and premonitory urges after combined therapy of THC and the antipsychotic amisulpride [41]. The patient did far better on this combination than on monotherapy with either THC or amisulpride.

In addition, in 2011, Brunnauer et al. [42] reported the case of a 42-year-old male with TS, who suffered from multiple motor and vocal tics as well as OCB. Treatment with 15 mg THC resulted in a 75% tic reduction. As this patient was a professional driver, his driving abilities were assessed by professional computerized tests. Interestingly, the patient's concentration and visual abilities improved after THC administration.

Finally, Jakubovski and Müller-Vahl [43] reported about a 16-year old patient with vocal tics resembling stuttering-like phenomena accompanied by multiple simple and complex vocal tics as well as simple motor tics. Apart from tics, he was also experiencing further psychiatric problems including rage attacks, sleeping problems, tic-related anxiety and shame about speaking in public, depressed mood, and OCB (e.g., ordering of pencils, not just right feeling, and rumination) resulting in difficulties concentrating. Due to treatment resistance and intolerable AEs after established therapeutic interventions, it was decided to implement treatment with vaporized THC (up to a maximum dose of 22.4–33.6 mg THC/day). This leads to an improvement of his tics including complex vocal tics resulting in improved speech fluency. Moreover, coexisting psychiatric conditions improved.

3.2.2. *Case studies using nabiximols*

The first case report about effective treatment with nabiximols in a patient with TS was published by Trainor et al. [44] in 2016. This 26-year-old male suffered from treatment-resistant TS with severe motor and vocal tics, OCD, SIB, and depression. Administration of 4 puffs nabiximols (=10.8 mg of THC and 10 mg cannabidiol (CBD)) resulted in a 85% reduction of motor and 90% reduction of vocal tics after 4 weeks of treatment measured via the Rush Video Tape Rating Scale [45] and a 35% tic improvement according to the YGTSS-TTS. No AEs were reported.

Another single case study using nabiximols was reported by Kanaan et al. [46]. This was a 22-year-old male with complex and severe treatment resistant TS. Nabiximols (up-titrated to 9 puffs/day = 24.3 mg THC and 22.5 mg CBD) resulted in a reduction of tics measured with YGTSS-TTS, Tourette's Syndrome Symptom List (TSSL), and Rush Video Tape Rating Scale, premonitory urges, and a general improvement of quality of life without causing clinically relevant AEs.

3.2.3. Case studies using medicinal cannabis

Recently, Jakubovski and Müller-Vahl published a case report of a patient with TS treated with medicinal cannabis [43]. He suffered from a rare form of TS: a severe, impairing and treatment resistant vocal blocking and stuttering-like vocal tics as well as palilalia. These symptoms significantly impaired social contacts and daily living. The 19-year old patient received medicinal cannabis at a dose of 0.1 g cannabis once daily. After 8 months of follow-up, the symptoms improved significantly, especially speech fluency, but also other tics. After cannabis inhalation, beneficial effects lasted for about one and a half hour. Although the acute effect resolved thereafter, he experienced an overall positive effect during most time of the day. Only at the beginning of the treatment, he experienced a "high sensation" that resolved later on.

3.2.4. Treatment of minors with Tourette syndrome using cannabis-based medicines

Until today, only three single case studies are available reporting about treatment of minors with TS using CBM. The first report was published by Hasan et al. [47] in 2010. They described a 15-year old adolescent with severe and treatment resistant TS and comorbid ADHD. In this boy, augmentation of preexisting medication with risperidone (1 mg), aripiprazole (10 mg), and methylphenidate (15 mg) with oral THC (gradually up-titrated to 15 mg/day during 9 weeks) resulted in a significant tic reduction (global score of the YGTSS (range, 0–100) decreased from 97 to 54) and improved quality of life. The only AE observed was mild and transient euphoria.

The first ever case report of a child with TS treated with CBM was published only recently by Szejko et al. [48]. This 7-year-old boy suffered from severe tics and comorbid ADHD, which prevented him to attend school and finally resulted in social isolation, depression, and suicidal ideation. As all previous therapies including behavioral interventions and various medications (including risperidone, aripiprazole, tiapride, methylphenidate, and guanfacine) turned out to be unsuccessful, THC was proposed as a therapy of last choice. THC (in combination with risperidone (2 mg/day) and guanfacine (2 mg/day)) were gradually up-titrated to a maximal dose of 29.4 mg/day. Follow-up for more than 4 months demonstrated not only a clinically relevant improvement of tics, but also of accompanying psychiatric symptoms resulting in overall improved quality of life and social performance. Despite the relatively high dose of THC, no AEs were reported.

Furthermore, there is another single case report available describing beneficial effects of a combined treatment with vaporized medicinal cannabis and oral THC in a 12-year-old boy with TS (unpublished data, under revision). The boy complained of severe motor tics causing

http://dx.doi.org/10.5772/intechopen.79895

significant insomnia. Therefore, the boy's parents—both of whom were medical doctors—decided to medicate their son with 0.02 g vaporized cannabis (Bedrocan® variety containing 22% THC and 1% CBD, corresponding to a dose equivalent of 4.4 mg THC). This resulted—according to their reports—in a tremendous symptom improvement. Because of a further tic increase, the family presented at our Tourette outpatient clinic. Since the family reported about an ongoing effect while using cannabis with a relevant tic decrease, we decided to implement a combined treatment with vaporized medicinal cannabis (up to 0.1 g cannabis per day, varieties Bedrocan® and Amnesia Haze®, corresponding to 22 mg THC/day) plus oral THC drops (up to 12.5 mg/day). This combined therapy resulted not only in a marked tic reduction, but also an improvement of premonitory urges without any AEs.

Thus, currently, the database for treatment of minors with TS using CBM is very limited. However, from available preliminary results, it is suggested that CBM is effective and well tolerated even in this age group. At present time, no long-term follow-up data are available, and therefore, no statement is possible about positive and possible negative long-term effects, in particular with respect to detrimental effects on the developing brain. From observational oncological studies in children, however, it is also suggested that controlled application of CBM is safe and well tolerated. It is unknown, whether in children with TS the risk for psychosis is increased after treatment with CBM comparable to the increased risk in healthy children after excessive recreational cannabis use. Assuming a dysfunction in the ECS in TS, it can also be speculated that CBM may have beneficial effects on the course of the disease.

3.2.5. Controlled trials using tetrahydrocannabinol

Up to this date, only two small controlled studies have been conducted in adult patients with TS using CBM. Both of them were performed by Müller-Vahl's group. Dr. Müller-Vahl is an internationally renowned expert in the field of TS and tic disorders. She introduced CBM in the treatment of TS, conducted the first randomized controlled trials in this group of patients in the early 2000s, and since then dedicated a large part of her research endeavors in this area. In both controlled studies, efficacy and safety of pure THC have been investigated. The first one, published in 2002 by Müller-Vahl et al. [48], was a randomized double-blind placebo-controlled cross-over single-dose trial using 5.0, 7.5 or 10 mg of THC. The trial included 12 adult TS patients with a mean age of 34 ± 13 years. Tic severity was assessed both via a self-rating (TSSL) and different examiner-rating scales (Shapiro Tourette's syndrome Severity Scale (STSSS) and YGTSS). The Tourette's syndrome Global Impression Scale (TS-CGI) was used to assess global disease severity. To assess changes in psychiatric comorbidities (including OCB, ADHD, and anxiety), the self-assessment of the TSSL was used. According to TSSL, there was a significant improvement of tics and OCB compared to placebo. According to examiner rating scales for the assessment of tic severity, there was an improvement in the subscore "complex motor tics" and a trend toward a reduction in the subscores "motor tics," "simple motor tics" and "vocal tics." The following AEs were recorded: headache, nausea, dizziness, tiredness, cheerfulness, dry mouth, anxiety, sensitivity to noise and light, ataxia and poor concentration, but no SAEs were reported. Plasma levels of the THC metabolite 11-hydroxy-delta-tetrahydrocannabinol correlated with tic reduction as assessed by TSSL.

In 2003, Müller-Vahl et al. published results of a randomized, double-blind, placebo-controlled follow-up trial [49]. In this study, 24 adult patients with TS were treated for a period of 6 weeks with up to 10 mg THC/day. Tic severity was evaluated at six different time points. For tic assessment, both self-rating scales as well as examiner rating scales were used (TSSL, YGTSS, STSSS, and Rush Video-Based Tic Rating Scale) [45]. Nearly all rating scales indicated a significant superiority of the THC arm compared to placebo at visits 3 and 4. The Rush Video-Based Tic Rating Scale also showed a significant difference or trends toward significant group differences at visits 2 and 4 for the items "motor tic intensity" and "motor tic frequency," respectively. Seven patients dropped out of the study, but only one due to AEs (restlessness and anxiety). Five patients in the THC group reported AEs (tiredness, dry mouth, dizziness and fuzziness), while three in the placebo group (tiredness, dizziness, anxiety, depression) in the absence of SAEs.

3.2.6. Efficacy of cannabis-based medicines in the treatment of psychiatric comorbidities in patients with Tourette syndrome

Up to 90% of patients with TS suffer from psychiatric comorbidities and studies investigating quality of life in these patients clearly demonstrate that most patients are more impaired by ADHD, OCD, and depression, respectively, than their tics. Thus, in the majority of patients with TS, effective treatment of comorbidities is even more important than treatment of tics. Until today, however, there is no treatment strategy known that improves both tics and comorbidities. Therefore, in patients with complex TS combined therapy using different treatment strategies in parallel is inevitable.

Interestingly, from all available case studies and controlled trials, it is suggested that CBM improves not only tics, but also psychiatric symptoms. Therefore, it can be speculated that CBM might be the first treatment strategy that is useful in the treatment of the complete spectrum of symptoms. More specifically, there is preliminary evidence that CBM also improves ADHD [39], OCB/OCD [40] impulsivity [43], depression [50], sleeping problems [51], and anxiety [43].

For example, in the retrospective survey by Abi-Jaoude et al. [39], all patients reported in addition to the tic improvement also an improvement of psychiatric symptoms after treatment with cannabis including sleeping disturbances, anxiety, OCB, impulsivity, irritability and rage attacks. With respect to comorbid ADHD, only one out of 13 patients demonstrated no improvement of ADHD symptoms. This data in patients with TS is in line with preliminary results in patients suffering from pure ADHD (without tics or TS). In 2017, Cooper et al. [52] published results of a randomized placebo-controlled pilot study using nabiximols in patients with ADHD. In this trial, 30 adults with ADHD were included, and cognitive performance was assessed using an objective assessment for inattention, hyperactivity, and impulsivity (Qb-Test). Although for the primary outcome, no significant difference was observed, several secondary outcomes demonstrated superiority of nabiximols compared to placebo with improvements in hyperactivity, impulsivity and inattention, respectively. In the active group, three mild AEs and one SAE (muscular spasms/seizures) were recorded, while in the placebo group, one SAE (cardiovascular problems) occurred.

Although most patients with TS treated with CBM report about an improvement of one or even more psychiatric comorbidities, larger controlled trials are needed to confirm these promising, but preliminary results.

3.2.7. Safety profile and influence on psychomotor functioning in patients with Tourette syndrome

From the available preliminary results, it is suggested that—on average—the AE profile of CBM in the treatment of patients with TS is very similar to that in other groups of patients. In line with data from recent meta-analyses including mixed patients' groups [52], for example, in the retrospective study by Abi-Jaoude et al. [53], a relatively high number of AEs were reported in patients with TS, but most AEs were mild and transient, respectively. Most often reported AEs after use of cannabis in patients with TS were a "feeling of high," decreased concentration, decreased short-term memory, increased anxiety, increased appetite, sedation, irritability, dry mouth and eyes, and wheezing.

Contrary to these reports from open uncontrolled studies, from preliminary controlled data, it is suggested that the impact of THC on neuropsychological performance in adults with TS may differ as compared to both healthy people and other patient groups. In two controlled studies investigating the effects of THC in patients with TS, additionally, neuropsychological tests were performed. In the first study [54], the influence of a single dose treatment of THC on neuropsychological performance was investigated. However, no negative impact of THC compared to placebo was found on verbal and visual memory, reaction time, intelligence, sustained attention, divided attention, and vigilance. In another study, Müller-Vahl et al. [55] investigated the influence of a 6-week THC treatment as compared to placebo on neuropsychological performance using different neuropsychological tests to assess verbal learning, attention, and memory. Again, THC had no detrimental effects on neuropsychological performance and immediate verbal memory span even improved after treatment with THC.

These results are completely in line with observations in two open uncontrolled single case studies. In 2007, Strohbeck-Kühner et al. [56] published a case of a 28 year-old male with ADHD (without TS), who benefitted from treatment with THC, and, moreover, his fitness to drive improved after treatment. A similar case was reported by Brunnauer et al. [42] some years later. They described an effective treatment with THC in a 42 year-old male. Furthermore, his driving ability (concentration and visual abilities) was better under treatment with THC as compared to the off-medication state. The authors, therefore, suggested that in TS, CBM such as THC may have beneficial effects on psychomotor functions related to driving performance. Thus, from this preliminary data, it is strongly suggested that the influence of CBM on neuropsychological performance in patients with TS may differ from effects in healthy people and other groups of patients.

Finally, until today, very little is known about safety of CBM in children and adolescents with TS [47–49]. However, from available preliminary case reports, it is suggested that in this group of patients CBM such as THC is well tolerated or even better tolerated than in adults. This observation is in line with reports in other groups of young patients. For example when using CBM in antineoplastic therapy [30] it has been suggested that CBM—even at high doses—are well tolerated in children.

3.2.8. Practical clues for the treatment of patients with Tourette syndrome using cannabis-based medicines

Despite lack of clear evidence, recent European [25] and Canadian treatment guidelines [28] for TS acknowledged available data and recommend CBM in otherwise treatment resistant adult patients with TS. Most experts suggest treatment with CBM, before taking surgical treatment with deep brain stimulation into consideration. Comparable to most other indications, until today it is unclear, which CBM is the most effective and best tolerated in patients with TS. However, from available data, it is suggested that pure CBD is not effective in the treatment of tics. Data obtained from both a retrospective and prospective survey performed at the Tourette outpatient clinic at Hannover Medical School, Germany, provide preliminary evidence that medicinal cannabis might be superior to pure THC and nabiximols (unpublished data). Currently, treatment with CBM in minors with TS should be only taken into consideration in otherwise treatment resistant and severely affected patients.

With respect to the dose, no clear recommendation can be given. In any case, starting dose should be low (corresponding to 2.5 mg THC/day) and up-titration should be slow, for example by 2.5 mg THC every 3–5 days. Maximal dose differs from patient to patient, but usually ranges from 0.1 to 1 g cannabis/day, corresponding to about 2.5–30 mg THC/day. However, in individual patients, maximal doses can be much higher.

An overview on all available studies investigating efficacy and safety of CBM in TS is given in **Table 1**.

Reference	**Number of patients (sex)**	**Age**	**Substance**	**Study design**	**Outcome**
Sandyk et al. 1988	3 (male)	15, 17, 39	*Cannabis sativa L.*	Case report	Reduction of tics, premonitory urges and self-injurious behavior; general relaxation; improvement of attention and hypersexuality
Hemming et al. 1993	1 (male)	36	*Cannabis sativa L.*	Case report	Symptom free
Müller-Vahl et al. 1998	64 (55 male, 9 female)	15-64	Medical cannabis	Case series	Tic reduction or remission; premonitory urges; improvement of OCB and ADHD
Müller-Vahl et al. 1999	1 (male)	25	THC	Case report	Tic reduction, premonitory urges; improvement of attention, impulse control, and OCB
Müller-Vahl et al. 2002a	1 (female)	24	THC (in combination with amisulpride)	Case report	Tic reduction, premonitory urges
Müller-Vahl et al. 2002b	24 (19 male, 5 female)	18-68	THC	Randomized double-blind parallel group placebo-controlled trial	Tic reduction; global improvement

Reference	Number of patients (sex)	Age	Substance	Study design	Outcome
Müller-Vahl et al. 2003b	12 (11 male, 1 female)	18-66	THC	Randomized double-blind placebo-controlled crossover trial	Tic reduction; improvement of OCB
Hasan et al. 2010	1 (male)	15	THC (in combination with aripiprazole and risperidone)	Case report	Tic reduction, improvement of quality of life; treatment with methylphenidate was tolerated without tic increase
Brunnauer et al. 2011	1 (male)	42	THC	Case report	Reduction of tics, improvement of concentration and visual perception
Trainor et al. 2016	1 (male)	26	Nabiximols	Case report	Reduction of motor and vocal tics
Abi-Jaoude et al. 2017	19 (16 males, 3 females)	18-51	Medical cannabis	Case series, structured interview	Reduction of tics
Jakubovski and Müller-Vahl. 2017	2 (male)	16, 19	THC, medical cannabis	Case report	Improvement of tics including complex vocal tics resulting in improved speech fluency, co-existing psychiatric conditions improved
Kanaan et al. 2017	1 (male)	22	Nabiximols	Case report	Reduction of tics, improvement of quality of life
Szejko et al. 2018	1 (male)	8	THC	Case report	Reduction of tics, improvement of comorbid psychiatric conditions (ADHD, depression), improvement of quality of life
Szejko et al. (submitted to Frontiers in Psychiatry)	1 (male)	12	THC, medical cannabis	Case report	Reduction of tics, improvement of sleeping problems

Table 1. Case studies employing CBM in TS.

4. Future directions

Larger well-designed controlled studies are urgently needed to confirm available preliminary results. Further studies should investigate not only the efficacy of CBM in the treatment of tics, but also their potency to improve typical psychiatric comorbidities in TS including ADHD, OCB, depression, anxiety, sleeping disorders, and rage attacks. Finally, the AE profile should be investigated in detail, since from available data, it is suggested that neuropsychological performance may improve—and not deteriorate—after treatment with CBM in this group of patients. So far, it is unknown, which CBM is the most effective and best tolerated in patients with TS. However, based on available reports, patients with TS seem to prefer CBM with median to high THC content.

Currently, a large randomized controlled trial in Germany is recruiting to further investigate efficacy and safety of nabiximols in patients with TS (ClinicalTrials.gov Identifier: NCT03087201). In this study, in addition, patients' fitness to drive will be investigated after treatment with nabiximols.

While all published studies investigated the effects of different synthetic or plant-derived cannabinoids in the treatment of TS, unpublished data from a single dose pilot study in 20 adult patients suggests that also modulators of the endocannabinoid system—such as inhibitors of the monoacylglycerol lipase (MGLL)— might be effective in the treatment of TS (ClinicalTrials.gov Identifier: NCT03058562).

5. Conclusions

There is increasing evidence that CBM might be a promising new treatment strategy for patients with TS. However, larger well-designed controlled studies are urgently needed to confirm preliminary results. However, already today, a substantial number of patients use CBM, either prescribed off-label or no-label under the guidance of the treating physician or as a self-medication without supervision of a medical doctor. Physicians, who treat patients with tic disorders and TS, should actively ask their patients about possible use of cannabis, since it is well known that many patients with TS use complementary or alternative treatments without informing their doctor [57]. If patients with TS report about (illegal) self-medication with cannabis, treating physicians should inform their patients about legal treatment options and available routes of intake without the risks associated with smoking.

Conflict of interest

KMV has received payment for consulting from Abide Pharmaceuticals and Fundacion Canna and support for research from GW and Almirall. She is carrying out studies in cooperation with Abide Pharmaceuticals, GW and Almirall. She is a member of the Scientific Advisory Board of Therapix and a second chairwoman of the International Association for Cannabinoid Medicine (IACM).

Author details

Natalia Szejko[1,2]*, Ewgeni Jakubovski[1] and Kirsten Müller-Vahl[1]

*Address all correspondence to: natalia.szejko@gmail.com

1 Clinic of Psychiatry, Social Psychiatry and Psychotherapy, Hannover Medical School, Germany, Hannover

2 Department of Neurology and Department of Bioethics, Medical University of Warsaw, Poland

References

[1] Robertson MM, Eapen V, Cavanna AE. The international prevalence, epidemiology, and clinical phenomenology of Tourette syndrome: A cross-cultural perspective. Journal of Psychosomatic Research. 2009;**67**:475-483

[2] Robertson MM. The Gilles de la Tourette syndrome: the current status. Archives of disease in childhood. Education and practice edition. 2012;**97**:166-175

[3] Leckman JF, Bloch MH, Sukhodolsky DG, Scahill L, King RA. Phenomenology of Tics and Sensory Urges: The Self Under Siege. In: Tourette Syndrome [Internet]. 2013. pp. 3-25. Available from: http://oxfordmedicine.com/view/10.1093/med/9780199796267.001.0001/med-9780199796267-chapter-1

[4] Sambrani T, Jakubovski E, Müller-Vahl KR. New insights into clinical characteristics of Gilles de la Tourette syndrome: Findings in 1032 patients from a single German center. Front Neuroscience. 2016;**10**(Sep)

[5] Bloch MH. Clinical Course and Adult Outcome in Tourette Syndrome. In: Tourette Syndrome. 2013

[6] Paschou P. The genetic basis of Gilles de la Tourette Syndrome. Neuroscience and Biobehavioral Reviews. 2013;**37**:1026-39

[7] Hoekstra PJ, Dietrich A, Edwards MJ, Elamin I, Martino D. Environmental factors in Tourette syndrome. Neuroscience and Biobehavioral Reviews. 2013;**37**:1040-9

[8] Hoekstra PJ. Perinatal Adversities and Tourette Syndrome. In: Tourette Syndrome [Internet]. 2013. pp. 156-167. Available from: http://oxfordmedicine.com/view/10.1093/med/9780199796267.001.0001/med-9780199796267-chapter-8

[9] Burd L, Severud R, Klug MG, Kerbeshian J. Prenatal and perinatal risk factors for Tourette disorder. Journal of Perinatal Medicine. 1999;**27**(4):295-302. Available from: http://www.ncbi.nlm.nih.gov/pubmed/10560082

[10] Murphy TK, Kurlan R, Leckman J. The immunobiology of Tourette's disorder, pediatric autoimmune neuropsychiatric disorders associated with Streptococcus, and related disorders: A way forward. Journal of Child and Adolescent Psychopharmacologyl [Internet]. 2010;**20**(4):317-331 Available from: http://www.ncbi.nlm.nih.gov/pubmed/20807070%5Cnhttp://www.pubmedcentral.nih.gov/articlerender.fcgi?artid=PMC4003464

[11] Wong DF, Singer HS, Brandt J, Shaya E, Chen C, Brown J, et al. D2-like dopamine receptor density in Tourette syndrome measured by PET. J NucÃ-Med. 1997;**38**:1243-1247

[12] Wong DF, Brasić JR, Singer HS, Schretlen DJ, Kuwabara H, Zhou Y, et al. Mechanisms of dopaminergic and serotonergic neurotransmission in Tourette syndrome: Clues from an in vivo neurochemistry study with PET. Neuropsychopharmacology: official publication of the American College of Neuropsychopharmacology. 2008 May;**33**(6):1239-1251

[13] Segura B, Strafella AP. Functional imaging of dopaminergic neurotransmission in tourette syndrome. International Review of Neurobiology. 2013;**112**:73-93

[14] Buse J, Schoenefeld K, Münchau A, Roessner V. Neuromodulation in Tourette syndrome: Dopamine and beyond. Neuroscience and Biobehavioral Reviews. 2013;**37**:1069-1084

[15] Yoon DY, Gause CD, Leckman JF, Singer HS. Frontal dopaminergic abnormality in Tourette syndrome: A postmortem analysis. Journal of the Neurological Sciences. 2007 Apr;**255**(1-2):50-56

[16] Alam M, Schwabe K, Lütjens G, Capelle HH, Manu M, von Wrangel C, et al. Comparative characterization of single cell activity in the globus pallidus internus of patients with dystonia or Tourette syndrome. Journal of Neural Transmission. 2015 May 1 [cited 2018 Jan 28];122(5):687-699. Available from: http://www.ncbi.nlm.nih.gov/pubmed/25081018

[17] Müller-Vahl KR, Berding G, Kolbe H, Meyer GJ, Hundeshagen H, Dengler R, et al. Dopamine D2 receptor imaging in Gilles de la Tourette syndrome. Acta Neurologica Scandinavica [Internet]. 2000;**101**(3):165-171. Available from: http://onlinelibrary.wiley.com/store/10.1034/j.1600-0404.2000.101003165.x/asset/j.1600-0404.2000.101003165.x.pdf?v=1&t=hlrwzw8u&s=a3434bae5ad56fdd5597fcf0c5d1fdc0e9a58942

[18] Müller-Vahl KR, Meyer GJ, Knapp WH, Emrich HM, Gielow P, Brücke T, et al. Serotonin transporter binding in Tourette syndrome. Neuroscience Letters. 2005 Sep;**385**(2):120-125

[19] Hartmann A, Worbe Y, Arnulf I. Increasing histamine neurotransmission in Gilles de la Tourette syndrome. Journal of Neurology. 2012;**259**:375-376

[20] Kanaan AS, Gerasch S, García-García I, Lampe L, Pampel A, Anwander A, et al. Pathological glutamatergic neurotransmission in Gilles de la Tourette syndrome. Brain. 2017;**140**(1):218-234

[21] Draper A, Stephenson MC, Jackson GM, Pépés S, Morgan PS, Morris PG, et al. Increased GABA contributes to enhanced control over motor excitability in tourette syndrome. Current Biology. 2014;**24**(19):2343-2347

[22] Ganos C, Hartmann A. Altered cholinergic neurotransmission in Tourette syndrome. Movement Disorders. 2015;**30**:638

[23] Sweeney D, Pickar D, Redmond DE, Maas J. Noradrenergic and dopaminergic mechanisms in gilles de la tourette syndrome. The Lancet. 1978;**311**:872

[24] Wang Z, Maia TV, Marsh R, Colibazzi T, Gerber A, Peterson BS. The neural circuits that generate tics in Tourette's syndrome. The American Journal of Psychiatry. 2011;**168**(12):1326-1337

[25] Plessen RV. European clinical guidelines for Tourette syndrome and other tic disorders. Part II: Pharmacological treatment. European Child and Adolescent Psychiatry. 2011;**20**:173-196

[26] Müller-Vahl KR, Cath DC, Cavanna AE, Dehning S, Porta M, Robertson MM, et al. European clinical guidelines for Tourette syndrome and other tic disorders. Part IV: Deep brain stimulation. European Child & Adolescent Psychiatry. 2011 Apr 29 [cited 2018 Jan 23];**20**(4):209-217 Available from: http://link.springer.com/10.1007/s00787-011-0166-4

[27] Verdellen C, Van De Griendt J, Hartmann A, Murphy T, Androutsos C, Aschauer H, et al. European clinical guidelines for Tourette syndrome and other tic disorders. Part III: Behavioural and psychosocial interventions. European Child & Adolescent Psychiatry. 2011;**20**(4):197-207

[28] Pringsheim T, Doja A, Gorman D, McKinlay D, Day L, Billinghurst L, et al. Canadian guidelines for the evidence-based treatment of tic disorders: Pharmacotherapy. Canadian Journal of Psychiatry. 2012;**57**:133-143

[29] Mechoulam R, Parker LA. The endocannabinoid system and the brain. Annual Review of Psychology [Internet]. 2013;**64**(1):21-47. Available from: http://www.annualreviews.org/doi/10.1146/annurev-psych-113011-143739

[30] Abrahamov A, Abrahamov A, Mechoulam R. An efficient new cannabinoid antiemetic in pediatric oncology. Life Sciences. 1995;**56**(23-24):2097-2102

[31] Giuffrida A, Parsons LH, Kerr TM, Rodríguez De Fonseca F, Navarro M, Piomelli D. Dopamine activation of endogenous cannabinoid signaling in dorsal striatum. Nature Neuroscience. 1999;**2**(4):358-363

[32] Di Marzo V, Hill MP, Bisogno T, Crossman AR, Brotchie JM. Enhanced levels of endogenous cannabinoids in the globus pallidus are associated with a reduction in movement in an animal model of Parkinson's disease. FASEB Journal [Internet]. 2000;**14**(10):1432-1438 Available from: http://www.ncbi.nlm.nih.gov/entrez/query.fcgi?cmd=Retrieve&db=PubMed&dopt=Citation&list_uids=10877836%5Cnhttp://www.fasebj.org/content/14/10/1432.full.pdf

[33] Müller-Vahl KR. Cannabinoids reduce symptoms of Tourette's syndrome. Expert Opinion on Pharmacotherapy [Internet]. 2003;**4**(10):1717-1725 Available from: http://www.tandfonline.com/doi/full/10.1517/14656566.4.10.1717

[34] Berding G, Müller-Vahl K, Schneider U, Gielow P, Fitschen J, Stuhrmann M, et al. [123I] AM281 single-photon emission computed tomography imaging of central cannabinoid CB1 receptors before and after Delta9-tetrahydrocannabinol therapy and whole-body scanning for assessment of radiation dose in Tourette patients. Biological Psychiatry. 2004 May 1;**55**(9):904-915

[35] Gadzicki D, Müller-Vahl KR, Heller D, Ossege S, Nöthen MM, Hebebrand J, et al. Tourette syndrome is not caused by mutations in the central cannabinoid receptor (CNR1) gene. American Journal of Medical Genetics Part B: Neuropsychiatric Genetics [Internet]. 2004;**127B**(1):97-103. Available from: http://www.ncbi.nlm.nih.gov/pubmed/15108190

[36] Hemming M, Yellowlees PM. Effective treatment of Tourette's syndrome with marijuana. Journal of Psychopharmacology. 1993;**7**(4):389-391

[37] Sandyk R, Bamford CR. Tourette syndrome. Pediatric Neurology. 1987

[38] Muller-Vahl KRK. Cannabinoids: Possible role in patho-physiology and therapy of Gilles de la Tourette syndrome. Acta Psychiatrica Scandinavica. 1998;**98**:502-506

[39] Abi-Jaoude E, Chen L, Cheung P, Bhikram T, Sandor P. Preliminary evidence on cannabis effectiveness and tolerability for adults with Tourette syndrome. Journal of Neuropsychiatry and Clinical Neurosciences [Internet]. 2017;appi.neuropsych. Available from: http://psychiatryonline.org/doi/10.1176/appi.neuropsych.16110310

[40] Muller-Vahl K, Schneider U, Kolbe H, Emrich HM. Treatment of Tourette's syndrome with delta-9-tetrahydrocannabinol [3]. American Journal of Psychiatry. 1999;**156**:495

[41] Muller-Vahl KRS. Combined treatment of Tourette syndrome with 9-THC and dopamine receptor antagonists. Journal of Cannabis Theraphy. 2002;**2**:145-154

[42] Brunnauer A, Segmiller FM, Volkamer T, Laux G, Müller N, Dehning S. Cannabinoids improve driving ability in a Tourette's patient. Psychiatry Research. 2011;**190**:382

[43] Jakubovski E, Müller-Vahl K. Speechlessness in Gilles de la Tourette Syndrome: Cannabis-based medicines improve severe vocal blocking tics in two patients. International Journal of Molecular Sciences. 2017;**18**(8)

[44] Trainor D, Evans L, Bird R. Severe motor and vocal tics controlled with Sativex®. Australasian Psychiatry. 2016;**24**(6):541-544

[45] Goetz CG, Pappert EJ, Louis ED, Raman R, Leurgans S. Advantages of a modified scoring method for the rush video-based tic rating scale. Movement Disorders [Internet]. 1999 May [cited 2018 Jan 28];**14**(3):502-506. Available from: http://www.ncbi.nlm.nih.gov/pubmed/10348478

[46] Kanaan AS, Jakubovski E, Müller-Vahl K. Significant tic reduction in an otherwise treatment-resistant patient with gilles de la tourette syndrome following treatment with nabiximols. Brain Science. 2017;**7**(5)

[47] Hasan A, Rothenberger A, Münchau A, Wobrock T, Falkai P, Roessner V. Oral 9-tetrahydrocannabinol improved refractory Gilles de la Tourette syndrome in an adolescent by increasing intracortical inhibition: A case report. Journal of Clinical Psychopharmacology. 2010;**30**(2):190-192

[48] Müller-Vahl KR, Schneider U, Koblenz A, Jöbges M, Kolbe H, Daldrup T, et al. Treatment of Tourette's syndrome with Delta 9-tetrahydrocannabinol (THC): A randomized crossover trial. Pharmacopsychiatry. 2002;**35**(2):57-61

[49] Müller-Vahl KR, Schneider U, Prevedel H, Theloe K, Kolbe H, Daldrup T, et al. 9-tetrahydrocannabinol (THC) is effective in the treatment of tics in Tourette syndrome: A 6-week randomized trial. The Journal of Clinical Psychiatry. 2003;**64**(4):459-465

[50] Martiny K. Novel augmentation strategies in major depression. Danish Medical Journal. 2017;**64**

[51] Belendiuk KA, Babson KA, Vandrey R, Bonn-Miller MO. Cannabis species and cannabinoid concentration preference among sleep-disturbed medicinal cannabis users. Addictive Behaviors. 2015;**50**:178-181

[52] Whiting PF, Wolff RF, Deshpande S, Di Nisio M, Duffy S, Hernandez AV, et al. Cannabinoids for medical use. JAMA [Internet]. 2015;**313**(24):2456. Available from: http://jama.jamanetwork.com/article.aspx? doi=10.1001/jama.2015.6358

[53] Kopera M, Trucco EM, Jakubczyk A, Suszek H, Michalska A, Majewska A, et al. Interpersonal and intrapersonal emotional processes in individuals treated for alcohol use disorder and non-addicted healthy individuals. Addictive Behaviors. 2018;**79**

[54] Müller-Vahl KR, Koblenz A, Jöbges M, Kolbe H, Emrich HM, Schneider U. Influence of treatment of Tourette syndrome with Δ9-tetrahydrocannabinol (Δ9-THC) on neuropsychological performance. Pharmacopsychiatry. 2001;**34**(1):19-24

[55] Müller-Vahl KR, Prevedel H, Theloe K, Kolbe H, Emrich HM, Schneider U. Treatment of tourette syndrome with delta-9-tetrahydrocannabinol (Δ9-THC): No influence on neuropsychological performance. Neuropsychopharmacology. 2003;**28**(2):384-388

[56] Strohbeck-Kuhner P, Skopp G, Mattern R. Fitness to drive in spite (because) of THC. Archiv für Kriminologie [Internet]. 2007;**220**(1-2):11-19 Available from: http://ovidsp.ovid.com/ovidweb.cgi?T=JS&CSC=Y&NEWS=N&PAGE=fulltext&D=med5&AN=17879702%5Cnhttp://imp-primo.hosted.exlibrisgroup.com/openurl/44IMP/44IMP_services_page?sid=OVID&isbn=&issn=0003-9225&volume=220&issue=1&date=2007&title=Archiv+fur+Kriminologie&a

[57] Kompoliti K, Fan W, Leurgans S. Complementary and alternative medicine use in Gilles de la Tourette syndrome. Movement Disorders [Internet]. 2009;**24**(13):2015-2019. Available from: http://www.ncbi.nlm.nih.gov/pubmed/19705358

Chapter 8

Cannabis Use Disorder

Iris Balodis and James MacKillop

Additional information is available at the end of the chapter

http://dx.doi.org/10.5772/intechopen.80344

Abstract

Extensive changes in cannabis regulation accompany changing public attitudes toward cannabis use and legalization. Cannabis use is more prevalent when the drug is legal; therefore, there is a substantial need for an evidence-based understanding of the risks associated with cannabinoids. The current chapter reviews the definition of CUD, its prevalence and associated conditions, and the contemporary understanding of its causes to inform policy, prevention efforts, and treatment of CUD in a dynamic and evolving legislative landscape. Studies are currently limited by an absence of standardized methods to characterize cannabis consumption levels as well as compound composition. Understanding the harms associated with cannabis use and CUD will be fundamental in informing policy and supporting clinicians.

Keywords: cannabis, addiction, withdrawal, prevalence, neurobiology, neurocognition, motivation, comorbidities

1. Introduction

The term 'cannabis' refers to any product from plants of the *cannabis* genus, including marijuana and hashish, which are used primarily for their reinforcing effects. The main psychoactive compound in cannabis is Δ^9-tetrahydrocannabinol (THC); however, more than 100 other cannabinoids have been identified [1]. Other compounds include cannabidiol, cannabinol and cannabigerol; there is some evidence for protective effects of cannabidiol on THC's effects [2–4]. In a major shift from the 'war on drugs' campaigns that characterized the 1980s, legalization of cannabis for medicinal and recreational purposes is spreading across Canada and the United States. These extensive changes in cannabis regulation accompany changing public attitudes toward cannabis use and legalization [5]. Cannabis use is more prevalent when the drug is legal [5], therefore with the widespread social and legislative changes, there is a substantial need for an evidence-based understanding of the risks associated with cannabinoids. Of particular concern is a potential rise in the development of cannabis use disorder (CUD), the psychiatric diagnosis of addiction to cannabis, and it is still unclear how legalization of the drug relates to the prevalence and severity of CUD [6]. Here we review the definition of CUD, its prevalence and associated conditions, and the contemporary understanding of its causes to inform policy, prevention efforts and treatment of CUD in a dynamic and evolving legislative landscape.

2. Definition of CUD

The fifth edition of the Diagnostic and Statistical Manual of Mental Disorders (DSM-5) [7] defines CUD as any 2 of 11 diagnostic criteria (**Table 1**), which include hazardous use of the drug (e.g. driving while under the influence), taking the drug in larger/longer amounts than intended, preoccupation with cannabis, unsuccessful efforts to cut down, drug tolerance, neglecting major roles to use, and social/interpersonal problems related to use. While the DSM-IV included two categories, including both abuse (putatively lower severity) and dependence (putatively higher severity), research supports a dimensional one-factor model, indicating that CUD can best be described as a unidimensional construct [8]. The number of endorsed criteria serves as a disorder severity marker: mild (2–3 criteria), moderate (4–5 criteria) and severe (6+ criteria) CUD [7]. Criteria for craving as well as withdrawal were added in the DSM-5, with 60% endorsement of craving and over 30% reporting withdrawal symptoms in past-year individuals with CUD [9].

3. Cannabis withdrawal syndrome

While it is popularly reported that there are no withdrawal effects from cannabis, there is evidence for withdrawal symptoms in CUD that are comparable to nicotine withdrawal in magnitude and consequences [10, 11]. The DSM-5 now includes a Cannabis Withdrawal Syndrome [7] which consists mostly of emotional and behavioral symptoms including anxiety, irritability, restlessness, depression, anger, as well as sleep, weight and appetite disturbances [12]. Less common physical symptoms include stomach pain, shakiness and sweating [12]. The clinical significance of the withdrawal syndrome was originally questioned; however, those symptoms are linked with increased functional impairment in normal daily activities [13]. The delayed onset of the withdrawal syndrome may explain why it is often overlooked: symptoms peak 2–3 days after cessation of heavy cannabis use and can last 2–3 weeks [12, 14]. Given the daily use of many individuals with CUD, they may not notice the symptoms. Withdrawal symptoms are nevertheless closely linked to relapse: most abstinent individuals experiencing withdrawal symptoms will take the drug to alleviate symptoms, thereby perpetuating cannabis use [15, 16]. The withdrawal syndrome is also important in medicinal cannabis use. Notably, cannabis withdrawal symptoms overlap with mood and anxiety disorder symptoms [7]—the very symptoms that some cannabinoid products are posited to treat. Many individuals cite mood modification as a motivation for cannabis use and are unaware that their short term use for symptomatic relief may result in a long-term withdrawal syndrome [17]. More

A. A problematic pattern of cannabis use leading to clinically significant impairment or distress.
B. Two (or more) of the following occurring within a 12-month period: 1. Cannabis is often taken in larger amounts or over a longer period than was intended. 2. Persistent desire or unsuccessful effort to cut down or control cannabis use. 3. A great deal of time is spent in activities necessary to obtain cannabis, use cannabis, or recover from its effects. 4. Recurrent cannabis use resulting in a failure to fulfill major role obligations at work, school, or home (e.g., repeated absences or poor work performance related to cannabis use; substance-related absences, suspensions, or expulsions from school; neglect of children or household). 5. Continued cannabis use despite having persistent or recurrent social or interpersonal problems caused or exacerbated by the effects of the substance. 6. Important social, occupational, or recreational activities are given up or reduced because of cannabis use. 7. Recurrent cannabis use in situations in which it is physically hazardous (e.g., driving an automobile or operating a machine when impaired). 8. Cannabis use is continued despite knowledge of having a persistent or recurrent physical or psychological problem that is likely to have been caused or exacerbated by the substance. 9. Tolerance, as defined by either or both of the following: a. a need for markedly increased amounts of cannabis to achieve intoxication or a desired effect; b. markedly diminished effect with continued use of the same amount of the substance. 10. Withdrawal, as manifested by either of the following: a. The characteristic withdrawal syndrome for cannabis (anxiety, irritability, restlessness, negative affect, as well as sleep and appetite disturbances); b. The same (or a closely related) substance is taken to relieve or avoid withdrawal symptoms. 11. There is craving or a strong desire or urge to use cannabis.

Table 1. Diagnostic criteria for cannabis use disorder in the Diagnostic and Statistical Manual of the American Psychiatric Association (5th edition).

generally, medicinal cannabis can be thought of as no different than other medications for which the pharmacology results in physiological dependence including a withdrawal syndrome (e.g., benzodiazepines and opioids), requiring clinical consideration and management. Indeed, the same is true for its abuse liability in the context of CUD.

4. Prevalence of cannabis use and cannabis use disorder (CUD)

Cannabis remains the most commonly used illicit* (*state/country-dependent) psychoactive drug. Large epidemiological studies show that ~43% of individuals in the US and Canada report having tried cannabis, with ~35% having tried it more than once [18–20]. Cannabis use is highest in adults (ages 18–44), with just over half reporting using cannabis [18]. Past-year cannabis use in emerging adult populations (18–24 years-olds) is around 33.3%, with daily use almost 4% in this age group [18, 19].

Cannabis use prevalence rates from 2002 to 2012 show overall increases across North America [5, 18, 19, 21] and, increases in use and frequency of use coincide with declining risk perceptions of the drug [5]. Nevertheless, cannabis use trends differ longitudinally across specific age groups. For example, since 2002, prevalence rates appear to have increased in adults aged 25–44 (from 14 to 15.6%), remained stable in 18–24 year olds (around 33%) and decreased in the 15–17 age range (from 28.5 to 20%) [18, 19].

Prevalence rates for cannabis use disorder (CUD) range from 2.9% up to 19%—with approximately 13 million individuals worldwide meeting criteria [9, 22, 23]. Severe lifetime CUD rates are around 2%, with rates peaking during the emerging adulthood period (~21 years of age) [9]. There are also sociodemographic differences in prevalence rates—lifetime CUD rates are almost twice as high in males versus females, in adults 18–29, with a mean age of onset in the early twenties [9]. Unmarried individuals and those with lower socio-economic status report higher CUD prevalence rates; however, education appears largely unrelated [9].

One large epidemiological study in the United States also suggests that CUDs doubled between 2002 and 2012 [21], but not all longitudinal studies report the same prevalence trends in CUD [5, 20, 21, 24]. Discrepant prevalence rates may relate to underreporting in earlier studies as social acceptance of cannabis use increases [25]. Indeed, there are notable sociocultural influences on harm perception and willingness to acknowledge CUD symptoms varies between legal cultures [26]. Endorsement of CUD criteria can differ between countries and may relate to legalization status. For example, reports of failed quit attempts and withdrawal symptoms differ between the US and Netherlands [26, 27].

Importantly, CUD is associated with high levels of disability, including social and emotional functioning and greater CUD severity is associated with increasing levels of disability [9]. Information on cannabis-related disability is fairly new, as many previous studies did not include cannabis when studying disease burdens, but newer studies demonstrating that CUD can produce more years with disability [28]. Disability can persist even after CUD remission, although the reason for this is not yet clear [29]. It is also important to note that cannabis use and misuse (more broadly than just CUD) are associated with significant economic costs. In Canada, the estimated economic burden of cannabis use was 2.8Bn in 2014 and cannabis costs exhibited the largest increase among substances from 2007 to 2014, a 19.1% increase [30].

Finally, it is important to contextualize cannabis with other psychoactive drugs. One way to quantify addiction liability across substances is to examine the proportion of individuals who develop a substance use disorder, such as CUD, relative to the number of individuals who have at least tried a given substance. Using this metric in the large National Epidemiologic Survey on Alcohol and Related Conditions (NESARC) cohort, fewer than one in ten (8.9%) individuals transitioned from any cannabis use to cannabis dependence (pre-DSM-5), which was lower than tobacco, alcohol, and cocaine [31]. Another way to contextualize relative risk is to consider the conditional probability between use and misuse (i.e., the proportion of active users of a given drug that have a diagnosable problem). Again, drawing on large-scale NESARC data, 7.96% of cannabis users met criteria for cannabis dependence, which was higher than alcohol (5.82%) but substantially lower than tobacco (46.13%), heroin (26.96%), and cocaine (23.91%) [32]. In an interesting study of addiction experts using a multi-criteria decision analysis to judge substance use harms, cannabis was ranked 8th out of 20, behind alcohol, heroin, crack cocaine, methamphetamine, cocaine, tobacco, and amphetamine (in that order). Collectively, these findings suggest that although cannabis is far from without risk, it can also be thought of as lower risk than a number of other psychoactive drugs, both legal and illegal.

5. Common comorbidities

Other comorbid conditions are common in CUD; in particular, high rates of depression, anxiety, substance use and personality disorders are consistently associated with CUD [5, 9]. Understanding associations between CUD and other disorders is important as it provides more information on course and progression of the disorder.

Other substance use disorders (SUDs) are most commonly associated with CUD, with greater lifetime use of illicit drugs, including sedative/tranquilizers, painkillers, cocaine stimulants, club-drugs, hallucinogens, inhalant/solvents, heroin and other prescription drugs [33]. Recent epidemiological studies suggest increasing links with stimulant-based substances including MDMA, methamphetamine and prescription stimulants such as Ritalin [33]. It is possible that cannabis and stimulant co-abuse patterns represent individuals counterbalancing each drug's pharmacokinetic effects; for example applying sedative effects of cannabis following stimulant use [33]. Individuals with CUD are also more likely to also be current smokers and report high rates of alcohol use [9, 33]. Longitudinal studies are now providing more support for a causal relationship between early cannabis use and CUD as well as substance use and other psychiatric disorders. One large study demonstrated consistent, dose-response characteristics between early cannabis use and the development of CUD, other illicit substance use, depression and suicide attempts [34]. Altogether consistent data show polydrug use with CUD even when controlling for other health and psychiatric factors present before or during adolescence [33, 34].

In terms of other conditions, personality disorders are highly comorbid, in particular increased rates of antisocial and borderline personality disorder are noted [9]. Anxiety disorders are also linked to CUD, with Post Traumatic Stress Disorder (PTSD) most highly associated, followed by general anxiety and panic disorder [9, 21]. Applying the CUD severity specifiers (mild, moderate, severe) shows that increasing CUD severity is associated with the increasing strength of associations with these psychiatric conditions [21]—similar to CUD, clinical problems also exist on a severity continuum [5].

Converging lines of preclinical, epidemiological and experimental studies demonstrate strong links between cannabinoids and psychosis. The exogenous cannabinoid hypothesis posits that cannabinoid exposure is linked to the development of psychosis [35]. In controlled human laboratory settings, THC and cannabis extract administration produces increased positive symptoms, (including delusions, suspiciousness and perceptual alterations), negative symptoms (including blunted affect, psychomotor retardation, reduced rapport), cognitive deficits (including learning, memory and attention),—some of which are related to schizophrenia including verbal recall impairment with increased "false positives" and "intrusions" [36]. In healthy individuals, these acute laboratory effects of cannabis are time-locked to drug administration, dose-related and transient [36].

Consistent with acute intoxication experiments, epidemiological studies also provide strong evidence for cannabis use increasing the risk for psychosis, even after adjusting for covariates [37]. While these studies have difficulty demonstrating a causal relationship with psychotic disorders, a growing number of longitudinal prospective studies are beginning to demonstrate these links [37]. There is still more research needed integrating neurobiology, epidemiology and psychopharmacology with particular compounds and potencies (including synthetic cannabinoids) to determine the magnitude and mechanisms of a causal effect [37]. Nevertheless, many individuals who use cannabis regularly do not develop psychotic disorders, therefore understanding those subgroups most at risk to propsychotic effects still needs to be clarified [35].

These findings have significant implications for treatment; high comorbidity rates underscore the fact that clinicians should screen for other conditions as these are likely present. Additionally, treatment approaches may need to target concurrent conditions. The co-relationship between CUD and other conditions is also important if CUD prevalence increases with legislative changes. While the causal relationship between these co-occurrences is not yet definitive, the close association nonetheless highlights important vulnerabilities and speaks to the importance of prevention and early intervention efforts.

6. Contemporary biopsychosocial model of etiology

Most individuals who try cannabis do not use it regularly or progress to CUD; therefore cannabis use alone is not sufficient to develop a CUD. Modern etiological theories of CUD emphasize neurophysiological adaptations that occur with persistent cannabis use, resulting in changes in cognition and motivation that recursively sustain drug-seeking, and important developmental features in which early cannabis use can create vulnerabilities for subsequent misuse and CUD.

6.1. Neurobiology and neurocognition

The endocannabinoid system in the brain modulates the activity of multiple neurotransmitters, including dopamine, through the cannabinoid receptor 1 (CB1) [38].

Most of the rewarding effects of cannabis are mediated through THC at the cannabinoid CB1 receptor in the brain [39–41]. These feelings of high relate to THC concentrations and can be blocked by a CB1 antagonist [42]. Additionally, there is evidence for the CB1 receptor in the development of dependence and in the withdrawal syndrome [39]. The brain responds to persistent cannabis consumption and the resulting circulating THC by homeostatically downregulating CB1 receptors [43]; full recovery of CB1 receptor density has been detected after one-month abstinence and substantial recovery has been detected as soon as 72-hours [43, 44].

Both the acute and chronic effects of cannabis on the central nervous system are not well-understood in humans. CB1 receptors are heavily expressed in the striatum, hippocampus, amygdala and prefrontal cortex (PFC) and it is mostly in these regions that regular cannabis users show altered neuroanatomy [45]. Understanding neuroanatomic alterations with cannabis use is complicated by this drug's composition changes in recent years including different cannabinoid compounds with unique neural effects [45]. Since the 1990s, THC potency has increased from 4 to 12%; simultaneously, the average concentration of THC to cannabidiol has increased almost 80 times, suggesting plants are now bred with much higher THC concentrations (based on confiscated cannabis materials) [46]. These compound alterations are important as preclinical evidence suggests neurotoxic effects of THC on CB1 rich areas [45]. In humans, volumetric reductions and gray matter density alterations are consistently noted in the hippocampus, which relate to duration of use and cannabis dosage [45, 47, 48]. There are also links with compound composition; THC levels are inversely related to volumetric reductions while higher THC/cannabidiol ratios are associated with reduced volume and gray matter [45]. There is some evidence for neuroprotective cannabidiol effects as individuals with high cannabidiol levels do not show hippocampal volume reductions, however the mechanisms by which cannabidiol might offset THC effects are currently unknown [45].

Outside of the hippocampus, neuroanatomic alterations are additionally noted in high-density CB1 areas including the amygdala and striatum, PFC, parietal cortex, insula and cerebellum [45]. Altogether, these neuroanatomic alterations may result from THC metabolites accumulating and producing neurotoxic effects, cannabinoid receptor adaptations and/or changes in cells or vascularity [45]. All of these CB1-rich areas serve core functions in memory, attention, learning and reward and cognitive control. The hippocampus, PFC and amygdala are central in cognitive processing, indeed behavioral/functional impairments are noted in memory, attention and learning in CUD [49].

6.2. Cognitive functioning

Although the findings are mixed, overall subtle neurocognitive deficits in executive function, memory and learning are found with cannabis exposure, however, long term cannabis effects, and whether they are reversible, are still unclear [49, 50]. The ability to hold and manipulate information is consistently impaired with acute cannabis administration, although few studies report long-term working memory problems [50–53]. Diminished prefrontal cortex and hippocampal activity are noted during memory tasks in heavy cannabis users [54].

Of particular relevance to cannabis is the role of impulsivity—a systematic review provides support for alterations in inhibitory control in heavy cannabis users [55].

There are mixed behavioral findings when examining attention and concentration in CUD as well as impulsive behaviors following acute administration, short-term and long-term abstinence [50]. Nevertheless several neuroimaging studies demonstrate reduced prefrontal, anterior cingulate and dorsolateral PFC activity during inhibitory control tasks [56–58]. Delay discounting, a behavioral economic measure of impulsivity reflecting preferences for smaller immediate rewards relative to larger delayed rewards, has been inconsistently associated with CUD, although a recent meta-analysis detected an overall small magnitude association [59]. This is consistent with greater impulsivity on this measure in relation to other forms of addiction, ADHD, and obesity [60–62].

Decision-making and risk-taking appear altered following acute cannabis administration as well as after short-term and longer-term abstinence [50]. It is yet unclear whether these effects are short-term or long-lasting or if these represent an exposure effect; while some studies report reversible findings following abstinence [63, 64] others report deficits even years after drug cessation, suggesting cumulative drug effects [65, 66]. Mixed findings again may relate to the changing compound profile of cannabis—most findings reported from acute intoxication experiments to date administer cannabis concentrations ~3% THC—significantly lower levels than the 12% rate often found in current samples [46]. Longitudinal studies with more potent drugs and more systematic control for cannabis use will be critical to clarify the effects. It is also possible that neurocognitive alterations exist prior to cannabis use; however, few longitudinal studies exist testing this hypothesis.

Clarifying neurocognitive impairments associated with CUD is important for understanding how the disorder progresses and impacts specific functions. To date, few studies examine how these impairments relate to recovery and abstinence. Understanding these impairments is also important for clinicians; particular deficits may put into question the usefulness of cognitive therapy [67] as specific cognitive functions may underlie learning adaptive responses and skills in behavioral therapies and avoiding relapse [50].

To date, functional neuroimaging studies examining the underlying neural substrates of these executive functions provide some evidence for altered processing [2, 50, 54, 56–58, 66]. Mixed findings may relate to the neuroimaging techniques employed, the constructs examined and the heterogeneity of characteristics in the samples studied.

6.3. Motivation and cannabis

One of the effects of chronic cannabis use in popular culture is changes in motivation. A recent longitudinal study showed cannabis use predicted lower persistence and initiative in college students [68]. Nevertheless, only a handful of studies have systematically examined cannabis' effects on motivation under controlled conditions. Laboratory studies of cannabis on motivation have found pro-motivational effects [69, 70], amotivational effects [71], or no effect [72]. These mixed findings may relate to problematic methodology, including differing cannabis doses (even within the same study), small sample numbers (e.g. N = 5), cross sectional designs, and differing compound composition over time. The heterogeneity of the cannabis users sampled in the studies is quite diverse; indeed, most human studies in cannabis users compare groups of cannabis users with varying levels of cannabis related problems (e.g. heavy, regular, occasional, light) to controls without assessing CUDs with rigorous diagnostic instruments. Additionally, some of the simple finger-tapping tasks that participants are asked to perform in the laboratory may not adequately capture the affected motivated behavior.

A recent study examining chronic effects of cannabis on reward learning, found that non-intoxicated individuals with CUD did not develop a response bias to reward-paired cues over time, suggesting an impaired ability to learn new rewards [73]. The neurobiology underlying impaired reward learning in CUD is currently not clear, including whether this is a predisposing factor or a result of heavy cannabis use. Nevertheless, the inability to form new reward associations lies at the core of an amotivational syndrome.

There is also evidence for heterogeneity of effects of different active cannabis concentrations and compounds. On another task examining effort-related decision-making, acute administration of cannabis with or without cannabidiol reduced the number of effortful choices for monetary reward compared to placebo [73]. Although the effortful choices were not differentially affected by the presence of cannabidiol in the compound, the investigators found that following cannabis administration with cannabidiol, the expected value of the reward (measured as the outcome value X the probability of receiving that outcome) increased the likelihood of making a high-effort choice. These results suggest that the presence of cannabidiol may affect THC's effects on processing expected value [73].

Amotivation in CUD may reflect that cannabis itself becomes a predominant motivator over other stimuli. One study investigated neural sensitivity to hedonic stimuli and showed that long-term daily users showed greater neural responses in reward networks to cannabis cues, relative to natural reward (fruit) cues [74]. Moreover, activity in frontostriatal temporal regions correlated with subjective reports of craving, THC metabolite levels as well as cannabis withdrawal scores. These findings suggest a hyper-responsivity and specificity of the brain's response to cannabis cues in heavy users. Additionally, the positive relationship between THC levels and neural response suggests that the latter may relate to cannabis use [74]. Another large longitudinal fMRI study prospectively examined striatal changes following cannabis use in youths at the ages of 20, 22, to 24 [75]. The striatum is a key node of the reward network that signals the motivational significance of a stimulus [76]. The results in youths showed that past-year cannabis use at each of the 3 scans related to striatal activation during reward anticipation, even when covarying for binge drinking or other drug use [75]. At the first scan, past-year cannabis use negatively correlated with striatal activation at Time 2, while past-year cannabis use at Time 2 was negatively associated with striatal activation at Time 3. Importantly, blunted striatal response was only present in those individuals with escalating drug use, suggesting that cannabis may be triggering these changes. Overall, this is the first study to show longitudinal associations between cannabis use and striatal activation during a nondrug reward anticipation task. More prospective studies are needed to evaluate whether an amotivational syndrome exists and the mechanisms by which it might develop.

6.4. Developmental influences

Given their increased drug experimentation, combined with a developing endocannabinoid system, adolescents represent a population particularly vulnerable to cannabis' effects [77, 78]. A meta-analysis of cognitive functioning in adolescents reported reduced cognitive functioning with frequent or heavy cannabis use, however, abstinence greater than 72 hours appears to diminish this effect [79].

To date, few neuroimaging studies examine adolescent populations with CUD. Adolescent chronic cannabis use is associated with greater performance-related activation in frontotemporal areas, despite similar performance, suggesting neuroadaptations, or greater neural effort to perform memory and inhibition tasks [56]. A recent prospective cohort study scanned adolescents as they performed a working memory task prior to and after their first cannabis exposure [80]. The researchers found that those youths that would go on to use cannabis by the age of 15 (follow up), showed increased frontoparietal activity at baseline relative to the non-using group—these neural differences remained unchanged or increased when examined longitudinally. This is the first study to demonstrate frontoparietal and neurocognitive alterations prior to cannabis use. The researchers also found that at 12 years of age (baseline), the adolescents who would go on to use cannabis by the age of 15 (follow-up) had significantly lower scores on the cognitive battery. The difference scores on the cognitive battery from baseline to follow-up did not change, suggesting no significant neurocognitive changes following cannabis initiation. This prospective cohort study is one of the first to demonstrate specific neurocognitive features that may exist prior to cannabis exposure.

Given the changing compound composition of cannabis, combined with increasing THC levels and availability, understanding the effects of cannabis use on the brain and on memory, learning and reward processing should be a priority in adolescents. Accordingly, the Adolescent Brain Cognitive Development (ABCD) study recently launched by the National Institute of Health in the United States will follow 10,000 children longitudinally with multiple measures of neural, cognitive and emotional functioning [81]. This prospective cohort study will provide much-needed information on the long-term effects of cannabis use.

7. Other harms from cannabis

With the exception of nicotine, smoked cannabis includes many of the same chemicals and carcinogens found in tobacco that can damage lung tissue [82]. Heavy cannabis smoking is associated with chronic bronchitis and inflammation/injury in the larger airways [82]. Findings for other types of lung diseases and cancers are mixed, given high rates of comorbid tobacco use in regular cannabis users. Some of the chronic respiratory effects appear reversible, particularly in those individuals who only smoke cannabis [83, 84]. The impact of cannabis use on lung health may also change, as other methods of intake are gaining popularity, such as vaping or edibles [82].

One of the largest public health concerns with legalization of cannabis use is the effect of the drug on driving. Driving simulation studies show a relationship between blood THC levels and impaired performance, particularly with reaction time and lane position variability (i.e., weaving) [85]. One study had occasional cannabis smokers perform a visuomotor tracking task while undergoing fMRI after taking low-dose THC and found decreased psychomotor skills as well as reduced activity in fronto-parietal areas [86]. After alcohol, cannabis is the most commonly reported drug in driving accidents and fatalities [87]. There is current ongoing research to better understand drug interactions, particularly with alcohol, as psychomotor impairments appear more severe when alcohol and cannabis are combined [85]. Indeed, greater information on the pharmacokinetic effects of cannabis on driving is needed, together with other drug interactions. One difficult problem for roadside testing remains that current cannabis detection through breath, saliva, blood or urine does not provide a reliable measure of recency or potency of use.

8. Future directions in CUD research

A fundamental question in cannabis research is whether observed alterations in neurobiology and cognition with heavy cannabis use persist with abstinence or whether they are reversible. The neurobiological studies are currently limited by an absence of standardized methods to characterize cannabis consumption levels as well as compound composition. The varying compounds in cannabis samples present a challenge to conducting systematic cannabis research; it is unknown how all of these might interact [28] and varying cannabinoid levels across studies may account for the diverse findings reported in the literature. Most studies rely on self-report measures of cannabis use and those that do toxicology analyses provide poor measures for quantifying exposure or the timeframe. Additionally, different measures of intake (i.e., inhaling, vaping, with/without tobacco) can also influence THC release/metabolism. Given all of the uncertainty between exposure parameters and neural substrates, many researchers are now calling for standardization of cannabis use metrics, particularly as the drug's effects appear more closely linked to dosage than duration of use [49]. Questions for future research include: (1) understanding CB1 receptor changes and relationships with reward, motivation, craving and abstinence, (2) clarifying cognitive and motivational alterations and whether these are precursors or consequences of CUD and (3) understanding the links between cannabis use and psychotic disorders. In this changing political, social, psychopharmacological and compositional landscape of cannabis, understanding the harms associated with cannabis use and CUD will be fundamental in informing policy and supporting clinicians.

Author details

Iris Balodis[1,2]* and James MacKillop[1,2]

*Address all correspondence to: balodisi@mcmaster.ca

1 Michael G. DeGroote Centre for Medicinal Cannabis Research, Master University/
St. Joseph's Healthcare Hamilton, Hamilton, ON, Canada

2 Peter Boris Centre for Addictions Research, McMaster University/St. Joseph's Healthcare Hamilton, Hamilton, ON, Canada

References

[1] Felder CC, Glass M. Cannabinoid receptors and their endogenous agonists. Annual Review of Pharmacology and Toxicology. 1998;**38**:179-200

[2] Bhattacharyya S et al. Opposite effects of delta-9-tetrahydrocannabinol and cannabidiol on human brain function and psychopathology. Neuropsychopharmacology. 2010;**35**(3):764-774

[3] Colizzi M, Bhattacharyya S. Does cannabis composition matter? Differential effects of Delta-9-tetrahydrocannabinol and cannabidiol on human cognition. Current Addiction Reports. 2017;**4**(2):62-74

[4] Zuardi AW et al. Action of cannabidiol on the anxiety and other effects produced by delta 9-THC in normal subjects. Psychopharmacology. 1982;**76**(3):245-250

[5] Compton WM et al. Marijuana use and use disorders in adults in the USA, 2002-14: Analysis of annual cross-sectional surveys. Lancet Psychiatry. 2016;**3**(10):954-964

[6] Budney AJ, Borodovsky JT. The potential impact of cannabis legalization on the development of cannabis use disorders. Preventive Medicine. 2017;**104**:31-36

[7] APA. Diagnostic and Statistical Manual of Mental Disorders. 5th ed. Washington, DC: American Psychiatric Association; 2013

[8] Hasin DS et al. DSM-5 criteria for substance use disorders: Recommendations and rationale. The American Journal of Psychiatry. 2013;**170**(8):834-851

[9] Hasin DS et al. Prevalence and correlates of DSM-5 cannabis use disorder, 2012-2013: Findings from the National Epidemiologic Survey on alcohol and related conditions-III. The American Journal of Psychiatry. 2016;**173**(6):588-599

[10] Vandrey RG et al. A within-subject comparison of withdrawal symptoms during abstinence from cannabis, tobacco, and both substances. Drug and Alcohol Dependence. 2008;**92**(1-3):48-54

[11] Budney AJ et al. Marijuana abstinence effects in marijuana smokers maintained in their home environment. Archives of General Psychiatry. 2001;**58**(10):917-924

[12] Budney AJ et al. Review of the validity and significance of cannabis withdrawal syndrome. The American Journal of Psychiatry. 2004;**161**(11):1967-1977

[13] Allsop DJ et al. Quantifying the clinical significance of cannabis withdrawal. PLoS One. 2012;**7**(9):e44864

[14] Davis JP et al. Cannabis withdrawal, posttreatment abstinence, and days to first cannabis use among emerging adults in substance use treatment: A prospective study. Journal of Drug Issues. 2016;**46**(1):64-83

[15] Budney AJ, Novy PL, Hughes JR. Marijuana withdrawal among adults seeking treatment for marijuana dependence. Addiction. 1999;**94**(9):1311-1322

[16] Haney M. The marijuana withdrawal syndrome: Diagnosis and treatment. Current Psychiatry Reports. 2005;**7**(5):360-366

[17] Hasin DS. US epidemiology of cannabis use and associated problems. Neuropsychopharmacology. 2018;**43**(1):195-212

[18] Rotermann M, Langlois K. Prevalence and correlates of marijuana use in Canada, 2012. Health Reports. 2015;**26**(4):10-15

[19] Rotermann M, Macdonald R. Analysis of trends in the prevalence of cannabis use in Canada, 1985 to 2015. Health Reports. 2018;**29**(2):10-20

[20] SAMHSA. Results from the 2012 National Survey on Drug Use and Health: Summary of national findings and detailed tables. In: SAaMHS Administration, editor. 2012. archive.samhs.gov/data/NSDUH/2012SummNatFindDetTables/Index.aspx

[21] Hasin DS et al. Prevalence of marijuana use disorders in the United States between 2001-2002 and 2012-2013. JAMA Psychiatry. 2015;**72**(12):1235-1242

[22] Farmer RF et al. Natural course of cannabis use disorders. Psychological Medicine. 2015;**45**(1):63-72

[23] UNODC. World Drug Report 2015. In: WDR Series, editor. Geneva: United Nations Office on Drugs and Crime; 2015

[24] Grucza RA et al. Discrepancies in estimates of prevalence and correlates of substance use and disorders between two national surveys. Addiction. 2007;**102**(4):623-629

[25] Grucza RA et al. Recent trends in the prevalence of marijuana use and associated disorders in the United States. JAMA Psychiatry. 2016;**73**(3):300-301

[26] Delforterie M et al. Functioning of cannabis abuse and dependence criteria across two different countries: The United States and The Netherlands. Substance Use & Misuse. 2015;**50**(2):242-250

[27] Reinarman C, Cohen PD, Kaal HL. The limited relevance of drug policy: Cannabis in Amsterdam and in San Francisco. American Journal of Public Health. 2004;**94**(5):836-842

[28] Degenhardt L et al. The global epidemiology and contribution of cannabis use and dependence to the global burden of disease: Results from the GBD 2010 study. PLoS One. 2013;**8**(10):e76635

[29] Rubio JM et al. Quality of life following remission of mental disorders: Findings from the National Epidemiologic Survey on Alcohol and Related Conditions. The Journal of Clinical Psychiatry. 2013;**74**(5):e445-e450

[30] Canadian Substance Use Costs and Harms Scientific Working Group C. Canadian substance use costs and harms (2007-2014). In: CIfSURatCCoSUa Addiction, editor. Ottawa, ON: Canadian Centre on Substance Use and Addiction; 2018

[31] Lopez-Quintero C et al. Probability and predictors of transition from first use to dependence on nicotine, alcohol, cannabis, and cocaine: Results of the National Epidemiologic

Survey on Alcohol and Related Conditions (NESARC). Drug and Alcohol Dependence. 2011;**115**(1-2):120-130

[32] Grant BF, Dawson DA, Moss HB. Disaggregating the burden of substance dependence in the United States. Alcoholism, Clinical and Experimental Research. 2011;**35**(3):387-388

[33] Hayley AC, Stough C, Downey LA. DSM-5 cannabis use disorder, substance use and DSM-5 specific substance-use disorders: Evaluating comorbidity in a population-based sample. European Neuropsychopharmacology. 2017;**27**(8):732-743

[34] Silins E et al. Young adult sequelae of adolescent cannabis use: An integrative analysis. Lancet Psychiatry. 2014;**1**(4):286-293

[35] Ranganathan M, Skosnik PD, D'Souza DC. Marijuana and madness: Associations between cannabinoids and psychosis. Biological Psychiatry. 2016;**79**(7):511-513

[36] Sherif M et al. Human laboratory studies on cannabinoids and psychosis. Biological Psychiatry. 2016;**79**(7):526-538

[37] Gage SH, Hickman M, Zammit S. Association between cannabis and psychosis: Epidemiologic evidence. Biological Psychiatry. 2016;**79**(7):549-556

[38] Castillo PE et al. Endocannabinoid signaling and synaptic function. Neuron. 2012;**76**(1): 70-81

[39] Cooper ZD, Haney M. Cannabis reinforcement and dependence: Role of the cannabinoid CB1 receptor. Addiction Biology. 2008;**13**(2):188-195

[40] Haney M et al. Factors influencing marijuana self-administration by humans. Behavioural Pharmacology. 1997;**8**(2-3):101-112

[41] Kelly TH et al. Are choice and self-administration of marijuana related to delta 9-THC content? Experimental and Clinical Psychopharmacology. 1997;**5**(1):74-82

[42] Huestis MA et al. Single and multiple doses of rimonabant antagonize acute effects of smoked cannabis in male cannabis users. Psychopharmacology. 2007;**194**(4):505-515

[43] Hirvonen J et al. Reversible and regionally selective downregulation of brain cannabinoid CB1 receptors in chronic daily cannabis smokers. Molecular Psychiatry. 2012;**17**(6):642-649

[44] D'Souza DC et al. Rapid changes in CB1 receptor availability in cannabis dependent males after abstinence from Cannabis. Biological Psychiatry: Cognitive Neuroscience and Neuroimaging. 2016;**1**(1):60-67

[45] Lorenzetti V, Solowij N, Yucel M. The role of cannabinoids in neuroanatomic alterations in cannabis users. Biological Psychiatry. 2016;**79**(7):e17-e31

[46] ElSohly MA et al. Changes in cannabis potency over the last 2 decades (1995-2014): Analysis of current data in the United States. Biological Psychiatry. 2016;**79**(7):613-619

[47] Cousijn J et al. Grey matter alterations associated with cannabis use: Results of a VBM study in heavy cannabis users and healthy controls. NeuroImage. 2012;**59**(4):3845-3851

[48] Rocchetti M et al. Is cannabis neurotoxic for the healthy brain? A meta-analytical review of structural brain alterations in non-psychotic users. Psychiatry and Clinical Neurosciences. 2013;**67**(7):483-492

[49] Nader DA, Sanchez ZM. Effects of regular cannabis use on neurocognition, brain structure, and function: A systematic review of findings in adults. The American Journal of Drug and Alcohol Abuse. 2018;**44**(1):4-18

[50] Crean RD, Crane NA, Mason BJ. An evidence based review of acute and long-term effects of cannabis use on executive cognitive functions. Journal of Addiction Medicine. 2011;**5**(1):1-8

[51] Hart CL et al. Effects of acute smoked marijuana on complex cognitive performance. Neuropsychopharmacology. 2001;**25**(5):757-765

[52] Tinklenberg JR et al. Marijuana and immediate memory. Nature. 1970;**226**(5251):1171-1172

[53] Verdejo-Garcia AJ et al. Differential effects of MDMA, cocaine, and cannabis use severity on distinctive components of the executive functions in polysubstance users: A multiple regression analysis. Addictive Behaviors. 2005;**30**(1):89-101

[54] Block RI et al. Effects of frequent marijuana use on memory-related regional cerebral blood flow. Pharmacology, Biochemistry, and Behavior. 2002;**72**(1-2):237-250

[55] Wrege J et al. Effects of cannabis on impulsivity: A systematic review of neuroimaging findings. Current Pharmaceutical Design. 2014;**20**(13):2126-2137

[56] Batalla A et al. Structural and functional imaging studies in chronic cannabis users: A systematic review of adolescent and adult findings. PLoS One. 2013;**8**(2):e55821

[57] Eldreth DA et al. Abnormal brain activity in prefrontal brain regions in abstinent marijuana users. NeuroImage. 2004;**23**(3):914-920

[58] Gruber SA, Yurgelun-Todd DA. Neuroimaging of marijuana smokers during inhibitory processing: A pilot investigation. Brain Research. Cognitive Brain Research. 2005;**23**(1):107-118

[59] Amlung M et al. Steep delay discounting and addictive behavior: A meta-analysis of continuous associations. Addiction. 2017;**112**(1):51-62

[60] Amlung M et al. Steep discounting of delayed monetary and food rewards in obesity: A meta-analysis. Psychological Medicine. 2016;**46**(11):2423-2434

[61] Jackson JN, Mac Killop J. Attention-deficit/hyperactivity disorder and monetary delay discounting: A meta-analysis of case-control studies. Biological Psychiatry: Cognitive Neuroscience and Neuroimaging. 2016;**1**(4):316-325

[62] MacKillop J et al. Delayed reward discounting and addictive behavior: A meta-analysis. Psychopharmacology. 2011;**216**(3):305-321

[63] Lyons MJ et al. Neuropsychological consequences of regular marijuana use: A twin study. Psychological Medicine. 2004;**34**(7):1239-1250

[64] Pope HG Jr et al. Neuropsychological performance in long-term cannabis users. Archives of General Psychiatry. 2001;**58**(10):909-915

[65] Auer R et al. Association between lifetime marijuana use and cognitive function in middle age: The coronary artery risk development in young adults (CARDIA) study. JAMA Internal Medicine. 2016;**176**(3):352-361

[66] Bolla KI et al. Dose-related neurocognitive effects of marijuana use. Neurology. 2002;**59**(9):1337-1343

[67] Verdejo-Garcia A et al. Clinical implications and methodological challenges in the study of the neuropsychological correlates of cannabis, stimulant, and opioid abuse. Neuropsychology Review. 2004;**14**(1):1-41

[68] Lac A, Luk JW. Testing the Amotivational syndrome: Marijuana use longitudinally predicts lower self-efficacy even after controlling for demographics, personality, and alcohol and cigarette use. Prevention Science. 2018;**19**(2):117-126

[69] Foltin RW et al. Motivational effects of smoked marijuana: Behavioral contingencies and low-probability activities. Journal of the Experimental Analysis of Behavior. 1990;**53**(1):5-19

[70] Mendelson JH et al. Operant acquisition of marihuana in man. The Journal of Pharmacology and Experimental Therapeutics. 1976;**198**(1):42-53

[71] Cherek DR, Lane SD, Dougherty DM. Possible amotivational effects following marijuana smoking under laboratory conditions. Experimental and Clinical Psychopharmacology. 2002;**10**(1):26-38

[72] Mello NK et al. The effects of marihuana use on operant behavior in man. Psychopharmacology Bulletin. 1976;**12**(4):7-9

[73] Lawn W et al. Acute and chronic effects of cannabinoids on effort-related decision-making and reward learning: An evaluation of the cannabis 'amotivational' hypotheses. Psychopharmacology. 2016;**233**(19-20):3537-3552

[74] Filbey FM et al. fMRI study of neural sensitization to hedonic stimuli in long-term, daily cannabis users. Human Brain Mapping. 2016;**37**(10):3431-3443

[75] Martz ME et al. Association of marijuana use with blunted nucleus accumbens response to reward anticipation. JAMA Psychiatry. 2016;**73**(8):838-844

[76] Pessoa L, Engelmann JB. Embedding reward signals into perception and cognition. Frontiers in Neuroscience. 2010:**4**

[77] Gogtay N et al. Dynamic mapping of human cortical development during childhood through early adulthood. Proceedings of the National Academy of Sciences of the United States of America. 2004;**101**(21):8174-8179

[78] Luna B et al. An integrative model of the maturation of cognitive control. Annual Review of Neuroscience. 2015;**38**:151-170

[79] Scott JC et al. Association of cannabis with cognitive functioning in adolescents and young adults: A systematic review and meta-analysis. JAMA Psychiatry. 2018;**75**(6):585-595

[80] Tervo-Clemmens B et al. Early cannabis use and neurocognitive risk: A prospective functional neuroimaging study. Biological Psychiatry: Cognitive Neuroscience and Neuroimaging. Aug 2018 ;**3**(8):713-725. DOI: 10.1016/j.bpsc.2018.05.004. Epub 29 May 2018

[81] Lisdahl KM et al. Adolescent brain cognitive development (ABCD) study: Overview of substance use assessment methods. Developmental Cognitive Neuroscience. 2018;**32**: 80-96

[82] Tashkin DP. Marijuana and lung disease. Chest. Sep 2018;**154**(3):653-663. DOI: 10.1016/j.chest.2018.05.005. Epub 17 May 2018. Review

[83] Hancox RJ et al. Effects of quitting cannabis on respiratory symptoms. The European Respiratory Journal. 2015;**46**(1):80-87

[84] Tashkin DP, Simmons MS, Tseng CH. Impact of changes in regular use of marijuana and/or tobacco on chronic bronchitis. COPD. 2012;**9**(4):367-374

[85] Hartman RL, Huestis MA. Cannabis effects on driving skills. Clinical Chemistry. 2013;**59**(3):478-492

[86] Battistella G et al. Weed or wheel! FMRI, behavioural, and toxicological investigations of how cannabis smoking affects skills necessary for driving. PLoS One. 2013;**8**(1):e52545

[87] Brady JE, Li G. Trends in alcohol and other drugs detected in fatally injured drivers in the United States, 1999-2010. American Journal of Epidemiology. 2014;**179**(6):692-699

Chapter 9

Bioligands Acting on the Cannabinoid Receptor CB1 for the Treatment of Withdrawal Syndrome Caused by *Cannabis sativa*

Jaderson Vieira Ferreira, Lenir Cabral Correa,
Daniel Castro da Costa and
Lorane Izabel da Silva Hage-Melim

Additional information is available at the end of the chapter

http://dx.doi.org/10.5772/intechopen.82184

Abstract

Every day, the questions about *Cannabis sativa* ability to cause chemical dependence are closed with the considerable increase in the demand for treatment of addicts to this plant. Most drug addicts submitted to treatment have difficulty in achieving and maintaining abstinence from *Cannabis* due to the appearance of symptoms as irritability, anxiety, desire to consume marijuana, decreased quality and quantity of sleep, and change in appetite, weight loss, and physical discomfort, besides emotional and behavioral symptoms. The neurobiological basis for the withdrawal syndrome, that is, withdrawal of *Cannabis*, was established after the discovery of the endogenous cannabinoid system, identification of CB1 and CB2 cannabinoid receptors, and demonstrations of precipitated removal with antagonists of these receptors. The chapter discusses the main studies currently conducted for the treatment of withdrawal syndrome based on bioligands that act directly on the CB1 cannabinoid receptor.

Keywords: receptor cannabinoid CB1, withdrawal syndrome, *Cannabis sativa*, drugs computer aided

1. Introduction

Cannabis sativa, commonly known as marijuana, is the illicit drug most consumed in many countries [1]. The form of *Cannabis* abuse is predominantly smoked, although it can be found in paste form called hashish, mixed with crack, or as *skunk*, which is a polymorphic form of marijuana [2] cultivated in special appearance and 7–25 times stronger than common marijuana causing greater psychotropic effects, as well as adverse effects such as triggering of schizophrenia [3].

Studies have found moderate evidence that there is a link between *Cannabis* use and in relation to the development of dependence and substance abuse such as alcohol and tobacco among other illicit drugs [4], and after a long discussion about the relevance of recent *Cannabis* withdrawal syndrome, this condition was added to the fifth version of the Diagnostic and Statistical Manual of Mental Disorders (DSM-5) [5]. This syndrome appears within 24 h after cessation of *Cannabis* use, reaches a peak in about days 2–6, and can last from 1 or 2 weeks. It affects 55–89% of regular *Cannabis* users. The *Cannabis* withdrawal syndrome is clinically defined by irritability, anger, nervousness, anxiety, sleep difficulties, decreased appetite or weight loss, restlessness, and mood depression, in addition to various physical symptoms such as abdominal pain, tremor, or sweating [6–8].

The evidence of *Cannabis* withdrawal syndrome is based on behavioral observations in animal studies [9], clinical observation of patients [10], or epidemiological surveys [11, 12]. However, the biological correlates of this phenomenon remain obscure, challenging the validity of the syndrome. This lack of knowledge is partly explained by the interindividual variability of delta 9-tetrahydrocannabinol (THC) metabolism [13] and the complexity of plasma-tissue exchanges [14].

In the last decades, many studies have been dedicated to discover and understand the diverse effects of cannabinoids on the organism whether therapeutic (with the relief of chronic pains and muscle spasms related to multiple sclerosis) [15, 16] or derived from the psychoactivity of *C. sativa*, originating the dependence and consequently the withdrawal syndrome [17]. These symptoms include physical discomforts such as headaches and stomach psychological symptoms accompanied by irritability, anxiety, sleep disturbances, decreased appetite/weight loss, restlessness, or depressed mood [18]. The chapter discusses the main studies currently conducted for the treatment of *Cannabis* withdrawal syndrome, that is, molecules which have their activity associated with some kind of interaction by structural complementarity beside the CB1 cannabinoid receptor.

2. Physiology

2.1. Cannabinoid receptor type 1 (CB1)

After the use of *Cannabis*, THC interacts with the CB1 cannabinoid receptor, inducing conformational changes in this receptor, the interaction with the residue of amino acid TRP356 and its surroundings being the activation trigger for the signaling [19]. Also, the binding site of the CB1 receptor comprises the amino acid residues Phenylalanine 174 (PHE174), Leucine 193 (LEU193), and Serine 383 (SER383) (**Figure 1**) that must be in contact or proximity to the preferred THC docking position [20].

The morphological differences between CB1 and CB2 cannabinoid receptors indicate that most cannabinoid compounds interact differently in both receptors [21], and the location of

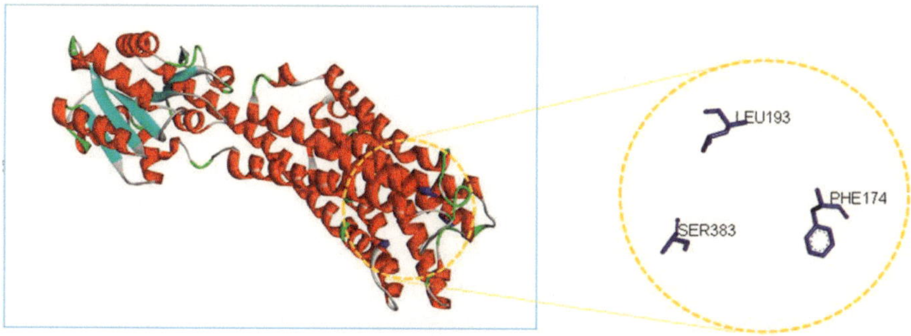

Figure 1. Amino acid residues present at the cannabinoid receptor binding site CB1.

CB1 receptors in the central nervous system is directly associated with the behavioral effects produced by cannabinoids [22, 23]. CB1 gene polymorphisms have been observed and their importance is still unknown, but it is suggested that they are linked to increased susceptibility to *C. sativa* dependence and neuropsychiatric disorders [24].

CB1 cannabinoid receptors are present in areas associated with motor control, emotional response, learning, memory, goal-oriented behaviors, energy homeostasis, and higher cognitive functions, among others [25]. In peripheral organs and tissues, CB1 receptors are expressed in low density and have potential implication to regulate inflammation and autoimmune diseases [26]. Unlike the standard of others neuroreceptor systems, levels of CB1 receptors in rats are increased in the transition from adolescence to adult age, a fact that suggests the propensity to search for cannabinoid compounds at this stage of life [27].

The CB1 receptor is a subfamily member of the G protein-coupled receptors (GPCRs) [28] and is predominantly present in the presynaptic terminal, although small amounts are present in peripheral nerves and its function seems to modulate the release of neurotransmitters such as dopamine, noradrenaline, glutamate, and serotonin in the synaptic cleft [29].

The inhibition of adenylate cyclase by psychoactive cannabinoids in more densely populated regions of CB1 receptors was initially identified in N18TG2 neuroblastoma cells and thereafter in many other preparations [30]. This inhibition causes modulation of intracellular cAMP concentration, thereby regulating protein kinase A (PKA) phosphorylation, fact that may result in large changes on cellular activity, such as regulation of K^+ channels undergoing PKA action in hippocampus [31].

Mitogen-activated protein kinases (MAP kinases) are important signal transduction enzymes involved in cell regulation to physiological functions of gene expression control, proliferation, and programmed cell death (apoptosis) [32]. Studies confirm a positive connection of CB1 receptors with MAP kinase, so that, *in vivo*, acute administration of Δ9-THC and CB1 cannabinoid receptor agonists (CP-55940, WIN 55,212-2, anandamide (AEA), and 2-O-arachidonoylglycerol (2-AG)) stimulates the MAP kinase of guinea pigs. Synaptic plasticity is considered as the capacity of rearrangement by the neural networks, constitutes an important mechanism to recover or adapt in case of injury, and provides the basis for most models of learning, memory, and development in neural circuits [33]. Brain-derived neurotrophic factor (BDNF) and Krox-24 gene have been recognized for their importance in synaptic plasticity and are prevented by the activation of MAP kinase [34], including studies that indicate that cannabinoid receptors alter this physiological process and may favor the induction of long-term depolarization (LTD) [35].

The voltage-dependent ion channels, mainly K^+ and Ca^{2+}, are modulated by CB1 receptors, suggesting that the release of gamma-aminobutyric acid (GABA), a neurotransmitter responsible for CNS inhibition, is mediated by the opening of these channels [36], thus influencing cognitive processes such as learning and memory [37].

Cerebral cortex neurons expressing the G-protein coupled receptors, called CCK receptors, are responsible for the release of the neuropeptide cholecystokinin (CCK) [38], whose action on the hypothalamus produces the sensation of satiety, and also express the CB1 receptors [39]. Activation of CB1 receptors also activates CCK receptors, thus inhibiting the release of CCK [40] and negatively influencing satiety [41].

Rich areas in CB1 receptors reveal a high expression of N-methyl D-aspartate (NMDA) receptors, a class of receptors involved in glutamate neurotransmission and therefore important in movement control and memory formation [42]. Cannabinoid substances have shown dual effects on NMDA receptor activity, influencing memory acquisition and learning mechanisms [43].

2.2. Cannabinoid receptor type 2 (CB2)

The main and most well-known location of CB2 receptors on human beings is in nonneuronal tissues, mainly in the immune system and hematopoietic cells. The exclusively peripheral location of the CB2 receptors was already questioned when, in 2006, their existence was confirmed in the nervous system, principally in neuronal, glial, and endothelial cells in the brain, although in lower proportions than the CB1 receptors [44]. As CB2 receptors has an important role in neuroinflammatory responses, neurodegenerative diseases such as multiple sclerosis, amyotrophic lateral sclerosis, and Alzheimer's disease become the subject of pharmaceutical studies in this regard [45], where the concentration of these receptors seems to be increased in specific brain regions related to these pathologies [46].

As with CB1 receptors, CB2 receptors are also coupled to G protein although their action seems to be part of a general protection system since its activation has no association with psychoactive effects. Agonist molecules of these receptors are being tested in neuropsychiatric, cardiovascular, and hepatic pathologies [47].

3. Chemical dependence and withdrawal syndrome

THC is a partial agonist of CB1 and CB2 receptors, although it is the interaction with CB1 receptors that is responsible for the psychoactive effects of *C. sativa* [40, 41]. CB1 receptors are found at high densities in the ventral tegmental area, nucleus accumbens, prefrontal cortex, hippocampus, amygdala, and cerebellum, whereas CB2 receptors are primarily located in immune cells [24, 41].

THC, as well as other CB1 receptor agonists, has inhibitory effects on the release of GABA and glutamate. Excitatory effects on dopamine (DA) are also evident, leading to an increase in the level of extracellular DA [42].

The chemical dependence on *C. sativa* develops in about 10% of the people who experience the plant, being more common and on higher levels of use at an early age [48]. Withdrawal syndrome was recognized and added to DSM-5 in 2014, mainly due to the increase with the number of treatment episodes to chronic users of *Cannabis* in the last years [49]. These treatments involve psychosocial approaches, but only 20% of patients achieve definitive abstinence [50], manifesting a clear need to develop effective treatments for this pathology.

Studies using positron emission tomography revealed a significantly lower availability of CB1 receptors between *Cannabis* smokers and nonsmokers, in which the level of downregulation correlated with the time of *Cannabis* use [46]. Interestingly, after a 30-day abstinence period, there was an increase in CB1 receptor availability to levels comparable to healthy controls [6, 51].

For the diagnosis of *C. sativa* withdrawal, it is necessary to have criteria such as (1) the development in specific syndrome of the substance due to cessation or reduction in use; (2) the syndrome causes clinically significant distress or impairment in social, occupational, or other important areas of functioning; and (3) the symptoms are not due to a general medical condition and are not better accounted for by another mental disorder [52].

Following the recognition by the ICD-10 (International Statistical Classification of Diseases and Related Health Problems) system of *Cannabis* withdrawal, the demand for treatment of *Cannabis* abuse has grown in several countries and a large proportion of adults and adolescents who participate in the outpatient treatments have difficulty in achieving and maintaining *Cannabis* withdrawal [53].

3.1. Symptoms of withdrawal syndrome

Experimental studies on *Cannabis* withdrawal in humans began in the 1970s and showed moderate withdrawal symptoms (such as transient nervousness) following cessation of marijuana use and more robust symptoms (restlessness, sleep problems, poor appetite, and disorientation). In the 1980s, new withdrawal symptoms were reported as decreased appetite/weight loss, hostility, irritability, mild nausea, lack of cooperation, restlessness, sleep EEG changes (increased REM sleep), and sleep/insomnia difficulties. These symptoms started within 5–6 h of the last dose and decreased by 96 h with a reduction in weight and sleep. Changes in EEG (i.e., increase in REM) are also observed [54, 55].

More recent studies have demonstrated *Cannabis* withdrawal syndrome associated with significantly increased outcomes of anxiety, depression, and irritability; decrease in sleep quality and quantity indices; and decreased food intake [56]. Symptoms such as stomach pain and decreased assessments of contentment, friendliness, language, sociability, and energy were also reported. Most of the mood symptoms begin within 48 h after cessation and appear to peak at day 3 or 4 of the withdrawal phases, and it is interesting to note that studies of oral THC use have not reported sleep disturbances during the withdrawal phases [57].

The symptoms reached the highest levels of aggression on days 3 and 7 of abstinence and lasted until day 28, being reported for up to 6 months after cessation of use, showing an effect transient. Among chronic and daily users, the appetite decreased after day 9 of abstinence, anxiety occurred between days 1 and 11, irritability was greatest on days 1–14, and the mood was lower on days 3–9 and was higher on days 1–10. Daily users have higher levels of anxiety, irritability, nervousness, restlessness, tremors, difficulty sleeping, stomach pain, strange dreams, excessive sweating, negative mood, physical symptoms, and decreased appetite during the abstinence period, suggesting reliable studies of *Cannabis* abstinence [58, 59].

4. Treatment of withdrawal syndrome

Although there are more than 160 million *Cannabis* users in the world, no pharmacological therapy currently available is considered adequate for the treatment of symptoms caused during the withdrawal syndrome. The known effects of withdrawal syndrome, which occur when drug use is deprived and disappear with the reintroduction of Δ9-THC [60], favor the recurrence of use by users attempting to stop. The main compounds that have activity on the cannabinoid receptor and mechanisms related to *Cannabis* withdrawal syndrome are as follows.

4.1. Agonist compounds

The involvement of the CB1 receptor with the development of dependence, as well as the expression of withdrawal symptoms, has already been evidenced in several animal experiments. Therefore, it is suggested that treatment with low doses of CB1 receptor agonists could reduce the severity of withdrawal symptoms [61]. Low doses of Δ9-THC were tested to improve withdrawal symptoms; however, these doses exhibited reinforcing properties in chronic *Cannabis* users, eliminating THC as a viable treatment [62].

The endocannabinoids AEA and 2-AG, which are low and high efficiency agonists for the CB1 receptor, respectively, as well as fatty acid amide hydrolase (FAAH) enzymes responsible for the degradation of AEA and monoacylglycerol lipase (MAGL) responsible for the degradation of 2-AG were proposed as mediating mechanisms of *Cannabis* withdrawal but lack further enlightening studies [6, 63].

4.1.1. Synthetic cannabinoids

These synthetic cannabinoid agonists present themselves as promising molecules, providing ample reduction in *Cannabis* withdrawal symptoms (mood, sleep, and food intake), both in the laboratory and in clinical settings. Unlike the isomer of THC and derived from the *Cannabis* plant, dronabinol, the synthetic cannabinoid nabilone (**Figure 2**) has potential to reduce self-administration of *Cannabis,* presenting as more promising for treatment [64].

Nabilone has more predictable side effects, and it is well tolerated among *Cannabis* users, better bioavailability, and longer duration of action than dronabinol, allowing the end of abstinence with a single daily dose [65]. In addition, nabilone produces non-*Cannabis* urinary

http://dx.doi.org/10.5772/intechopen.82184

biomarkers that allow monitoring of abstinence through the use of standard urine toxicology during nabilone maintenance, but this consistently decreases *Cannabis* self-administration in the laboratory, ensuring that testing occurs in a clinical setting [66].

4.1.2. *α2a adrenergic receptor agonist*

Preclinical data have demonstrated that abstinence of cannabinoid is associated with adrenergic hyperactivity [67], and that α2 receptors agonists decrease the withdrawal symptoms of THC. Therefore, the α2a adrenergic receptor agonist, lofexidine (**Figure 3**), has been tested, and its use has improved sleep during the abstinence period and decreased *Cannabis* relapse [68] but is poorly tolerated even at less frequent doses and at lower target dose (0.6 mg three times a day), with 40% of patients presenting dizziness and fatigue [69]. Another α2-adrenergic agonist, guanfacine hydrochloride (**Figure 3**), which improves memory performance in humans, was tested on the hypothesis that nocturnal administration of this drug would reduce *Cannabis* withdrawal while producing little evidence of sedation or hypotension. Daily administration of the compound significantly reduced irritability, produced small but significant decreases in blood pressure and heart rate, however was well tolerated, producing no sedation, dizziness, or altered food intake observed with lofexidine. Due to these results, guanfacine hydrochloride stands out as one of the first non-cannabinoid agonists to reduce *cannabis* abstinence-related irritability [64, 70].

Despite reductions in certain withdrawal symptoms, guanfacine did not reduce self-administration of *Cannabis* and did not worsen abstinence-related anorexia and weight loss but did not

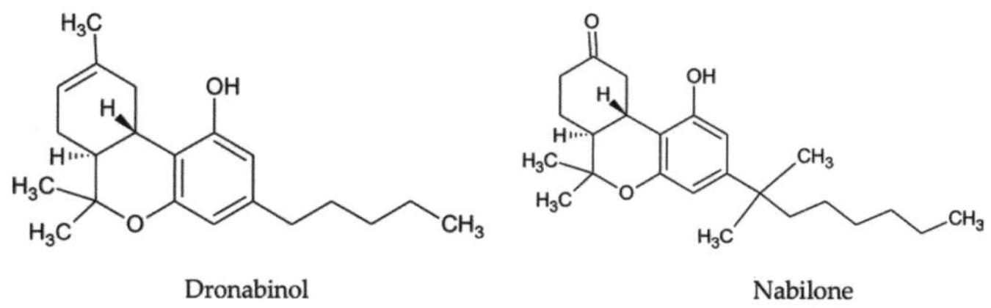

Figure 2. Chemical structure of isomer of THC, dronabinol and synthetic cannabinoid, and nabilone.

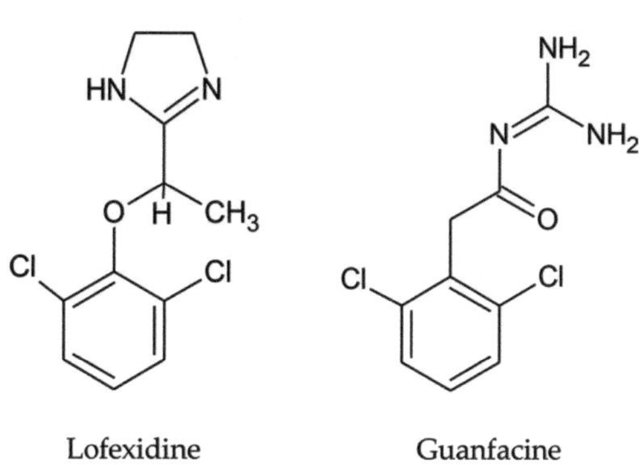

Figure 3. Chemical structure of α2a adrenergic receptor agonist.

improve both. In contrast, lofexidine decreased self-administration of *Cannabis* in the laboratory after abstinence but worsened the performance of psychomotor tasks [68].

4.1.3. *Nabiximols*

Nabiximols are used to treat muscle spasticity associated with multiple sclerosis. These produce little intoxication, tolerance, or abstinence. They are oral spray medications containing THC, cannabidiol (CBD), and various terpenoids (**Figure 4**) derived from *C. sativa* plants. Once CBD attenuated the paranoia and euphoria associated with THC studies, nabiximols were used to treat *Cannabis* withdrawal and observed that they attenuated abstinence symptoms and improved patient compliance to treatment, as well as reducing irritability and depression of the users [71].

The indirect CBD agonist, which has a relatively low affinity for CB1 and CB2 receptors, inhibits AEA reuptake and hydrolysis while maintaining CB1 receptor stimulation, thus potentiating endocannabinoid transmission and emerging as an alternative treatment for the abstinence syndrome of *C. sativa* [72]. It is a compound with no significant adverse effects even with chronic

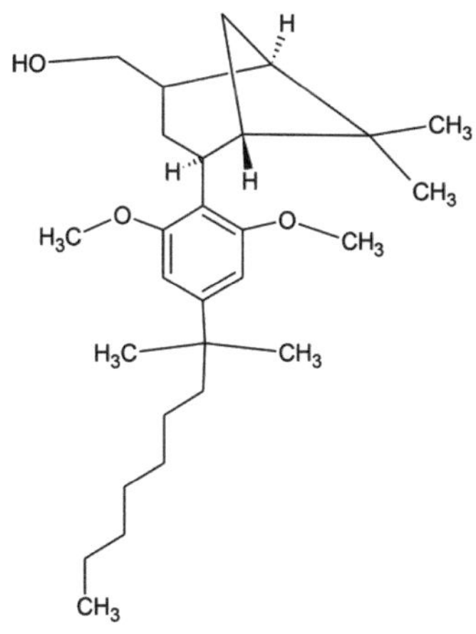

Nabiximols

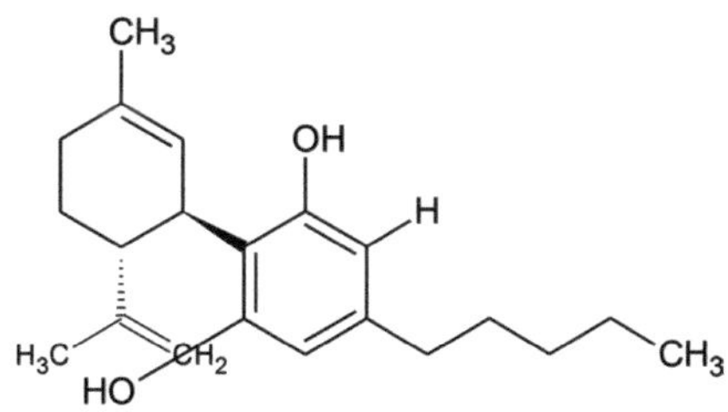

Cannabidiol (CBD)

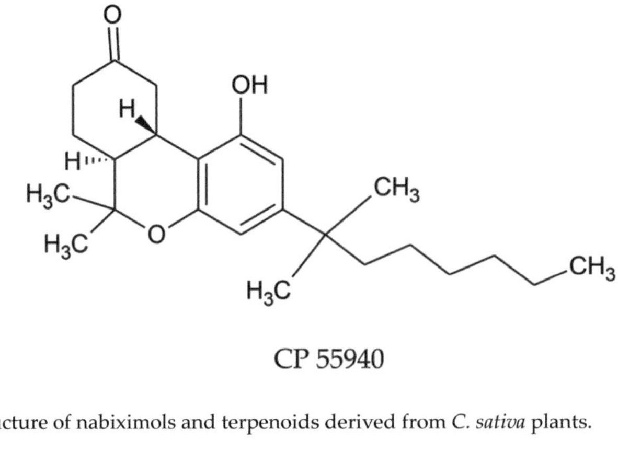

CP 55940

Figure 4. Chemical structure of nabiximols and terpenoids derived from *C. sativa* plants.

and high dose use. Due to this property on the endocannabinoid system, CBD has several pharmacological effects, including anxiolytic, antipsychotic, neuroprotective, antiinflammatory, and antiemetic actions, favoring its use in the treatment of *Cannabis* withdrawal syndrome [73, 74].

Comparative studies of the use of nabiximols and dronabinol concluded that they did not produce significant cognitive or psychomotor adverse effects and showed a similar or lower reinforcement potential than dronabinol at lower doses [71, 75]. However, high doses of both drugs exhibited some potential for a booster. This fact highlights the need for careful monitoring related to drug administration during future studies and clinical practice for treatment of dependence and abstinence from *Cannabis* with nabiximols.

4.2. Antagonists

The use of CB1 cannabinoid receptor antagonists is more related to the treatment of *C. sativa* dependence than to the treatment of withdrawal syndrome triggered by the withdrawal of this use in chronic users, as much as characteristic symptoms of withdrawal syndrome such as insomnia, dysphoria, and anxiety manifesting with the use of the CB1 receptor antagonist, rimonabant (also known as SR 141716A) (**Figure 5**) [8]. For this reason, the rimonabant, previously used in the treatment of obesity, was removed from the market in 2008, but it is useful in inducing signs of withdrawal in *Cannabis*-dependent individuals. One of the explanations is that the neural circuits involved with the serotonergic, noradrenergic, and dopaminergic systems have been shown to be sensitive to CB1 receptor antagonists [76, 77].

It is important to mention that the endogenous opioid system also contributes to the dependence of *Cannabis* because it also has G protein-coupled membrane receptors [78], and users of opioid-dependent *Cannabis* are less likely to experience withdrawal symptoms. Opioid receptor antagonists, such as naltrexone, reduce self-administration of *C. sativa* and their subjective positive effects in chronic plant users [79].

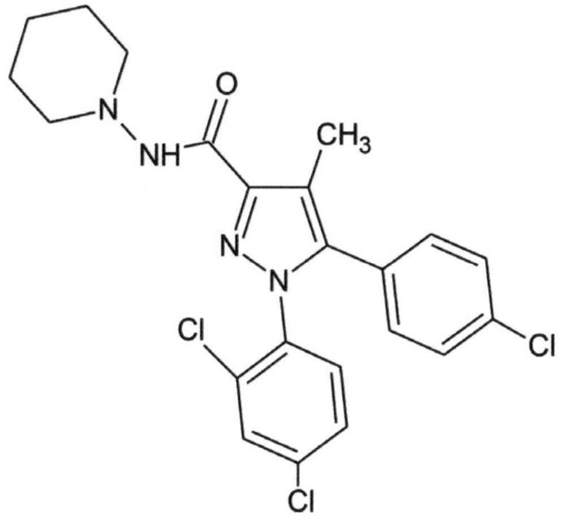

Figure 5. Chemical structure of SR 141716A.

5. New studies on the treatment of withdrawal syndrome

There are no drugs approved for the treatment of addiction or withdrawal syndrome of *Cannabis*. Pharmacotherapy in these cases is focused exclusively on symptoms such as increased anxiety, insomnia, loss of appetite, migraine, and irritability. We disclose these symptoms being a result of desensitization of CB1 receptors by THC studies advancing toward the development of compounds that act selectively at this receptor. There are four main chemical classes of exogenous cannabinoid ligands under study: (a) classical cannabinoids such as Δ9-THC, AM2389, cannabinol, nabilone, HU-210, and other tricyclic terpenoid derivatives, such as Δ9-tetrahydrocannabivarin (Δ9-THCV) (**Figure 6**), which contains a polar benzopyran moiety attached to a hydrophilic (*n*-pentyl) alkyl terminus [80]; (b) the nonclassical cannabinoids CP 55,940, HU-308 (**Figure 7**) and other bicyclic and tricyclic analogs of Δ9-THC without the pyran ring of classical cannabinoids [81]; (c) the aminoalkylindoles WIN55,212-2, JWH-018, JWH-073, and AM1241 (**Figure 8**), which differ in structure, lipophilicity, and binding activity at cannabinoid receptors compared to nonclassical cannabinoids [82]; and (d) biarylpyrazole ligands such as rimonabant and AM251 antagonists, which are selective for the CB1 receptor, and SR144528 (**Figure 9**), which is selective for the CB2 receptor [83].

5.1. *In vivo* and *in vitro*

It is known that because cannabinoid receptors, when bound by agonists or antagonists, have the potential to treat a variety of pathologies such as pain, neurodegeneration, obesity, tumors,

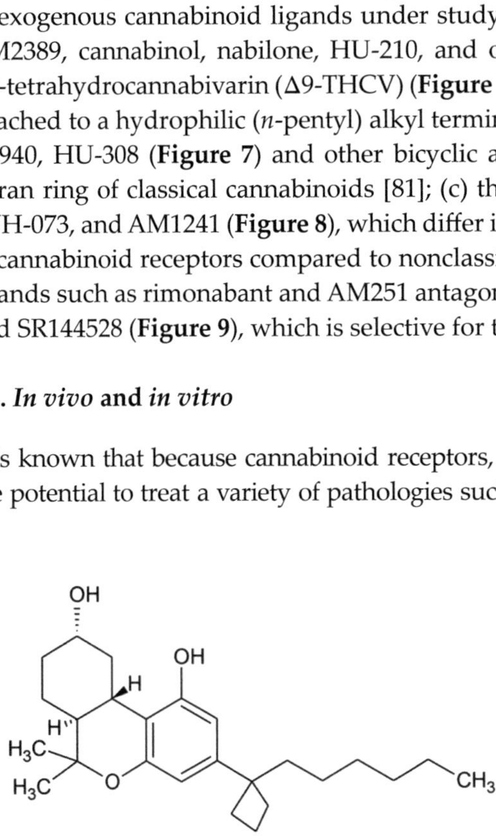

AM2389

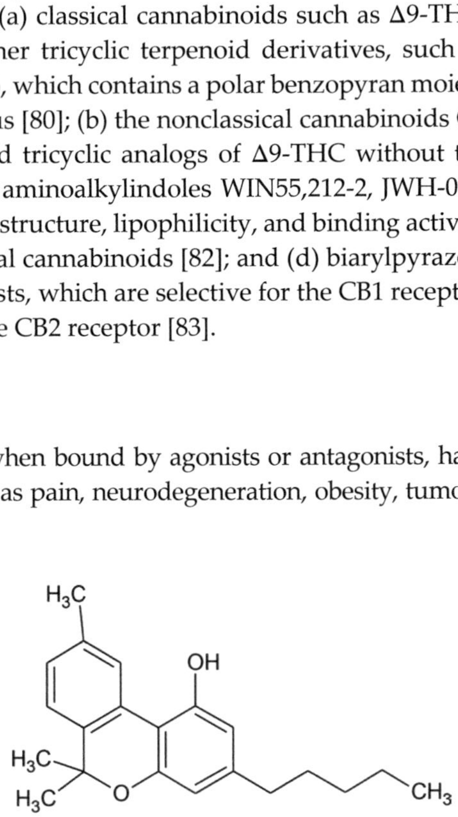

Canabinol

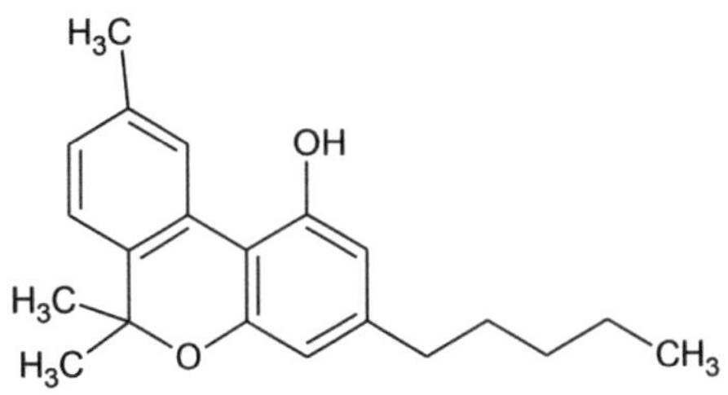

HU – 210

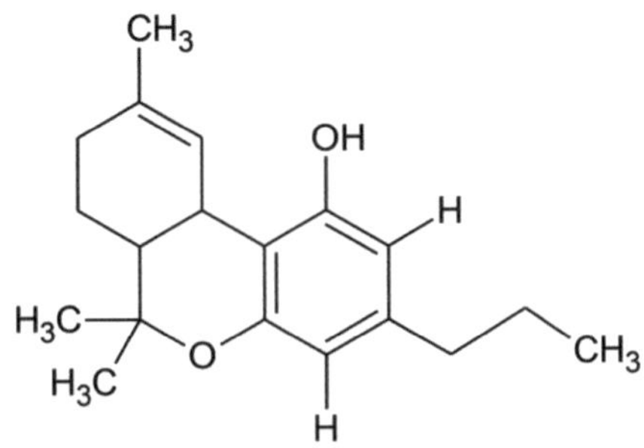

Δ^9-Tetrahydrocannabivarin (Δ^9-THCV)

Figure 6. Chemical structure of classical cannabinoids.

chemical dependency, and immune function, it is important to develop in vitro bioassays activity determination and the function of these receptors [84]. The *in vitro* assays established in the studies related to CB1 and CB2 receptors involve the use of membranes or tissues containing

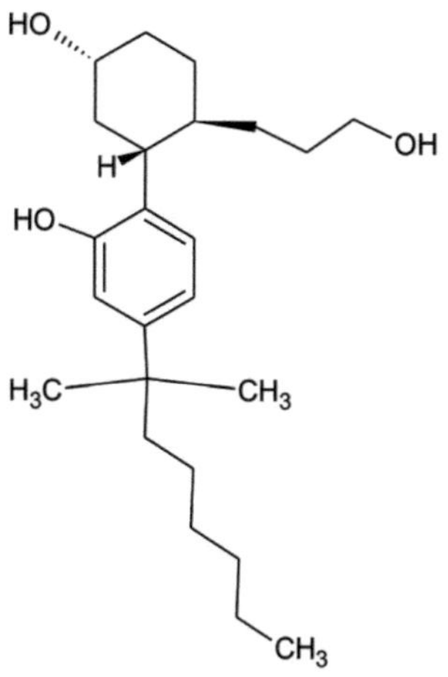

CP55,940

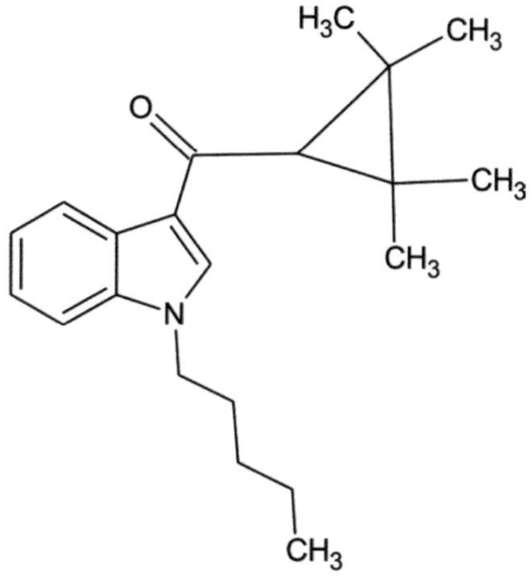

HU 308

Figure 7. Chemical structure of the non-classical cannabinoids.

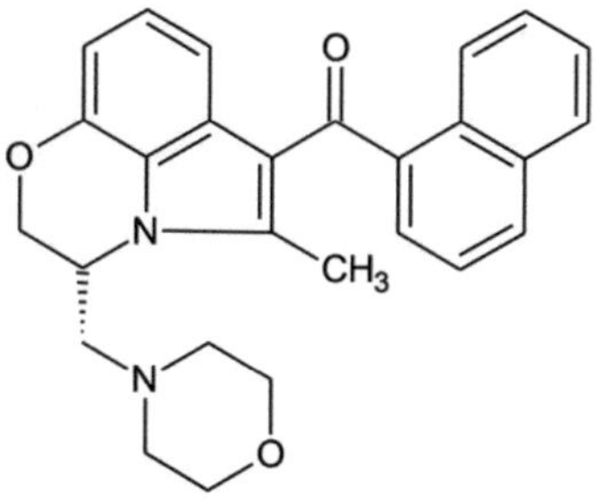

WIN55,212-2

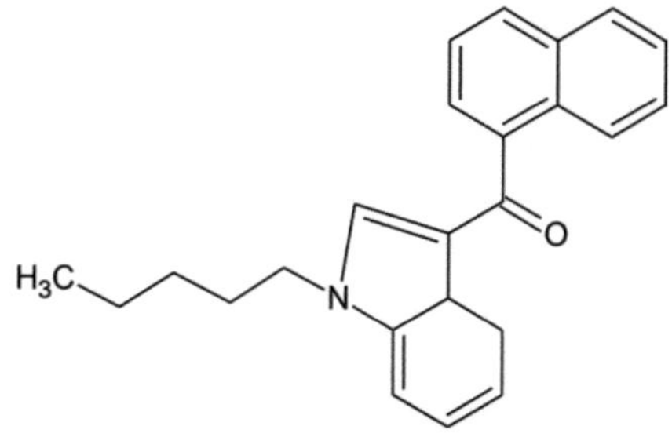

JWH-018

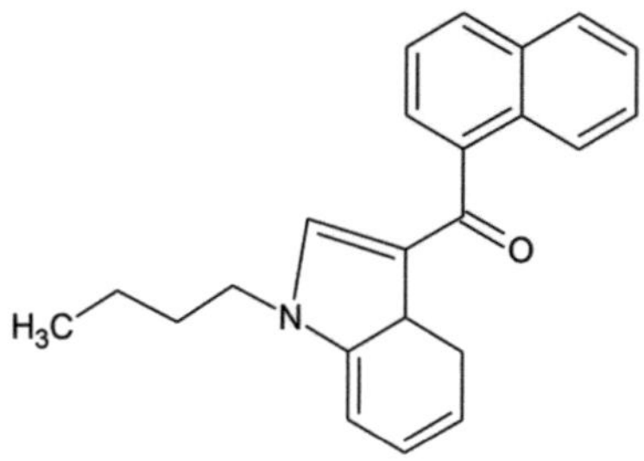

JWH-073

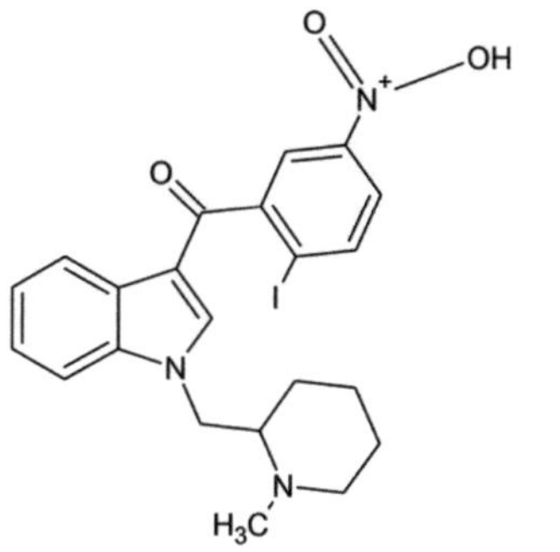

AM1241

Figure 8. Chemical structure of the aminoalkylindoles.

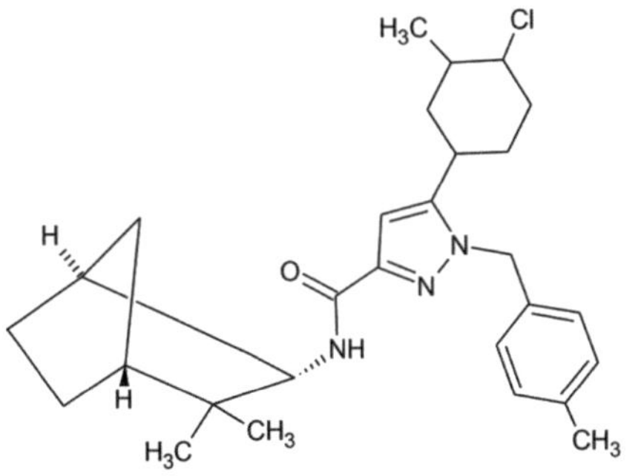

SR144528

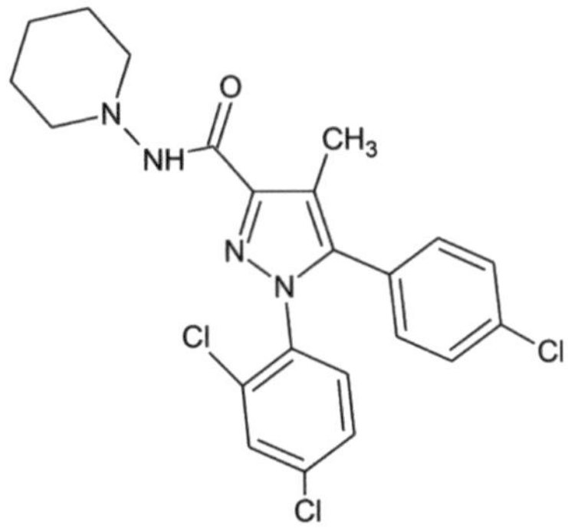

AM 251

Figure 9. Chemical structure of the biarylpyrazole ligands such as rimonabant and AM251 antagonists.

these receptors [85]. Of particular note is the assay using radiolabeled CB1 or CB2 receptors with [^{3}H] CP55940 (**Figure 10**) and bioassays with preparations of nerve-smooth muscle where the ability of the molecule under study to produce inhibition or excitation of cannabinoid receptors is verified [86].

In vitro functional bioassays measure the effects of synthetic cannabinoids and their metabolites in relation to cannabinoid receptor signaling CB1/CB2, evaluating the production of cyclic ATP and elevation of intracellular calcium. In the middle of the last century, initial studies on the effects of cannabinoids used Gayer's tests (found at the time as a useful test for the effects of THC [87]), where corneal areflexia was measured in rabbits, catatonia in mice, and increased defecation and aggressiveness in rats stressed by REM sleep deprivation [88]. In mice, high-dose catalepsy with Δ9-THC was also observed [95]. In rodents, the main bioassay is the measurement of locomotor activity, rectal temperature, and analgesia (in the tail or hot plate test) [89].

The sum of the various symptoms observed in the initial studies originated characteristic effects in laboratory animals called cannabinoid tetrad and being characterized by hypothermia, analgesia, catalepsy, and locomotor suppression [90]. This tetrad is widely used nowadays because, since the data obtained through its observation are qualitatively consistent, it is common to evaluate the dose-dependence relation of cannabinoids quickly and without any specific training of the animals, a fact that is configured as an advantage [89].

The Δ9-THC dependency/withdrawal modeling studies are based on the cannabinoid tetrad in which The triggered effects are verified with the administration of cannabinoid antagonist (usually rimonabant), and precipitation withdrawal symptoms, being, in general, the synthetic cannabinoids such as UR-144 (**Figure 11**), responsible to promote effects greater than that of Δ9-THC [91].

Studies in rats revealed that individual enzyme activity mainly related to the genetic polymorphisms of cytochrome P450 enzymes in the phase I metabolism of cannabinoids has an important role in determining the response of an individual on the use of cannabinoids [92]. Thus, an individual may experience attenuated effects and other individual effects exacerbated by

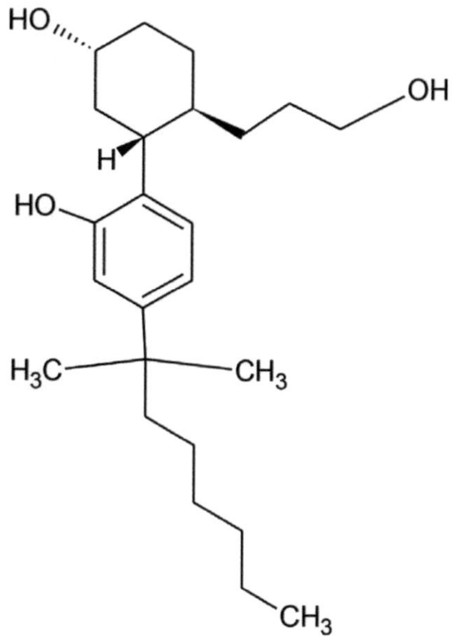

Figure 10. Chemical structure of the CP55940.

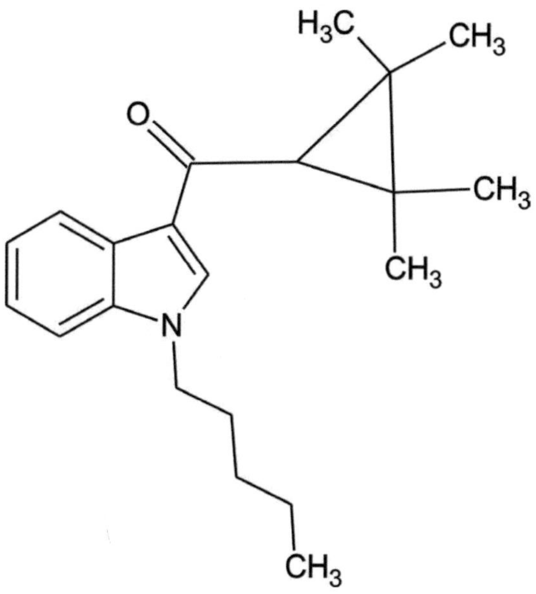

Figure 11. Chemical structure UR-144.

cannabinoids, depending on the liver enzyme profile that favors the formation of antagonistic or agonist metabolites, respectively [93].

Technological refinement has led to the use of new techniques and different experimental models [94] in the studies of compounds in potential for reinforcement, with the search for new targets and biomarkers [95]. Among the experimental models emerges the *Danio rerio (Zebrafish)*, a small fish, because it has the facility of genetic manipulation and the biology of its development [96]. *Zebrafish* is particularly useful for measuring changes in the development of the nervous system [97], and its measures of sensorimotor plasticity, emotional function, cognition, and social interaction have been used to characterize the adverse effects of drug abuse such as Δ9-THC [98, 99] due to phylogenetic analyzes, which reveal the endocannabinoid system as highly conserved between *Zebrafish* and mammals [100].

Tolerance and cross-tolerance tests for cannabinoids are also performed *in vivo*, although studies indicate that not all effects of cannabinoids are developed during these tests, for example, adrenocorticotropic hormone (ACTH) secretion is not observed in rodents during these tests, indicating low reliability and the need for greater improvement *in vivo* methods used in this sense [101, 102].

5.2. *In silico*

There are several computational methods; among them, homology modeling is being used in cannabinoid studies [103], considering that the drugs utilized during the withdrawal syndrome of *C. sativa* act at a symptomatic level. The resolution of the crystalline structure of the CB1cannabinoid receptor is recent [19], and this fact favored *in silico* studies that evolve toward the planning of molecules that act as selective agonists of this receptor, mainly studies related to better understanding of the interaction and the relation structure-activity of

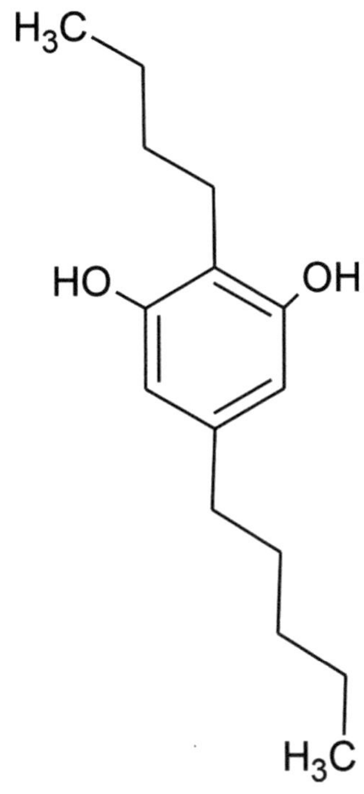

Figure 12. Chemical structure of Stemphol.

synthetic cannabinoids [104]. A study can be mentioned where computational tools were used, with the objective of proposing drug candidates for the treatment of the abstinence syndrome based on the natural ligands of this receptor. A particular compound derived from marine fungi, stemphol (**Figure 12**) [105], presented positive predictions regarding pharmacokinetic and toxicological properties for a human CB1 receptor ligand, in addition to having a relatively simple molecular structure. Due to these computational results and the recent crystallographic elucidation of the cannabinoid CB1 receptor [20], experimental studies are being conducted for the development of candidate pharmacotherapeutic alternatives for the treatment of *C. sativa* withdrawal syndrome [106].

6. Conclusion

Studies on cannabinoids were stimulated after the characterization and structural elucidation of Δ9-THC in the 1960s, and later on, the discovery of the cannabinoid system represented by CB1/CB2 receptors and binding substances to these receptors. Many *in vitro, in vivo,* and *in silico* trials have been developed in the last decades, and advances mainly regarding the mechanism of addiction, abuse, and withdrawal syndrome have been achieved. However, with the use of cannabinoid-based drugs and the chemical development of synthetic cannabinoids, further studies into these mechanisms are relevant, especially considering that Δ9-THC is a low-efficacy cannabinoid compared to the "new cannabinoids."

It is expected in the future that the investigations will deepen the knowledge on the mechanisms of the cannabinoids, especially those that cause chemical dependence, both as cannabinoid system and as noncanabinoid physiological systems. In this way, it is possible to increase the knowledge about the different classes of these substances and, therefore, favor the development of new models and improvement of the tests currently used in the studies related to *C. sativa*.

Author details

Jaderson Vieira Ferreira, Lenir Cabral Correa, Daniel Castro da Costa
and Lorane Izabel da Silva Hage-Melim*

*Address all correspondence to: loranehage@gmail.com

Laboratory of Pharmaceutical and Medicinal Chemistry (PharMedChem),
Federal University of Amapá, Macapá, Brazil

References

[1] Degenhardt L, Chiu WT, Sampson N, Kessler RC, Anthony JC, Angermeyer M, et al. Toward a global view of alcohol, tobacco, cannabis, and cocaine use: Findings from the WHO world mental health surveys. PLoS Medicine. 2008;**5**(7):1053-1067

[2] Datwyler S, Weiblen GD. Genetic variation in hemp and marijuana (*Cannabis sativa* L.) according to amplified fragment length polymorphisms. Journal of Forensic Sciences. 2006;**51**(2):371-375

[3] Di Forti M, Murray RM. Cannabis, skunk and spice: The evolving risk of psychosis. Schizophrenia Studies. 2014;**153**:S31. Available from: http://linkinghub.elsevier.com/retrieve/pii/S0920996414701045

[4] Lachenmeier DW, Rehm J. Comparative risk assessment of alcohol, tobacco, cannabis and other illicit drugs using the margin of exposure approach. Scientific Reports. 2015;**5**(1):8126. Available from: http://www.nature.com/articles/srep08126

[5] Kerridge BT, Pickering R, Chou P, Saha TD, Hasin DS. DSM-5 cannabis use disorder in the National Epidemiologic Survey on Alcohol and Related Conditions-III: Gender-specific profiles. Addictive Behaviors. 2018;**76**:52-60. Available from: https://www-sciencedirect-com.ez7.periodicos.capes.gov.br/science/article/pii/S0306460317302721

[6] Schlienz NJ, Budney AJ, Lee DC, Vandrey R. Cannabis withdrawal: A review of neurobiological mechanisms and sex differences. Current Addiction Reports. 2017;**4**(2):75-81. Available from: https://link-springer-com.ez7.periodicos.capes.gov.br/content/pdf/10.1007%2Fs40429-017-0143-1.pdf

[7] D'Souza DC, Cortes-Briones JA, Ranganathan M, Thurnauer H, Creatura G, Surti T, et al. Rapid changes in cannabinoid 1 receptor availability in cannabis-dependent male subjects after abstinence from cannabis. Biological Psychiatry: Cognitive Neuroscience and Neuroimaging. 2016;**1**(1):60-67. Available from: https://www-sciencedirect-com.ez7.periodicos.capes.gov.br/science/article/pii/S2451902215000099

[8] Bonnet U, Preuss U. The cannabis withdrawal syndrome: Current insights. Substance Abuse and Rehabilitation. 2017;**8**:9-37. Available from http://www.ncbi.nlm.nih.gov/pubmed/28490916

[9] Hesse M, Thylstrup B. The cannabis withdrawal syndrome-symptoms and time course. In: Handbook of Cannabis and Related Pathologies: Biology, Pharmacology, Diagnosis, and Treatment. London: Elsevier; 2017. pp. 1066-1073. Available from: http://linkinghub.elsevier.com/retrieve/pii/B9780128007563001289

[10] Volkow ND, Swanson JM, Evins AE, DeLisi LE, Meier MH, Gonzalez R, et al. Effects of cannabis use on human behavior, including cognition,motivation, and psychosis: A review. JAMA Psychiatry. American Medical Association. 2016;**73**:292-297. Available from: http://archpsyc.jamanetwork.com/article.aspx?doi=10.1001/jamapsychiatry.2015.3278

[11] De Luca MA, Di Chiara G, Cadoni C, Lecca D, Orsolini L, Papanti D, et al. Cannabis; epidemiological, neurobiological and psychopathological issues: An update. CNS & Neurological Disorders—Drug Targets. 2017;**16**(5):598-609. Available from: http://www.eurekaselect.com/151581/article

[12] Hasin DS. US Epidemiology of Cannabis Use and Associated Problems. Neuropsychopharmacology. Vol. 43. New York: Nature Publishing Group; 2018. p. 195-212. Available from: http://www.nature.com/doifinder/10.1038/npp.2017.198

[13] Awasthi R, An G, Donovan MD, Boles Ponto LL. Relating observed psychoactive effects to the plasma concentrations of delta-9-tetrahydrocannabinol and its active metabolite: An effect-compartment modeling approach. Journal of Pharmaceutical Sciences. 2018;**107**(2):745-755. Available from: https://www-sciencedirect-com.ez7.periodicos.capes.gov.br/science/article/pii/S0022354917306329

[14] Dinis-Oliveira RJ. Metabolomics of Delta-9-tetrahydrocannabinol: Implications in Toxicity. Drug Metabolism Reviews. Vol. 48. London: Taylor & Francis; 2016. pp. 80-87. Available from: http://www.tandfonline.com/doi/full/10.3109/03602532.2015.1137307

[15] Viera AJ, Neutze DM. Diagnosis of secondary hypertension: An age-based approach. American Family Physician. 2010;**82**(12):1471-1478

[16] Lynch ME, Ware MA. Cannabinoids for the Treatment of Chronic Non-Cancer Pain: An Updated Systematic Review of Randomized Controlled Trials. Journal of Neuroimmune Pharmacology. Vol. 10. Washington: Springer US; 2015. pp. 293-301. Available from: http://link.springer.com/10.1007/s11481-015-9600-6

[17] Panagis G. Cannabinoid reward and dependence: Focus on the main psychoactive ingredients of marijuana in preclinical studies. In: Handbook of Cannabis and Related Pathologies: Biology, Pharmacology, Diagnosis, and Treatment. London: Elsevier; 2017. p. 659-670. Available from: http://linkinghub.elsevier.com/retrieve/pii/B978012800756300079X

[18] Bonnet U, Borda T, Scherbaum N, Specka M. Abstinence phenomena of chronic cannabis-addicts prospectively monitored during controlled inpatient detoxification (Part II): Psychiatric complaints and their relation to delta-9-tetrahydrocannabinol and its metabolites in serum. Drug and Alcohol Dependence. 2015;**155**:302-306. Available from: http://www.ncbi.nlm.nih.gov/pubmed/25127704

[19] Hua T, Vemuri K, Pu M, Qu L, Han GW, Wu Y, et al. Crystal structure of the human cannabinoid receptor CB1. Cell. 2016;**167**(3):750-762.e14

[20] Shao Z, Yin J, Chapman K, Grzemska M, Clark L, Wang J, et al. High-resolution crystal structure of the human CB1 cannabinoid receptor. Nature. 2016;**540**(7634):1-20. Available from: http://www.nature.com/doifinder/10.1038/nature20613

[21] Song ZH, Slowey CA, Hurst DP, Reggio PH. The difference between the CB(1) and CB(2) cannabinoid receptors at position 5.46 is crucial for the selectivity of WIN55212-2 for CB(2). Molecular Pharmacology. 1999;**56**(4):834-840. Available from: http://www.molpharm.org

[22] Sierra S, Luquin N, Rico AJ, Gómez-Bautista V, Roda E, Dopeso-Reyes IG, et al. Detection of cannabinoid receptors CB1 and CB2 within basal ganglia output neurons in macaques: Changes following experimental parkinsonism. Brain Structure and Function. 2015;**220**(5):2721-2738. Available from: http://link.springer.com/10.1007/s00429-014-0823-8

[23] Onaivi ES, Ishiguro H, Liu Q-R. Cannabinoid CB2 receptor mechanism of *Cannabis sativa* L. In: *Cannabis sativa* L—Botany and Biotechnology. Cham: Springer International Publishing; 2017. pp. 227-247. Available from: http://link.springer.com/10.1007/978-3-319-54564-6_10

[24] Zhang P-W, Ishiguro H, Ohtsuki T, Hess J, Carillo F, Walther D, et al. Human cannabinoid receptor 1: 5′ exons, candidate regulatory regions, polymorphisms, haplotypes and association with polysubstance abuse. Molecular Psychiatry. 2004;**9**(10):916-931

[25] Araque A, Castillo PE, Manzoni OJ, Tonini R. Synaptic functions of endocannabinoid signaling in health and disease. Neuropharmacology. 2017;**124**:13-24. DOI: 10.1016/j.neuropharm.2017.06.017

[26] Sido JM, Nagarkatti PS, Nagarkatti M. Role of Endocannabinoid Activation of Peripheral CB1 Receptors in the Regulation of Autoimmune Disease. International Reviews of Immunology. Vol. 34. London, New York: Informa Healthcare; 2015. pp. 403-414. Available from: http://www.tandfonline.com/doi/full/10.3109/08830185.2014.921165

[27] Verdurand M, Nguyen V, Stark D, Zahra D, Gregoire MC, Greguric I, et al. Comparison of cannabinoid CB(1) receptor binding in adolescent and adult rats: A positron emission tomography study using [F]MK-9470. International Journal of Molecular Imaging. 2011;**2011**:548123. Available from: http://www.ncbi.nlm.nih.gov/pubmed/22187642%5Cnhttp://www.ncbi.nlm.nih.gov/pmc/articles/PMC3236487/pdf/IJMI2011-548123.pdf

[28] Mallipeddi S, Janero DR, Zvonok N, Makriyannis A. Functional selectivity at G-protein coupled receptors: Advancing cannabinoid receptors as drug targets. Biochemical Pharmacology. 2017;**128**:1-11. DOI: 10.1016/j.bcp.2016.11.014

[29] Howlett AC. International union of pharmacology. XXVII. Classification of cannabinoid receptors. Pharmacological Reviews. 2002;**54**(2):161-202. Available from: http://pharmrev.aspetjournals.org/cgi/doi/10.1124/pr.54.2.161

[30] Howlett AC. Cannabinoid inhibition of adenylate cyclase. Biochemistry of the response in neuroblastoma cell membranes. Molecular Pharmacology. 1985;**27**(4):429-436

[31] Mu J, Zhuang SY, Hampson RE, Deadwyler SA. Protein kinase-dependent phosphorylation and cannabinoid receptor modulation of potassium A current (IA) in cultured rat hippocampal neurons. Pflügers Archiv: European Journal of Physiology. 2000;**439**(5):541-546. Available from: http://www.ncbi.nlm.nih.gov/pubmed/10764212

[32] Chang L, Karin M. Mammalian MAP kinase signalling cascades. Nature. 2001;**410**(6824):37-40

[33] Abbott LF, Nelson SB. Synaptic plasticity: Taming the beast. Nature Neuroscience. 2000;**3**(November):1178-1183

[34] Augustin SM, Lovinger DM. Functional relevance of endocannabinoid-dependent synaptic plasticity in the central nervous system. ACS Chemical Neuroscience. 2018;**9**(9):2146-2161. Available from: http://pubs.acs.org/doi/10.1021/acschemneuro.7b00508

[35] Auclair N, Otani S, Soubrie P, Crepel F. Cannabinoids modulate synaptic strength and plasticity at glutamatergic synapses of rat prefrontal cortex pyramidal neurons. Journal of Neurophysiology. 2000;**83**(6):3287-3293

[36] Lile JA, Fogel JS, Kelly TH. The role of γ-aminobutyric acid in the interoceptive effects of oral Δ9-tetrahydrocannabinol in humans. In: Handbook of Cannabis and Related Pathologies: Biology, Pharmacology, Diagnosis, and Treatment. London: Elsevier; 2017. pp. 770-778. Available from: http://linkinghub.elsevier.com/retrieve/pii/B9780128007563000909

[37] Howlett AC, Breivogel CS, Childers SR, Deadwyler SA, Hampson RE, Porrino LJ. Cannabinoid physiology and pharmacology: 30 years of progress. Neuropharmacology. 2004;**47**:345-358. Available from: http://linkinghub.elsevier.com/retrieve/pii/S0028390804002205

[38] Volk DW, Lewis DA. The Role of Endocannabinoid Signaling in Cortical Inhibitory Neuron Dysfunction in Schizophrenia. Biological Psychiatry. Vol. 79. London: Elsevier; 2016. pp. 595-603. Available from: http://www.ncbi.nlm.nih.gov/pubmed/26210060

[39] Davies SN, Pertwee RG, Riedel G. Functions of cannabinoid receptors in the hippocampus. Neuropharmacology. 2002;**42**(8):993-1007

[40] Beinfeld MC, Connolly K. Activation of CB1 cannabinoid receptors in rat hippocampal slices inhibits potassium-evoked cholecystokinin release, a possible mechanism contributing to the spatial memory defects produced by cannabinoids. Neuroscience Letters. 2001;**301**(1):69-71

[41] Smith GP, Jerome C, Cishing BJ, Eterno R, Simansky KJ. Abdominal vagotomy blockes the satiety effct of cholecystokinin in the rat. Science. 1981;**213**(13):1036-1037

[42] Zhang X, Feng ZJ, Chergui K. Induction of cannabinoid- and N-methyl-D-aspartate receptor-mediated long-term depression in the nucleus accumbens and dorsolateral striatum is region and age dependent. International Journal of Neuropsychopharmacology. 2014;**18**(4):1-9. Available from: https://academic.oup.com/ijnp/article-lookup/doi/10.1093/ijnp/pyu052

[43] Demuth DG, Molleman A. Cannabinoid signalling. Life Sciences. 2006;**78**(6):549-563

[44] Lu HC, MacKie K. An introduction to the endogenous cannabinoid system. Biological Psychiatry. 2016;**79**(7):516-525. DOI: 10.1016/j.biopsych.2015.07.028

[45] Gómez-Gálvez Y, Palomo-Garo C, Fernández-Ruiz J, García C. Potential of the cannabinoid CB2 receptor as a pharmacological target against inflammation in Parkinson's disease. Progress in Neuro-Psychopharmacology and Biological Psychiatry. 2016;**64**:200-208. DOI: 10.1016/j.pnpbp.2015.03.017

[46] Di Marzo V, Stella N, Zimmer A. Endocannabinoid signalling and the deteriorating brain. Nature Reviews Neuroscience. 2015;**16**(1):30-42. DOI: 10.1038/nrn3876

[47] Bossong MG, van Hell HH, Jager G, Kahn RS, Ramsey NF, Jansma JM. The endocannabinoid system and emotional processing: A pharmacological fMRI study with {increment}9-tetrahydrocannabinol. European Neuropsychopharmacology. 2013;**23**(12):1687-1697. DOI: 10.1016/j.euroneuro.2013.06.009

[48] Degenhardt L, Stockings E, Patton G, Hall WD, Lynskey M. The Increasing Global Health Priority of Substance Use in Young People. The Lancet Psychiatry. Vol. 3. London: Elsevier; 2016. pp. 251-264. Available from: https://www-sciencedirect-com.ez7.periodicos.capes.gov.br/science/article/pii/S2215036615005088

[49] Davis JP, Smith DC, Morphew JW, Lei X, Zhang S. Cannabis withdrawal, posttreatment abstinence, and days to first cannabis use among emerging adults in substance use treatment: A prospective study. Journal of Drug Issues. 2016;**46**(1):64-83. Available from: http://journals.sagepub.com/doi/10.1177/0022042615616431

[50] Blanco C, Hasin DS, Wall MM, Flórez-Salamanca L, Hoertel N, Wang S, et al. Cannabis use and risk of psychiatric disorders. JAMA Psychiatry. 2016;**73**(4):388. Available from: http://archpsyc.jamanetwork.com/article.aspx?doi=10.1001/jamapsychiatry.2015.3229

[51] Hirvonen J, Goodwin RS, Li CT, Terry GE, Zoghbi SS, Morse C, et al. Reversible and regionally selective downregulation of brain cannabinoid CB1receptors in chronic daily cannabis smokers. Molecular Psychiatry. 2012;**17**(6):642-649. Available from: http://www.nature.com/articles/mp201182

[52] Miller NS, Oberbarnscheidt T, Gold MS. Marijuana addictive disorders and DSM-5 substance-related disorders. Journal of Addiction Studies & Therapy. 2017;**11**:2-8. Available from: https://www.omicsonline.org/open-access/marijuana-addictive-disorders-and-dsm5-substancerelated-disorders-2155-6105-S11-013.php?aid=84734

[53] Brezing CA, Levin FR. The Current State of Pharmacological Treatments for Cannabis Use Disorder and Withdrawal. Neuropsychopharmacology. Vol. 43. New York: Nature Publishing Group; 2018. pp. 173-194. Available from: http://www.nature.com/doifinder/10.1038/npp.2017.212

[54] Herrmann ES, Weerts EM, Vandrey R. Sex differences in cannabis withdrawal symptoms among treatment-seeking cannabis users. Experimental and Clinical Psychopharmacology. 2015;**23**(6):415-421. Available from: http://doi.apa.org/getdoi.cfm?doi=10.1037/pha0000053

[55] Budney AJ, Hughes JR, Moore BA, Vandrey R. Review of the validity and significance of cannabis withdrawal syndrome. American Journal of Psychiatry. 2004;**161**(11):1967-1977

[56] De Aquino JP, Sherif M, Radhakrishnan R, Cahill JD, Ranganathan M, D'Souza DC. The psychiatric consequences of cannabinoids. Clinical Therapeutics. 2018;**40**(9):1448-1456. Available from: https://ac.els-cdn.com/S0149291818301061/1-s2.0-S0149291818301061-main.pdf?_tid=5b233e6c-c49a-43b6-b7c4-2976ac96ce15&acdnat=1526569968_c2402e4dfe4c86b4bae285609f244460

[57] Virani A, Bezchlibnyk-Butler K. Clinical Handbook of Psychotropic Drugs. 2012. 431 p. Available from: https://books.google.com.br/books?hl=pt-BR&lr=&id=TJ0nDwAAQBAJ&oi=fnd&pg=PP2&dq=More+recent+studies+have+evidenced+cannabis+withdrawal+syndrome+associated+with+significantly+increased+outcomes+of+anxiety,+depression,+and+irritability%3B+decrease+in+sleep+

[58] Zehra A, Burns J, Liu CK, Manza P, Wiers CE, Volkow ND, et al. Cannabis addiction and the brain: A review. Journal of Neuroimmune Pharmacology. 2018;**13**(4):438-452. Available from: http://link.springer.com/10.1007/s11481-018-9782-9

[59] Jacobus J, Squeglia LM, Escobar S, McKenna BM, Hernandez MM, Bagot KS, et al. Changes in marijuana use symptoms and emotional functioning over 28-days of monitored abstinence in adolescent marijuana users. Psychopharmacology. 2017;**234**(23-24): 3431-3442. Available from: http://link.springer.com/10.1007/s00213-017-4725-3

[60] Hines LA, Morley KI, Strang J, Agrawal A, Nelson EC, Statham D, et al. Onset of opportunity to use cannabis and progression from opportunity to dependence: Are influences consistent across transitions? Drug and Alcohol Dependence. 2016;**160**:57-64. Available from: http://linkinghub.elsevier.com/retrieve/pii/S037687161600003X

[61] Panlilio LV, Goldberg SR, Justinova Z. Cannabinoid Abuse and Addiction: Clinical and Preclinical Findings. Clinical Pharmacology and Therapeutics. Vol. 97. Hoboken: Wiley-Blackwell; 2015. pp. 616-627. Available from: http://doi.wiley.com/10.1002/cpt.118

[62] Crippa JAS, Hallak JEC, Machado-de-Sousa JP, Queiroz RHC, Bergamaschi M, Chagas MHN, et al. Cannabidiol for the treatment of cannabis withdrawal syndrome: A case report. Journal of Clinical Pharmacy and Therapeutics. 2013;**38**(2):162-164. Available from: http://doi.wiley.com/10.1111/jcpt.12018

[63] Lutz B, Marsicano G, Maldonado R, Hillard CJ. The Endocannabinoid System in Guarding Against Fear, Anxiety and Stress. Nature Reviews Neuroscience. Vol. 16. New York: Nature Publishing Group; 2015. pp. 705-718. Available from: http://www.nature.com/articles/nrn4036

[64] Haney M, Cooper ZD, Bedi G, Herrmann E, Comer SD, Reed SC, et al. Guanfacine decreases symptoms of cannabis withdrawal in daily cannabis smokers. Hoboken. Addiction Biology. 2018:**23**. DOI: 10.1111/adb.12621

[65] Bedi G, Foltin RW, Gunderson EW, Rabkin J, Hart CL, Comer SD, et al. Efficacy and tolerability of high-dose dronabinol maintenance in HIV-positive marijuana smokers: A controlled laboratory study. Psychopharmacology. 2010;**212**(4):675-686. Available from: http://link.springer.com/10.1007/s00213-010-1995-4

[66] Herrmann ES, Cooper ZD, Bedi G, Ramesh D, Reed SC, Comer SD, et al. Effects of zolpidem alone and in combination with nabilone on cannabis withdrawal and a laboratory model of relapse in cannabis users. Psychopharmacology. 2016;**233**(13):2469-2478. Available from: http://www.ncbi.nlm.nih.gov/pubmed/27085870

[67] Mendiguren A, Aostri E, Pineda J. Regulation of noradrenergic and serotonergic systems by cannabinoids: Relevance to cannabinoid-induced effects. Life Sciences. 2018;**192**(July):115-127. Available from: http://linkinghub.elsevier.com/retrieve/pii/S0024320517306069

[68] Haney M, Hart CL, Vosburg SK, Comer SD, Reed SC, Foltin RW. Effects of THC and lofexidine in a human laboratory model of marijuana withdrawal and relapse.

Psychopharmacology. 2008;**197**(1):157-168. Available from: http://link.springer.com/10.1007/s00213-007-1020-8

[69] Levin FR, Mariani JJ, Pavlicova M, Brooks D, Glass A, Mahony A, et al. Dronabinol and lofexidine for cannabis use disorder: A randomized, double-blind, placebo-controlled trial. Drug and Alcohol Dependence. 2016;**159**:53-60. DOI: 10.1016/j.drugalcdep.2015.11.025

[70] Mathai DS, Holst M, Rodgman C, Haile CN, Keller J, Hussain MZ, et al. Guanfacine attenuates adverse effects of dronabinol (THC) on working memory in adolescent-onset heavy cannabis users: A pilot study. The Journal of Neuropsychiatry and Clinical Neurosciences. 2017;**30**(1):66-76. Available from: https://psychiatryonline.org/doi/10.1176/appi.neuropsych.16120328

[71] Allsop DJ, Copeland J, Lintzeris N, Dunlop AJ, Montebello M, Sadler C, et al. Nabiximols as an agonist replacement therapy during cannabis withdrawal: A randomized clinical trial. JAMA Psychiatry. 2014;**71**(3):281-291

[72] Elmes MW, Kaczocha M, Berger WT, Leung KN, Ralph BP, Wang L, et al. Fatty acid-binding proteins (FABPs) are intracellular carriers for Δ9-tetrahydrocannabinol (THC) and cannabidiol (CBD). Journal of Biological Chemistry. 2015;**290**(14):8711-8721. Available from: http://www.ncbi.nlm.nih.gov/pubmed/25666611

[73] Blessing EM, Steenkamp MM, Manzanares J, Marmar CR. Cannabidiol as a Potential Treatment for Anxiety Disorders. Neurotherapeutics. Vol. 12. Washington: Springer US; 2015. pp. 825-836. Available from: http://link.springer.com/10.1007/s13311-015-0387-1

[74] Burstein S. Cannabidiol (CBD) and its analogs: A review of their effects on inflammation. Bioorganic and Medicinal Chemistry. 2015;**23**(7):1377-1385. DOI: 10.1016/j.bmc.2015.01.059

[75] Trigo JM, Lagzdins D, Rehm J, Selby P, Gamaleddin I, Fischer B, et al. Effects of fixed or self-titrated dosages of Sativex on cannabis withdrawal and cravings. Drug and Alcohol Dependence. 2016;**161**:298-306. Available from: http://www.ncbi.nlm.nih.gov/pubmed/26925704

[76] Hillard CJ. Cannabinoids and endocannabinoids. In: Encyclopedia of Psychopharmacology. Berlin, Heidelberg: Springer Berlin Heidelberg; 2015. pp. 329-336. Available from: http://link.springer.com/10.1007/978-3-642-36172-2_42

[77] Becker JAJ, Kieffer BL, Le Merrer J. Differential behavioral and molecular alterations upon protracted abstinence from cocaine versus morphine, nicotine, THC and alcohol. Addiction Biology. 2017;**22**(5):1205-1217. Available from: http://doi.wiley.com/10.1111/adb.12405

[78] Befort K. Interactions of the opioid and cannabinoid systems in reward: Insights from knockout studies. Frontiers in Pharmacology. Vol. 6. Strasbourg: Frontiers; 2015. p. 6. Available from: http://journal.frontiersin.org/Article/10.3389/fphar.2015.00006/abstract

[79] Haney M, Ramesh D, Glass A, Pavlicova M, Bedi G, Cooper ZD. Naltrexone maintenance decreases cannabis self-administration and subjective effects in daily cannabis smokers.

Neuropsychopharmacology. 2015;**40**(11):2489-2498. Available from: http://www.ncbi.nlm.nih.gov/pubmed/25881117

[80] Janero DR, Makriyannis A. Terpenes and Lipids of the Endocannabinoid and Transient-receptor-potential-channel Biosignaling Systems. ACS Chemical Neuroscience. Vol. 5. Washington: American Chemical Society; 2014. pp. 1097-1106. Available from: http://pubs.acs.org/doi/10.1021/cn5000875

[81] Varga B, Kassai F, Szabó G, Kovács P, Fischer J, Gyertyán I. Pharmacological comparison of traditional and non-traditional cannabinoid receptor 1 blockers in rodent models in vivo. Pharmacology Biochemistry and Behavior. 2017;**159**(December):24-35. DOI: 10.1016/j.pbb.2017.06.012

[82] Koller VJ, Ferk F, Al-Serori H, Mišík M, Nersesyan A, Auwärter V, et al. Genotoxic properties of representatives of alkylindazoles and aminoalkyl-indoles which are consumed as synthetic cannabinoids. Food and Chemical Toxicology. 2015;**80**:130-136. DOI: 10.1016/j.fct.2015.03.004

[83] Dang D-K, Shin E-J, Mai A-T, Jang C-G, Nah S-Y, Jeong JH, et al. Genetic or pharmacological depletion of cannabinoid CB1 receptor protects against dopaminergic neurotoxicity induced by methamphetamine in mice. Free Radical Biology and Medicine. 2017;**108**(October):204-224. DOI: 10.1016/j.freeradbiomed.2017.03.033

[84] Husni AS, McCurdy CR, Radwan MM, Ahmed SA, Slade D, Ross SA, et al. Evaluation of phytocannabinoids from high-potency *Cannabis sativa* using in vitro bioassays to determine structure-activity relationships for cannabinoid receptor 1 and cannabinoid receptor 2. Medicinal Chemistry Studies. 2014;**23**(9):4295-4300.Available from: http://link.springer.com/10.1007/s00044-014-0972-6

[85] Pertwee R. Pharmacological actions of cannabinoids. European Neuropsychopharmacology. 2010;**20**:S205. Available from: http://link.springer.com/10.1007/3-540-26573-2_1

[86] Pertwee RG. The pharmacology of cannabinoid receptors and their ligands: An overview. International Journal of Obesity. 2006;**30**:S13-S18. Available from: www.nature.com/ijo

[87] Carlini EA, Santos M, Claussen U, Bieniek D, Korte F. Structure activity relationship of four tetrahydrocannabinols and the pharmacological activity of five semi-purified extracts of *Cannabis sativa*. Psychopharmacologia. 1970;**18**(1):82-93. Available from: http://link.springer.com/10.1007/BF00402387

[88] Karniol IG, Carlini EA. Pharmacological interaction between cannabidiol and δ9-tetrahydrocannabinol. Psychopharmacologia. 1973;**33**(1):53-70. Available from: http://link.springer.com/10.1007/BF00428793

[89] Järbe TUC, Gifford RS. "Herbal Incense": Designer Drug Blends as Cannabimimetics and Their Assessment by Drug Discrimination and Other In Vivo Bioassays. Life Sciences. Vol. 97. London: Pergamon; 2014. pp. 64-71. Available from: https://www-sciencedirect-com.ez7.periodicos.capes.gov.br/science/article/pii/S0024320513003986

[90] Gurney SMR, Scott KS, Kacinko SL, Presley BC, Logan BK, Grove W. Pharmacology, toxicology, and adverse effects of synthetic cannabinoid drugs pharmacology, toxicology, and adverse effects of synthetic cannabinoid drugs. Forensic Science Review. 2014;**26**(1):53-78. Available from: http://www.chm.uri.edu/forensics/Gurney_PharmToxAdverseEffectsSynCannDrugs_ForScReview_2014.pdf

[91] Kaizaki-Mitsumoto A, Hataoka K, Funada M, Odanaka Y, Kumamoto H, Numazawa S. Pyrolysis of UR-144, a synthetic cannabinoid, augments an affinity to human CB1 receptor and cannabimimetic effects in mice. The Journal of Toxicological Sciences. 2017;**42**(3):335-341. Available from: https://www.jstage.jst.go.jp/article/jts/42/3/42_335/_article

[92] Zelasko S, Arnold WR, Das A. Endocannabinoid Metabolism by Cytochrome P450 Monooxygenases. Prostaglandins and Other Lipid Mediators. Vol. 116-117. London: Elsevier; 2015. pp. 112-123. Available from: https://www.sciencedirect.com/science/article/pii/S1098882314000744

[93] Tai S, Fantegrossi WE. Synthetic cannabinoids: Pharmacology, behavioral effects, and abuse potential. Current Addiction Reports. 2014;**1**(2):129-136. Available from: http://link.springer.com/10.1007/s40429-014-0014-y

[94] Doke SK, Dhawale SC. Alternatives to animal testing: A review. Saudi Pharmaceutical Journal: SPJ: The Official Publication of the Saudi Pharmaceutical Society. 2015;**23**(3):223-229. Available from: http://www.sciencedirect.com/science/article/pii/S1319016413001096

[95] Anderson DC, Kodukula K. Biomarkers in pharmacology and drug discovery. Biochemical Pharmacology. 2014;**87**(1):172-188. DOI: 10.1016/j.bcp.2013.08.026

[96] Kamstra JH, Aleström P, Kooter JM, Legler J. Zebrafish as a model to study the role of DNA methylation in environmental toxicology. Environmental Science and Pollution Studies. 2015;**22**(21):16262-16276

[97] Bailey J, Oliveri A, Levin ED. Zebrafish model systems for developmental neurobehavioral toxicology. Birth Defects Studies Part C—Embryo Today: Reviews. 2013;**99**(1):14-23

[98] Oltrabella F, Melgoza A, Nguyen B, Guo S. Role of the endocannabinoid system in vertebrates: Emphasis on the zebrafish model. Development Growth and Differentiation. 2017;**59**(4):194-210

[99] Krug RG, Clark KJ. Elucidating cannabinoid biology in zebrafish (*Danio rerio*). Gene. 2015;**570**(2):168-179. DOI: 10.1016/j.gene.2015.07.036

[100] Klee EW, Schneider H, Clark KJ, Cousin MA, Ebbert JO, Hooten WM, et al. Zebrafish: A model for the study of addiction genetics. Human Genetics. 2012;**131**(6):977-1008. Available from: http://link.springer.com/10.1007/s00439-011-1128-0

[101] Hillard CJ. Endocannabinoids and the endocrine system in health and disease. In: Endocannabinoids. Cham: Springer; 2015. pp. 317-339. Available from: http://link.springer.com/10.1007/978-3-319-20825-1_11

[102] Panlilio LV, Justinova Z. Preclinical Studies of Cannabinoid Reward, Treatments for Cannabis Use Disorder, and Addiction-Related Effects of Cannabinoid Exposure. Neuropsychopharmacology. Vol. 43. New York: Nature Publishing Group; 2018. pp. 116-141. Available from: http://www.nature.com/doifinder/10.1038/npp.2017.193

[103] Singh P, Ganjiwale A, Howlett AC, Cowsik SM. In silico interaction analysis of cannabinoid receptor interacting protein 1b (CRIP1b)—CB1 cannabinoid receptor. Journal of Molecular Graphics and Modelling. 2017;**77**:311-321. Available from: https://www.sciencedirect.com/science/article/pii/S1093326317305260

[104] Paulke A, Proschak E, Sommer K, Achenbach J, Wunder C, Toennes SW. Synthetic cannabinoids: In silico prediction of the cannabinoid receptor 1 affinity by a quantitative structure-activity relationship model. Toxicology Letters. 2016;**245**:1-6. Available from: https://www.sciencedirect.com/science/article/pii/S0378427416300017

[105] Xu J, Liu P, Li X, Gan L, Wang P. Novel stemphol derivatives from a marine fungus Pleospora sp. Natural Product Studies. 2018;**32**:1-7. Available from: https://www.tandfonline.com/doi/full/10.1080/14786419.2018.1452005

[106] Ferreira JV, Chaves GA, Marino BLB, Sousa KPA, Souza LR, Brito MFB, et al. Cannabinoid type 1 receptor (CB1) ligands with therapeutic potential for withdrawal syndrome in chemical dependents of *Cannabis sativa*. ChemMedChem. 2017;**12**(16):1408-1416

Chapter 10

Pediatric Dosing Considerations for Medical *Cannabis*

Jane Alcorn, Stephanie Vuong, Fang Wu,
Blair Seifert and Andrew Lyon

Additional information is available at the end of the chapter

http://dx.doi.org/10.5772/intechopen.85399

Abstract

For patients who fail conventional therapies, ability to access medical *Cannabis* may offer a therapeutic alternative that addresses their unmet clinical need. However, a paucity of clinical trial evidence has led to ambiguous pediatric dosing guidelines for medical *Cannabis*, a situation further complicated by the impact of developmental maturation of the pharmacokinetic (PK) and pharmacodynamic (PD) processes governing drug effect and dosing requirements. The pediatric population is very heterogeneous, and dissimilar developmental trajectories result in important differences in the rate and extent of cannabinoid absorption, distribution, elimination, and response both between and within pediatric age group classifications. These developmental changes will require the prescribing caregiver to consider age-specific dosage regimens that may demand continual modification as the child ages. The chapter that follows emphasizes the impact of age-related changes in PK and PD processes as important considerations in pediatric dosing recommendations for medical *Cannabis*.

Keywords: medical *Cannabis*, dosing, pediatric, ontogeny, pharmacokinetics

1. Introduction

Optimal dose selection is fundamental to appropriate clinical care. A comprehensive understanding of drug pharmacokinetics (PK) and pharmacodynamics (PD) and the factors that can influence the drug exposure-response (PK-PD) relationship is important to facilitate the optimization of dosage regimens. In the pediatric patient, though, normal growth and maturation complicates dose selection and optimization. Experience has demonstrated that the usual practice of adjusting dose size according to body weight often results in inappropriate pediatric doses as this practice ignores the impact of developmental changes on drug PK and PD

IntechOpen

processes. To ensure appropriate clinical care, then, dosing recommendations need to consider age-related changes in PK and PD. This becomes particularly important for new therapeutics, which have limited clinical trial data and experience of use in the pediatric population.

Medical *Cannabis* herbal extracts are being considered as new therapeutics for the management of pediatric conditions refractory to standard of care therapies. With no DIN (Drug Identification Number) designation, though, these herbal extracts have limited safety and efficacy data in the pediatric population. The small number of clinical pharmacology trials with pharmaceutical grade cannabinoid products as well as anecdotal use lends some support for medical *Cannabis* in such conditions, but no rational pediatric dosing recommendations are available for these products. The known age-related changes in drug PK and PD, differences further complicated by existing comorbidities and concurrent medications likely to influence drug PK and PD, have left treating caregivers uncertain and reluctant to recommend an appropriate medical *Cannabis* dosage regimen to their patient. A greater understanding of the developmental changes in cannabinoid PK and PD, though, may help to mitigate these uncertainties.

This chapter will mainly address issues of developmental maturation of PK and PD processes as key determinants of medical *Cannabis* herbal extract dosage regimens (henceforth referred to as *Cannabis* extracts). The chapter will first summarize the therapeutic applications for *Cannabis* extracts in pediatric populations. It then will highlight the key physiological determinants of PK and PD that undergo change with postnatal maturation and how such changes might lead to age-related cannabinoid PK and PD differences based on current understandings from adult populations. Superimposed with normal developmental programming, dose selection must also consider the influence of pharmacogenetics, disease, and drug-cannabinoid interactions, and these are briefly discussed. This chapter will underscore developmental maturation of PK and PD processes as paramount to considerations of medical *Cannabis* dosing of the pediatric patient.

2. Therapeutic applications

Many studies report the use of *Cannabis* to aid treatment of a diverse range of health conditions and symptoms. Although *Cannabis'* medical use dates back centuries with the first written records in China and India around 2900 BC and 900 BC, respectively, *Cannabis* was introduced to western medicine only in the nineteenth century [1, 2]. Today, potential indications for medical *Cannabis* include appetite stimulation, chronic pain, spasticity from multiple sclerosis or paraplegia, depression, anxiety, sleep problems, psychosis, glaucoma, Tourette's syndrome, epilepsy, dementia, cancer, post-traumatic stress disorder, and osteoarthritis [3]. Δ^9-Tetrahydrocannabinol (THC) and cannabidiol (CBD) are the most extensively studied cannabinoids for medical use. Individually, these cannabinoids have demonstrated therapeutic benefit and pharmaceutical grade products are available on the market today. However, CBD's ability to modulate THC's well-known intoxicating activity along with a growing body of evidence for an entourage effect among the many cannabinoids of the *Cannabis* plant may extend therapeutic benefit beyond the purified cannabinoid leading to greater interest in the use of *Cannabis* herbal extract preparations [4]. Such entourage properties may explain the varied therapeutic applications of *Cannabis* over the centuries.

Limited information is available on the therapeutic use of *Cannabis* in pediatric patients. *Cannabis* is usually considered when the clinical condition becomes intractable to other types of treatments [5]. This is seen, for example, in treatment of children with refractory epileptic encephalopathy, in particular Lennox-Gastaut syndrome and Dravet syndrome [6]. However, studies supporting medical *Cannabis* suffer from small sample sizes and lack of dose standardization with variations in dose size, formulation, and frequency of administration. These limitations make it difficult to extrapolate data to the larger pediatric population [7]. Furthermore, *Cannabis* extract use has predated the usual pharmacology and toxicology testing applied to other marketed drugs. With virtually no toxicity and efficacy data, dose-plasma concentration-response data, and information on *Cannabis*-drug interactions, the prescribing caregiver is apprehensive to recommend a *Cannabis* extract dosage regimen to a pediatric patient. This inability to define age-appropriate dosage regimens has compromised the acceptability of medical *Cannabis* as a viable therapeutic for pediatric medical conditions.

3. Pediatric dosing considerations

3.1. Medical cannabis dosage forms

Commercially available medical *Cannabis* includes the purified pharmaceutical preparations and the herbal extracts. The extracts contain well-defined proportions of the major psychoactive cannabinoids, THC and CBD, and poorly documented quantities of other cannabinoids and terpenoids [4, 8, 9]. Nonmedical or recreational *Cannabis* have unknown contents of THC, CBD, and other components and should be avoided when used for medical benefit. Much of the anecdotal and observational human trial data usually correlates therapeutic benefit with content of THC or CBD or some ratio of THC to CBD [10]. Given the differences in the pharmacology of THC and CBD, different THC:CBD ratios are promoted within the range of possible clinical indications for medical *Cannabis*. For the pediatric patient, the choice of THC:CBD ratio, though, must acknowledge the known dose-related intoxicating effects of THC and the potential for adverse neurodevelopmental effects with cannabinoid exposure [11]. As well, the selection of *Cannabis* product should consider the presence of the secondary components that often contribute to the more unique characteristics of *Cannabis* extracts [4]. Little is known about the pharmacology of these secondary cannabinoids and terpenes and age-related differences in their PK and PD properties [4, 9]. With the current absence of product quality control on the composition of these other active *Cannabis* components, dose optimization of *Cannabis* extracts for different pediatric indications will need to principally focus on the specific THC:CBD ratio for now.

At present, age-appropriate formulations of *Cannabis* extracts are limited to oil-based oral products. Oral dosing is a challenging route of administration in the pediatric population as issues with incomplete dose ingestion and product refusal negatively impact therapeutic outcomes [12, 13]. Often formulation development considers the adult patient and when used in the pediatric patient can be associated with reduced therapeutic efficacy and safety. For example, some excipients commonly used in adult formulations have well known safety concerns in the pediatric patient such as the common pharmaceutical formulation excipients propylene glycol, benzyl alcohol, and ethanol [14]. As well, factors such as ability to swallow, taste, texture, and smell that determine acceptability of an oral dosage formulation undergo developmental changes such that acceptable formulations in one pediatric age group may not be acceptable in another age group [12, 13]. Currently, medical *Cannabis* companies are actively pursuing product formulation development. Whether these efforts consider the unique requirements of the pediatric patient is uncertain, which will necessitate the treating caregiver to exercise caution when considering *Cannabis* product formulations for their pediatric patients.

3.2. Current dosing guidelines

Medical *Cannabis* dosing guidelines are largely unavailable for the pediatric patient. Such guidelines, though, should consider specific age strata since development and maturation result in age-dependent dosing requirements [15]. Recommended pediatric age strata are: pre-term newborn infants (born at less than 36 weeks of gestation), term newborn infants (age 0 to <28 days), infants and toddlers (age 28 days to 23 months; infants >28 days to 12 months and toddlers >12 months to 23 months), children (age 2–11 years; preschool children 2–5 years and school age children 6–11 years), and adolescents (12–18 years). As with other drugs, the safety and effectiveness of the cannabinoids likely will vary between the different age strata. Consequently, pediatric clinical trials that determine plasma cannabinoid concentration-effect relationships, efficacy, and safety within specific age strata will be required to develop optimal age-specific dosing recommendations.

In the absence of pediatric PK and clinical trial data, adult data become a starting point for pediatric dose selection. For simplicity, doses may be normalized to body weight and, in some cases, to body surface area. Dose scaling by body weight (or body surface area) requires dose adjustment according to the patient's clinical state and clinical response until a dose is titrated to appropriate effect. This process could take some time to identify an appropriate dosage regimen for the pediatric patient, if at all. Furthermore, given possible ceiling effects of the cannabinoids, where dosing beyond a certain amount per body weight may not yield further pharmacological benefit, this approach has risk of adverse therapeutic outcomes.

Other approaches exist to improve upon the simple extrapolation of body weight-adjusted adult doses. Allometric scaling approaches use body surface or body weight ratios and allometric models to extrapolate adult doses to the pediatric patient [16]. An important limitation of this approach is an assumption of a linear correlation between demographic covariates and the dose, which is not the case for the pediatric patient due to developmental maturation of PK and PD processes [16–18]. Children differ not only in body weight but also show changes in body composition, organ size, and maturation, which influence PK as well as result in differences in the therapeutic window (range of exposure concentrations that result in drug efficacy) due to PD changes with age. The use of exponential scaling factors adjusted by body size (and age) to predict dosages in pediatric patients is also limited by the complexity of these modeling approaches that precludes general application to many drugs [16–18]. Hence, we seem left with the current self-titration dosing model where doses, based on weight adjusted adult doses, begin low to moderate and are increased slowly, along with adjustments in dosing interval, until the desired effect is achieved [19]. This empirical "trial-and-error" approach will not likely result in optimal dosing guidelines for the different pediatric age strata due to diverse developmental periods within this population [20, 21].

3.3. Accounting for growth and development in dosage selection

Changes in body size and maturation of the physiological and biochemical processes determining PK and PD must be considered during dosage selection. Normal growth results in a decreasing ratio of body weight to body surface area with age making it difficult to recommend dosing according to patient body weight or body surface area consistent with adult guidelines [22]. For example, in an analysis of pediatric patients, dosing adjustments of hydrophobic drugs (cannabinoids are hydrophobic) based on body weight provided better clinical outcomes in patients between 1 month and 1 year of age, while dosing based on body surface area was best in older children [18]. As well, within and between the age strata maturational changes in PK and PD processes occur at considerably different rates and patterns suggesting that dosage adjustments with long-term therapy may be necessary to ensure efficacy and avoid risk of adverse events [23, 24]. Other clinical and demographic variables such as puberty, which bring hormonal changes known to influence PK in adolescents, and the patient's clinical state, are known to influence dosing requirements [25]. Only with a greater understanding of the impact of such factors can we hope to rationally identify doses for different pediatric populations, particularly in the absence of robust clinical data. The following section addresses a key determinant of dosing requirements, the age-related changes in the PK processes acting upon a dose exposure.

4. Ontogeny of pharmacokinetic processes

4.1. Exposure and exposure route

For many drugs, dosage regimens are designed to attain and maintain drug concentrations within a therapeutic window, the range of concentrations that produce a desired effect. Pediatric therapeutic windows may be quite different from the adult due to PD differences, such as receptor ontogeny (maturation of receptor number and functionality), and organ specific distributional differences resulting in different tissue concentrations of drug to elicit pharmacological activity. Such differences can result in differences in efficacy and toxicity which brings into question use of pediatric therapeutic ranges based on adult clinical data. However, the absence of dose-concentration-response data in children results in a void of evidence that risks the development of arbitrary therapeutic ranges. This was evident with theophylline for neonatal apnea where the therapeutic range adopted in the early 1980s was inadequate and a considerable number of neonates were under-dosed [26]. Understanding the therapeutic range of the cannabinoids for the different pediatric age-strata will be necessary to optimize dosing guidelines for *Cannabis* products. This will necessitate the use of population PK/PD modeling approaches with medical *Cannabis* extracts and a greater understanding of the age-related changes in PK and PD processes governing drug effect.

The attainment of plasma concentrations within the therapeutic window depends on route of administration, dosing frequency, size of dose, and the PK acting on the administered dose. Knowledge of the volume of distribution (V_d) is necessary in the design of a loading dose (the dose needed to quickly produce therapeutic concentrations, C_{Ther}), where V_d and the bioavailable dose (F × Dose) determine the plasma concentration (Eq. (1)). Following a chronic dosing regimen, the mean steady state therapeutic concentration ($C_{SS,Ther}$) is the result of the bioavailable dose, dosing interval (τ), and systemic clearance (Cl_S) (Eq. (2)).

$$C_{Ther} = \frac{F \times \text{Loading Dose}}{V_d} \quad (1)$$

$$C_{SS,Ther} = \frac{F \times {}^{Dose}/_{\tau}}{Cl_S} \quad (2)$$

With extravascular dosing (e.g., oral dosing), compounds must undergo absorption into the systemic circulation. Typically, less than 100% of the administered dose becomes available to the systemic circulation as presystemic mechanisms can limit the fraction of the oral dose that enters the systemic circulation as an unmodified compound (i.e., bioavailability (F)). Once absorbed into the blood supply, compounds distribute to the tissues of the body while systemic clearance mechanisms function to eliminate the compound. Hence, systemic exposure is determined by the extent of absorption (bioavailability) and by the efficiency of the systemic clearance mechanisms, while organ specific exposure additionally depends upon tissue distribution properties of the compound. Age-related changes occur with all these PK processes such that a standard dosage regimen will produce different systemic and tissue-specific exposure levels during pediatric development.

4.2. Oral absorption

The most common route of administration for pediatric patients is the oral route. The rate and extent of oral absorption is determined by the interaction of the physicochemical properties of the cannabinoid and its formulation with the physiological processes governing absorption. With oral ingestion of cannabinoids, time (T_{max}) to maximum concentrations (C_{max}) varies on average from 1 to 6 h, and bioavailability is low and quite variable (4–12%) in adults due to extensive first pass effects [27, 28]. As well, first-pass metabolism following an oral administration results in production of active metabolites (e.g., 11-hydroxy-THC, 7-hydroxy-CBD) with potent psychoactive effects that contribute to the pharmacology of the cannabinoids [27]. Age-related differences in T_{max}, C_{max}, and F may cause important differences in the onset and intensity of effect of an oral cannabinoid dose.

Growth and maturation of gastrointestinal absorption processes variably influence both absorption rate and extent (i.e., bioavailability), a key determinant of the effective dose.

pH dependent passive diffusion, biliary excretion, and gastrointestinal (GIT) transit times undergo considerable change with maturation [29]. Gastric pH is high at birth, becomes acidic in the first 24 h, returns to neutral pH values within the first 10 days of life, and subsequently decreases to adult pH levels within the first year or two of life [16]. Intestinal tract pH tends to be similar with the adult at all pediatric age groups [30]. Although impact of pH is likely limited on cannabinoid bioavailability (as these are neutral compounds), the higher gastric pH might reduce the extent of THC degradation [31]. Biliary excretion, though, is lower in the neonate (2–4 mM) than the adult (5–6 mM) in the first weeks of life, which is due to immaturity of the hepatic transporters responsible for their biliary excretion rather than ability to synthesize bile salts [32, 33]. As hydrophobic molecules, this may reduce cannabinoid bioavailability due to lower GIT solubilization in the first months of life. Gastrointestinal motility is also reduced at birth and gastric emptying and intestinal peristaltic function likely become similar to adults in the first weeks of life [34, 35]. This suggests T_{max} is likely to be similar with adults within a month of birth, although differences in motility may not influence C_{max}.

Other gastrointestinal physiological factors that have importance on the extent of absorption (i.e., bioavailability) include gastrointestinal permeability and first pass effects. All cannabinoids undergo passive permeation across the gastrointestinal epithelium. Intestinal permeability is initially high at birth given the leakiness of the epithelial tight junctions, but with junction closure within the first week of birth overall permeability becomes lower than adult due to a smaller intestinal absorptive surface area [36]. Passive transport mechanisms likely reach adult values within 4 months of birth. First-pass effects have a longer maturational trajectory. First pass effects include the activity of microbiota and gut luminal enzymes, enzymes and transporters of the gastrointestinal epithelia and liver. In adults, the low and variable bioavailability of CBD and THC is due to pre-systemic elimination by cytochrome P450 enzymes, principally CYP3A4 and CYP2C's, expressed in the intestinal and hepatic epithelium [37]. Intestinal and hepatic CYP3A4 expression and hepatic CYP2C expression principally contribute to considerable first-pass metabolism and the low oral bioavailability of cannabinoids [38]. With development, hepatic CYP2C expression reaches adult levels by 6 months, exceeds adult levels in childhood, and returns to adult levels after puberty [39]. CYP3A4 undergoes a slower maturation with considerable increases in the first 6 months but does not reach adult levels until after 2 years of age [40, 41]. CYP3A4 activity also exceeds the adult in early childhood and returns to adult levels after puberty. Their developmental maturation suggests bioavailability is likely to be higher in neonates and infants until these enzymes reach adult expression levels. The xenobiotic transporters also contribute to first-pass effects. THC is a substrate of efflux transporters including p-glycoprotein (MDR1) and BCRP, while CBD only inhibits these efflux transporters. These transporters undergo rapid ontogeny in the first 6 months of life to reach adult values by 2 years of age, but may not contribute to age-related differences in bioavailability beyond 6 months of age [42]. The immaturity of these transporters can further enhance THC bioavailability relative to the adult.

Bacterial activity within the gastrointestinal tract lumen may influence first pass metabolism. Whether cannabinoids undergo bacterial metabolism is unknown, but glucuronide metabolites may undergo deconjugation in the gut lumen. Children from 3 to 15 years of age showed no differences in activity of bacterial enzymes such as beta-glucuronidase, beta-glucosidase, and other enzymes and intestinal bacterial colonies approach adult characteristics by 1–4 years of age [43]. The gastrointestinal microbiome also influences the regulation of drug metabolizing enzymes and transporters, but information in the pediatric patient is lacking. A multitude of factors can influence the microbiome including age, disease, diet, and drug exposure, and our understanding of their impact during development is limited.

Overall, postnatal development of pH, gastrointestinal motility, and first-pass mechanisms should reach maturity by 5 years of age [17] at which time the rate and extent of oral absorption should have similarity to adult estimates. The variable rate and pattern of maturation, though, will lead to large ranges in T_{max}, C_{max}, and bioavailability estimates between the different pediatric age classes. Since variability in blood concentrations is principally inversely proportional to oral bioavailability, we may expect important differences in the oral dose requirements needed to attain equivalent plasma concentrations and therapeutic responses. Variable bioavailability will challenge treating caregivers on advising doses indicated by age, and individualization of dosage regimens will remain necessary. This expectation, though, creates opportunity for development of pediatric dosage formulations that considers both the potential age influences on cannabinoid liberation from the dosage formulation and the need to provide higher and more consistent oral bioavailability. Effective oral formulations promise more consistent dosage recommendations and reductions in the risk of under- or overdosing.

4.3. Distribution

Age-related differences in the extent of tissue distribution (i.e., volume of distribution, V_d) will impact intensity and duration of cannabinoid activity. In adults, the high plasma protein binding characteristics (>97% bound in the adult) [44] of the cannabinoids result in a small central V_d (2.5–3 L). The cannabinoids undergo rapid and extensive distribution into lipophilic tissues (e.g., brain and adipose) and the highly perfused tissues (e.g., heart, lung, and liver) resulting in a large steady state V_d with reports ranging from 2.5–3 to 10 L/kg [27, 45]. The slow redistribution of cannabinoids from tissues, in particular adipose, as well as enterohepatic recirculation lead to long half-lives ranging from 1.5 to 5 days or longer for THC and 1–2 days for CBD, and even longer for the metabolites [27, 45]. Since the V_d is an important determinant of half-life, which, in turn, is used to guide the dosing interval, the expected age-related differences in cannabinoid V_d are likely to lead to differences in half-lives between the pediatric age strata and a possible need to consider such differences in the dosing interval.

Body composition, plasma and tissue protein binding, and physicochemical characteristics of the cannabinoids will influence the extent of their distribution (i.e., V_d). For many compounds, V_d demonstrates a linear relationship with body size. In the pediatric population, body size can change from less than 1 kg to up to 100 kg or more with development. Consequently, V_d expressed on a per body weight basis will show tremendous variability in the pediatric population. Ratio of fat, muscle, and intracellular and extracellular water also changes with maturation. At birth, total body water is 75%, and total body water-to-fat ratio is the highest in neonates and young infants with total body water reaching adult values by 6 months [46]. However, older infants and toddlers tend to have the highest fat-to-body water ratio only to reach adult ratios in later childhood [46]. Although higher body fat to water ratio may suggest higher V_d for the hydrophobic cannabinoids in these age groups, studies with other highly lipophilic drugs suggest that the V_d was not different between adults and infants [47]. Past infancy, then, the V_d might be similar between children and adults for the cannabinoids [47]. The lipophilic nature of the cannabinoids, though, raise concerns with childhood obesity and whether obese children should be dosed based on actual or ideal body weights [48].

Plasma protein binding is an important physiological determinant of V_d and the unbound fraction in the blood. In adults, cannabinoids bind extensively to lipoproteins and albumin where the unbound fraction can range from 1 to 5% [44, 45]. In the pediatric population, the plasma levels of albumin and alpha$_1$-acid glycoprotein, the two major plasma binding proteins, are lower at birth and increase gradually to reach adult values by 1–3 years of age [49]. Lipoprotein and triglyceride levels also rise gradually during the first year of life, with further increases in childhood and adolescence [50]. Consequently, neonates and infants might exhibit lower bound fractions of the cannabinoids due to lower lipoprotein and albumin concentrations. These age dependent increases in plasma proteins might also mean higher distribution volumes in the neonate and infant and a lower C_{max}.

With high binding characteristics, seemingly small differences in binding, though, may result in large differences in the availability of cannabinoids to bind to their therapeutic targets. The unbound concentration is known to better reflect the pharmacodynamics of highly bound drugs [51], and a greater unbound fraction coupled with a lower elimination capacity for the cannabinoids (see section below) would enhance the availability of cannabinoids at their pharmacological sites of action. This can result in more intense pharmacological or toxicological responses and possibly a need to adjust doses to ensure equivalent PD responses. In addition to the amount of protein available for binding, binding affinity shows age-related changes. The presence of endogenous competitors for plasma protein binding sites, such as bilirubin and free fatty acids, is higher in the neonate [52], and along with exogenous competitors (e.g., co-administered drugs) may further increase the unbound cannabinoid concentration with subsequent enhancements in their pharmacological or adverse effects. Either way this might necessitate a dose reduction.

Relevant to the cannabinoids is the possible influence of age-related differences in the volume of the brain and the permeability of the blood-brain-barrier. Brain volume is larger in younger children and approaches adult values at 4–6 years of age [53]. THC but not CBD is a substrate for P-glycoprotein (P-gp, ABCB1) and breast cancer resistance protein (BCRP, ABCG2) [54], while both cannabinoids inhibit P-gp and BCRP activity [55, 56]. These transporters function to limit permeation of THC and other drug substrates across the blood-brain-barrier and expedite their elimination from the brain, while CBD brain uptake and removal is not influenced by these transporters [54]. This might suggest a longer residence time of CBD in brain tissue relative to THC and a potential disconnect between plasma levels and the psychoactive effects of these compounds. As an inhibitor of efflux transporters, CBD might also modulate brain disposition of THC, which could explain, in part, its known ability to modulate THC psychoactive effects [57]. Important cannabinoid-drug interactions might ensue with co-administration of other efflux transporter substrates with a concomitant risk for brain accumulation of these drugs and potential adverse effects. Finally, known pharmacogenetic polymorphisms in these transporters result in reduced activity, which may enhance brain penetration and residence, increase the psychoactive effects, and, in turn, risk *Cannabis* dependence or possibly brain disorders [58]. Although ontogeny of these transporters at the blood-brain-barrier is unknown, developmental maturation of the efflux transporters may result in a developmental vulnerability to THC use.

4.4. Elimination

The lipophilic cannabinoids are eliminated primarily through hepatic metabolic clearance. Hepatic clearance depends on three physiological determinants, plasma protein binding, hepatic blood flow, and intrinsic clearance (the overall ability of the liver to metabolize a compound). The cannabinoids appear to fall within the class of intermediate to high extraction ratio compounds (systemic clearance ranging from 600 to 1190 mL/min for THC and 960 to 1560 mL/min for CBD) [59, 60], suggesting that hepatic clearance is influenced variably by hepatic blood flow, intrinsic clearance, and plasma protein binding or predominantly by the hepatic blood flow at the highest hepatic clearance values. All determinants undergo developmental maturation. Hepatic metabolic clearance of the cannabinoids principally involves cytochrome P450 enzyme-mediated metabolism. The metabolites generated from P450 enzyme reactions may undergo further phase II enzyme conjugation reactions for their subsequent renal or biliary excretion. An understanding of the contribution of Phase I and II enzymes is important as the rate and pattern of their maturation tend to follow different developmental trajectories.

Cannabinoids are principally metabolized by CYP3A4, CYP2C9, and CYP2C19 [45, 61]. As a superfamily of enzymes, the developmental trajectories of P450 enzymes are grouped into three characteristic classes [62]. CYP3A4 and CYP2C enzymes are class II enzymes, where enzymes are expressed at low levels at birth and gradually increase postnatally to achieve adult values within a year or two of age [62]. For instance, CYP2C19 activity is less than one-third adult values at birth, surges to 50% of adult activity in the first month of postnatal life, and reaches adult values at 1 year of age [39]. After 1 year, the hepatic clearance of CYP2C19 substrates show similarity to adult values [62]. Although CYP3A4 is the most abundant hepatic P450 enzyme in the adult, the predominant CYP3A isoform at birth is CYP3A7, while CYP3A4 expression is only 10% of adult levels [62, 63]. A developmental switch is observed such that CYP3A4 activity increases concomitantly with reductions in CYP3A7 activity. By 1 year of age, CYP3A4 activity is 75% adult levels, while CYP3A7 activity is considerably reduced [62, 63]. Although the two isoforms share 95% identity in their nucleotide sequence, differences in substrate specificities are noted for the two isoforms as well as a lower metabolism rate by CYP3A7 [64]. No study has evaluated the metabolic activity of CYP3A7 against CBD and THC, but CBD was identified as an inhibitor of this CYP3A isoform [65].

CBD, THC, and their respective metabolites also undergo phase II metabolism principally by the UDP-glucuronosyltransferase (UGT) enzymes. UGT1 and UGT2 families are involved in drug metabolism and typically more than one isoform contributes to the metabolism of a single compound [66]. Generally, the UGT enzymes have 25% activity in young infants relative to adult levels with adult levels achieved within 6–30 months of birth [66]. However, individual UGT enzymes undergo different maturation patterns leading to considerable variability reported in the glucuronidation capacity of newborns and infants.

The developmental pattern of the major cannabinoid metabolizing enzymes suggests that systemic clearance and oral bioavailability may change throughout the pediatric period. Neonates and infants may demonstrate lower systemic clearance and higher oral bioavailability due to reductions in hepatic metabolism, but adolescents may have similar values to the adult. Interesting children ages 2–12 may require larger weight adjusted doses. In a mechanistic-based analysis, for drugs almost solely eliminated by CYP3A4 children required higher (~2 times) doses corrected for body weight relative to the younger child and adult, although similar weight-corrected doses between children and adults were required for drugs eliminated solely by CYP2C19 or UGT isoforms to achieve equivalent plasma concentrations [17]. Given the contribution of both P450 enzymes to the elimination of cannabinoids, higher weight adjusted doses may be required in children relative to the adult due to higher systemic clearance or first-pass metabolism.

Quantitatively and qualitatively P450 and UGT enzymes show considerable variation in their developmental maturation both within and between the age strata. A consequence of this variation may be altered cannabinoid metabolite profiles relative to the adult. After oral administration in the adult, extensive first-pass metabolism results in the production of high circulating levels of bioactive hydroxylated metabolites of CBD and THC [27]. These active metabolites contribute to the pharmacology of *Cannabis* herbal extracts. A further consideration is the genetic polymorphism of P450 and UGT enzymes which divides the population into poor metabolizers and fast metabolizers (e.g., CYP2C's) or results in extensive variability in metabolic rates (e.g., CYP3A4) [67]. The impact of genetic polymorphism in the different pediatric age classifications is unknown. A few drugs with available data suggest that phenotype does not relate to genotype at birth, but enzyme maturation will eventually result in phenotype-genotype relationships similar to the adult. Hence, postnatal maturation of P450 and UGT enzymes has considerable influence on therapeutic efficacy and toxicity because metabolism determines oral bioavailability, hepatic metabolic clearance, and the active metabolite profile.

Renal and biliary excretion mediates the elimination of the cannabinoid phase I and II enzyme metabolites. Elimination by the kidney occurs by glomerular filtration and tubular secretion. Neonates are born with reduced glomerular and tubular function, which is further compromised in the preterm neonate due to incomplete nephrogenesis [68]. Profound anatomical and functional changes in the kidney occur following birth that include enhancements in renal blood flow, redistribution of blood flow in the kidney, improvements in glomerular filtration efficiency, and the growth and maturation of renal tubules and tubular processes. These changes result in rapid attainment of renal elimination function within the first year of age [68]. Maturation of glomerular filtration processes precedes tubular processes, such that glomerular filtration rate reaches adult levels by 6 months of age and tubular reabsorption and excretion processes mature to adult levels by 1 year of age [68]. The excretion rate in toddlers and preschool children, though, can exceed adult levels but subsequently returns to adult levels in childhood [68]. The anatomical and functional immaturity of the kidney and the discordance in the maturation of glomerular and tubule function can contribute to considerable interindividual variability in renal elimination in pediatric patients.

4.5. Transporters

Transporters are categorized into ATP-Binding Cassette (ABC) and Solute Carrier (SLC) families. ABC proteins are efflux transporters expressed apically at tissue-blood interfaces and function to limit penetration of compounds into these tissues. Maturation of ABC transporters can result in a developmental vulnerability to THC use. ABC transporter ontogeny as well as genetic variation (polymorphisms) is known to influence treatment response to drugs and increase risk for psychiatric disorders in pediatric populations as a result of altered disposition to the brain [69]. For example, the common P-glycoprotein (ABCB1) genetic variant C3435T, which results in altered p-glycoprotein expression, was associated with increased risk of *Cannabis* dependence [58]. As well, transporter ontogeny and genetic polymorphisms can contribute to the interindividual variability in response to *Cannabis*. In general, the ontogeny of ABC and SLC transporters is poorly known.

5. Ontogeny of pharmacodynamic processes

Dosing considerations of the pediatric patient not only need to acknowledge the impact of age-related changes in PK processes, but also the maturation of the endocannabinoid system and how this will influence PD and the relationship between exposure and response. Very little data, though, are available from human clinical studies on the developmental maturation of the endocannabinoid system and how these may influence cannabinoid pharmacology. What is known is that the endocannabinoid system is expressed early in fetal life and plays a critical role in normal neurological development. Cannabinoid receptor populations and levels of the enzyme systems and endocannabinoids are dynamic in pediatric development particularly during adolescence [70]. Some data suggest daily high dose exposure to THC may pose a risk to normal neurological development, although the data are not available for CBD [71].

The lack of data on PD ontogeny and age-specific exposure-response relationships risks development of inappropriate therapeutic ranges. In the absence of any data, the treating caregiver may apply therapeutic ranges in adults or older pediatric age groups to younger pediatric age classes on the assumption of a similar exposure-response relationship to help inform dose selection [72]. Yet drawing from examples with other drugs, changes in receptor density expression with maturation have altered the efficacy and safety of drugs in children, such as reduced PD sensitivity to propofol resulting in overdosing and subsequently myocardial failure, metabolic acidosis, multiorgan failure, and death [73]. Given that the endocannabinoid system undergoes continued development, therapeutic windows are likely to be different among the different pediatric age strata.

6. Other factors

6.1. Safety and adverse effects

The toxicity of cannabinoids is generally considered quite low. In adults, cannabinoids have a number of central nervous system effects that include intoxication, appetite stimulation, disruption of psychomotor behavior, short-term memory impairment, antinociceptive actions, and anti-emesis. Lethal doses are unknown, but the size of a single lethal dose is likely to be very high. The apparent low toxicity in adults, though, cannot necessarily translate to a low adverse effect potential in pediatric patients. Very little information exists on the pediatric specific adverse effects of *Cannabis*. Further, its use as an adjunct therapy in conditions such as pediatric seizure creates uncertainty—are the reported adverse effects the result of the cannabinoid or due to a cannabinoid-drug interaction? Experience with other drugs suggests that the immature physiological system predisposes pediatric patients to an increased risk for adverse effects [74]. It is these examples that highlight the concern among the treating caregiver of the safety of *Cannabis* use in pediatric patients. Unfortunately, the typical short-term clinical trial is inadequate to determine safety of medical *Cannabis* on growth and maturation. Pharmacovigilance over the long-term will be necessary, and this will require reevaluation of the original cohort of patients in clinical trials years after termination of the trial.

6.2. Pharmacokinetic and pharmacodynamic interactions

In pediatric patients, medical *Cannabis* is typically administered as an add-on to standard of care therapies. This practice can result in clinically relevant competitive interactions involving metabolic enzymes, transporters, or plasma protein binding sites, and at times pharmacological receptors. Cannabinoids are known to inhibit the metabolism of drugs that share the same P450 enzymes, with inhibition constants in the low micromolar range [37]. Conversely, drug substrates of CYP2C and CYP3A4 can slow the metabolism of the cannabinoids. A well-known interaction is the co-administration of CBD with clobazam in refractory pediatric epilepsy where CBD is reported to increase clobazam and norclobazam (active metabolite) circulating concentrations due to inhibition of CYP2C19 [75]. Interactions between CBD and THC are also possible. CBD is known to competitively decrease the metabolism of THC resulting in its persistence in the body [76]. Higher ratios of CBD:THC can attenuate THC-induced effects and can produce more THC active metabolites [77]. P450 enzyme induction is possible in all pediatric age classes and can result in clinically significant enhancements in the elimination of cannabinoids and shorter half-lives. Without dosage regimen adjustments, enzyme induction and inhibition can result in concentrations outside the therapeutic window.

Other PK and PD interactions of concern include interactions at efflux transporters and impact of disease. The exposure-response relationship can be affected by clinically relevant interactions at the efflux transporters expressed at the blood brain barrier. Such interactions can alter the brain distribution of the pharmacologically active cannabinoid fraction to enhance cannabinoid response at a given *Cannabis* dose. Although our understanding of the impact of disease on cannabinoid PK and PD is very limited, clear examples exist where dosing recommendations depend upon the specific comorbidity under treatment. As well, some childhood diseases result in unique pathophysiological changes not present in the adult precluding a simple extrapolation of dose from adult experience. In the absence of data, pediatric patients will need close monitoring to ensure effective, safe therapy in the presence of disease and other comorbidities.

6.3. Perspectives on the use of medical cannabis in pediatric populations

We face a clinical and ethical dilemma in the use of medical *Cannabis* in pediatric populations. Product quality, limited age-appropriate formulations, the lack of PK and efficacy data spanning the specific pediatric age categories, the possible adverse effects of *Cannabis* on normal growth and development, and limited pediatric-specific safety data cause considerable uncertainty regarding the use of medical *Cannabis* and identification of an appropriate dosage regimen. It is not surprising that treating caregivers hesitate to give medical authority for use. Just as the regulatory agencies have identified a critical need for pediatric data in new drug development, so must the medical *Cannabis* field recognize the danger of inadequate safety and efficacy data and inadequate regulation of *Cannabis* product quality. To realize the full advantages of medical *Cannabis*, well-powered and rigorous clinical trials will be needed. Ethical justification for such studies should weigh toward benefit of the need to understand its safety and effectiveness in different pediatric age strata. Such studies must acknowledge the impact of physiological maturation and clinical variables on dose requirements and have sufficient power to enable evaluation of these factors on cannabinoid PK and PD. In fact, our current knowledge of the impact of maturation on PK and exposure-response relationships invalidates the practice of empirical methods for dose selection despite their simplicity for treating caregivers. Pediatric clinical trials for medical *Cannabis* should be considered mandatory and such trials should focus on both PK and the target PD outcome. Finally, a framework for assessing and reporting adverse effects and benefits should accompany the use of medical *Cannabis* in the pediatric population. Eventually, these studies will make possible the development of pediatric dosage regimens that are safe and precisely address the therapeutic need. Until then, the treating caregiver can rationally approach dose selection in different pediatric age groups with an understanding of the impact of growth and maturation on cannabinoid PK and PD.

Author details

Jane Alcorn[1]*, Stephanie Vuong[1], Fang Wu[2], Blair Seifert[3] and Andrew Lyon[2]

*Address all correspondence to: jane.alcorn@usask.ca

1 College of Pharmacy and Nutrition, University of Saskatchewan, Saskatoon, Saskatchewan, Canada

2 Department of Pathology and Laboratory Medicine, University of Saskatchewan and Saskatchewan Health Authority, Saskatoon, Saskatchewan, Canada

3 Department of Pharmacy Services, Royal University Hospital, Saskatchewan Health Authority, Saskatoon, Saskatchewan, Canada

References

[1] Brand JE, Zhao Z. Cannabis in chinese medicine: Are some tradition indications referenced in ancient literature related to cannabinoids? Frontiers in Pharmacology. 2017; **8**(108):1-11

[2] Kuddus M, Ginawi IAM, AL-Hazimi A. Cannabis sativa: An ancient wild plant of India. Emirates Journal of Food and Agriculture. 2013;**25**:735-745

[3] Lough S. Growing the evidence base for medical cannabis. CMAJ. 2015;**187**(13):955-956

[4] Russo EB. Taming THC: Potential cannabis synergy and phytocannabinoid-terpenoid entourage effects. British Journal of Pharmacology. 2011;**163**(7):1344-1364

[5] Ananth P, Ma C, Al-Sayegh H, Kroon L, Klein V, Wharton C, et al. Provider perspectives on use of medical marijuana in children with cancer. Pediatrics. 2018;**141**(1):e20170559

[6] Devinsky O, Patel AD, Thiele EA, Wong MH, Appleton R, Harden CL, et al. Randomized, dose-ranging safety trial of cannabidiol in Dravet syndrome. Neurology. 2018;**90**(14): e1204-e11

[7] Efron D, Freeman J. Medical cannabis for paediatric developmental-behavioural and psychiatric disorders. Journal of Paediatrics and Child Health. 2018;**54**(7):715-717

[8] Marcu JP. An overview of major and minor phytocannabinoids. In: Preedy VR, editor. Neuropathology of Drug Addictions and Substance Misuse. Boston, MA: Elsevier Academic Press: Amsterdam; 2016

[9] Pavlovic R, Nenna G, Calvi L, Panseri S, Borgonovo G, Giupponi L, et al. Quality traits of "cannabidiol oils": Cannabinoids content, terpene fingerprint and oxidation stability of European commercially available preparations. Molecules. 2018;**23**(5):1230

[10] Pertwee RG, Cascio MG. Known pharmacological actions of delta-9-tetrahydrocannabinol and of four other chemical constituents of cannabis that activate cannabinoid receptors. In: Pertwee RG, editor. Handbook of Cannabis. Oxford, UK: Oxford University Press; 2014. pp. 115-136

[11] Crane NA, Schuster RM, Fusar-Poli P, Gonzalez R. Effects of cannabis on neurocognitive functioning: Recent advances, neurodevelopmental influences, and sex differences. Neuropsychology Review. 2013;**23**(2):117-137

[12] Lawless H. Sensory development in children: Research in taste and olfaction. Journal of the American Dietetic Association. 1985;**85**(5):577-582, 585

[13] Ventura AK, Worobey J. Early influences on the development of food preferences. Current Biology. 2013;**23**(9):R401-R408

[14] Salunke S, Brandys B, Giacoia G, Tuleu C. The STEP (Safety and Toxicity of Excipients for Paediatrics) database: Part 2—The pilot version. International Journal of Pharmaceutics. 2013;**457**(1):310-322

[15] FDA U. E11(R1) addendum: Clinical investigation of medicinal products in the pediatric population. 2018. https://www.fda.gov/ucm/groups/fdagov-public/@fdagov-drugs-gen/documents/document/ucm530012.pdf

[16] Bartelink IH, Rademaker CM, Schobben AF, van den Anker JN. Guidelines on paediatric dosing on the basis of developmental physiology and pharmacokinetic considerations. Clinical Pharmacokinetics. 2006;**45**(11):1077-1097

[17] Anderson GD, Lynn AM. Optimizing pediatric dosing: A developmental pharmacologic approach. Pharmacotherapy. 2009;**29**(6):680-690

[18] Johnson TN. The problems in scaling adult drug doses to children. Archives of Disease in Childhood. 2008;**93**(3):207-211

[19] MacCallum CA, Russo EB. Practical considerations in medical cannabis administration and dosing. European Journal of Internal Medicine. 2018;**49**:12-19

[20] Baber N, Pritchard D. Dose estimation for children. British Journal of Clinical Pharmacology. 2003;**56**(5):489-493

[21] Kearns GL, Abdel-Rahman SM, Alander SW, Blowey DL, Leeder JS, Kauffman RE. Developmental pharmacology—Drug disposition, action, and therapy in infants and children. The New England Journal of Medicine. 2003;**349**(12):1157-1167

[22] Lack JA, Stuart-Taylor ME. Calculation of drug dosage and body surface area of children. British Journal of Anaesthesia. 1997;**78**(5):601-605

[23] Alcorn J, McNamara PJ. Ontogeny of hepatic and renal systemic clearance pathways in infants: Part I. Clinical Pharmacokinetics. 2002;**41**(12):959-998

[24] Allegaert K, Verbesselt R, Naulaers G, van den Anker JN, Rayyan M, Debeer A, et al. Developmental pharmacology: Neonates are not just small adults. Acta Clinica Belgica. 2008;**63**(1):16-24

[25] Rodman JH. Pharmacokinetic variability in the adolescent: Implications of body size and organ function for dosage regimen design. The Journal of Adolescent Health. 1994; **15**(8):654-662

[26] Gilman JT, Gal P. Inadequacy of FDA dosing guidelines for theophylline use in neonates. Drug Intelligence & Clinical Pharmacy. 1986;**20**(6):481-484

[27] Grotenhermen F. Clinical pharmacokinetics of cannabinoids. Journal of Cannabis Therapeutics. 2003;**3**(1):3-51

[28] Ohlsson A, Lindgren JE, Wahlen A, Agurell S, Hollister LE, Gillespie HK. Plasma delta-9 tetrahydrocannabinol concentrations and clinical effects after oral and intravenous administration and smoking. Clinical Pharmacology and Therapeutics. 1980;**28**(3):409-416

[29] Mooji MG, de Koning BA, Huijsman ML, de Wildt SN. Ontogeny of oral drug absorption processes in children. Expert Opinion on Drug Metabolism & Toxicology. 2012; **8**:1293-1303

[30] Yu G, Zheng QS, Li GF. Similarities and differences in gastrointestinal physiology between neonates and adults: A physiologically based pharmacokinetic modeling perspective. The AAPS Journal. 2014;**16**(6):1162-1166

[31] Garrett ER, Hunt CA. Physiochemical properties, solubility, and protein binding of delta9-tetrahydrocannabinol. Journal of Pharmaceutical Sciences. 1974;**63**(7):1056-1064

[32] Brouwer KL, Aleksunes LM, Brandys B, Giacoia GP, Knipp G, Lukacova V, et al. Human ontogeny of drug transporters: Review and recommendations of the pediatric transporter working group. Clinical Pharmacology and Therapeutics. 2015;**98**(3):266-287

[33] Poley JR, Dower JC, Owen CA Jr, Stickler GB. Bile acids in infants and children. The Journal of Laboratory and Clinical Medicine. 1964;**63**:838-846

[34] Bisset WM, Watt JB, Rivers RP, Milla PJ. Ontogeny of fasting small intestinal motor activity in the human infant. Gut. 1988;**29**(4):483-488

[35] Bonner JJ, Vajjah P, Abduljalil K, Jamei M, Rostami-Hodjegan A, Tucker GT, et al. Does age affect gastric emptying time? A model-based meta-analysis of data from premature neonates through to adults. Biopharmaceutics & Drug Disposition. 2015;**36**(4):245-257

[36] van Elburg RM, Fetter WP, Bunkers CM, Heymans HS. Intestinal permeability in relation to birth weight and gestational and postnatal age. Archives of Disease in Childhood. Fetal and Neonatal Edition. 2003;**88**(1):F52-F55

[37] Stout SM, Cimino NM. Exogenous cannabinoids as substrates, inhibitors, and inducers of human drug metabolizing enzymes: A systematic review. Drug Metabolism Reviews. 2014;**46**(1):86-95

[38] Paine MF, Khalighi M, Fisher JM, Shen DD, Kunze KL, Marsh CL, et al. Characterization of interintestinal and intraintestinal variations in human CYP3A-dependent metabolism. The Journal of Pharmacology and Experimental Therapeutics. 1997;**283**(3):1552-1562

[39] Koukouritaki SB, Manro JR, Marsh SA, Stevens JC, Rettie AE, McCarver DG, et al. Developmental expression of human hepatic CYP2C9 and CYP2C19. The Journal of Pharmacology and Experimental Therapeutics. 2004;**308**(3):965-974

[40] Johnson TN, Tanner MS, Taylor CJ, Tucker GT. Enterocytic CYP3A4 in a paediatric population: Developmental changes and the effect of coeliac disease and cystic fibrosis. British Journal of Clinical Pharmacology. 2001;**51**(5):451-460

[41] Stevens JC, Hines RN, Gu C, Koukouritaki SB, Manro JR, Tandler PJ, et al. Developmental expression of the major human hepatic CYP3A enzymes. The Journal of Pharmacology and Experimental Therapeutics. 2003;**307**(2):573-582

[42] Johnson TN, Thomson M. Intestinal metabolism and transport of drugs in children: The effects of age and disease. Journal of Pediatric Gastroenterology and Nutrition. 2008;**47**(1):3-10

[43] Matamoros S, Gras-Leguen C, Le Vacon F, Potel G, de La Cochetiere MF. Development of intestinal microbiota in infants and its impact on health. Trends in Microbiology. 2013;**21**(4):167-173

[44] Widman M, Agurell S, Ehrnebo M, Jones G. Binding of (+)- and (minus)-delta-1-tetrahydrocannabinols and (minus)-7-hydroxy-delta-1-tetrahydrocannabinol to blood cells and plasma proteins in man. The Journal of Pharmacy and Pharmacology. 1974;**26**(11):914-916

[45] Huestis MA. Human cannabinoid pharmacokinetics. Chemistry & Biodiversity. 2007;**4**(8): 1770-1804

[46] Bechard LJ, Wroe E, Ellis K. Body composition and growth. In: Duggan CW, Watkins JB, Walker WA, editors. Nutrition in Pediatrics: Basic Science, Clinical Applications. Hamilton: BC Decker Inc; 2008. pp. 20-40

[47] Anderson GD. Children versus adults: Pharmacokinetic and adverse-effect differences. Epilepsia. 2002;**43**(Suppl 3):53-59

[48] Kendrick JG, Carr RR, Ensom MH. Pediatric obesity: Pharmacokinetics and implications for drug dosing. Clinical Therapeutics. 2015;**37**(9):1897-1923

[49] Sethi PK, White CA, Cummings BS, Hines RN, Muralidhara S, Bruckner JV. Ontogeny of plasma proteins, albumin and binding of diazepam, cyclosporine, and deltamethrin. Pediatric Research. 2016;**79**(3):409-415

[50] Asayama K, Miyao A, Kato K. High-density lipoprotein (HDL), HDL2, and HDL3 cholesterol concentrations determined in serum of newborns, infants, children, adolescents, and adults by use of a micromethod for combined precipitation ultracentrifugation. Clinical Chemistry. 1990;**36**(1):129-131

[51] Greenblatt DJ, Sellers EM, Koch-Weser J. Importance of protein binding for the interpretation of serum or plasma drug concentrations. Journal of Clinical Pharmacology. 1982;**22**(5-6):259-263

[52] Nau H, Luck W, Kuhnz W. Decreased serum protein binding of diazepam and its major metabolite in the neonate during the first postnatal week relate to increased free fatty acid levels. British Journal of Clinical Pharmacology. 1984;**17**(1):92-98

[53] Fernandez E, Perez R, Hernandez A, Tejada P, Arteta M, Ramos JT. Factors and mechanisms for pharmacokinetic differences between pediatric population and adults. Pharmaceutics. 2011;**3**(1):53-72

[54] Brzozowska N, Li KM, Wang XS, Booth J, Stuart J, McGregor IS, et al. ABC transporters P-gp and Bcrp do not limit the brain uptake of the novel antipsychotic and anticonvulsant drug cannabidiol in mice. PeerJ. 2016;**4**:e2081

[55] Holland ML, Lau DT, Allen JD, Arnold JC. The multidrug transporter ABCG2 (BCRP) is inhibited by plant-derived cannabinoids. British Journal of Pharmacology. 2007; **152**(5):815-824

[56] Holland ML, Panetta JA, Hoskins JM, Bebawy M, Roufogalis BD, Allen JD, et al. The effects of cannabinoids on P-glycoprotein transport and expression in multidrug resistant cells. Biochemical Pharmacology. 2006;**71**(8):1146-1154

[57] Klein C, Karanges E, Spiro A, Wong A, Spencer J, Huynh T, et al. Cannabidiol potentiates Delta(9)-tetrahydrocannabinol (THC) behavioural effects and alters THC pharmacokinetics during acute and chronic treatment in adolescent rats. Psychopharmacology. 2011;**218**(2):443-457

[58] Benyamina A, Bonhomme-Faivre L, Picard V, Sabbagh A, Richard D, Blecha L, et al. Association between ABCB1 C3435T polymorphism and increased risk of cannabis dependence. Progress in Neuro-Psychopharmacology & Biological Psychiatry. 2009;**33**(7):1270-1274

[59] Ohlsson A, Lindgren JE, Andersson S, Agurell S, Gillespie H, Hollister LE. Single-dose kinetics of deuterium-labelled cannabidiol in man after smoking and intravenous administration. Biomedical & Environmental Mass Spectrometry. 1986;**13**(2):77-83

[60] Ohlsson A, Lindgren JE, Wahlen A, Agurell S, Hollister LE, Gillespie HK. Single dose kinetics of deuterium labelled delta 1-tetrahydrocannabinol in heavy and light cannabis users. Biomedical Mass Spectrometry. 1982;**9**(1):6-10

[61] Jiang R, Yamaori S, Takeda S, Yamamoto I, Watanabe K. Identification of cytochrome P450 enzymes responsible for metabolism of cannabidiol by human liver microsomes. Life Sciences. 2011;**89**(5-6):165-170

[62] Hines RN. Ontogeny of human hepatic cytochromes P450. Journal of Biochemical and Molecular Toxicology. 2007;**21**(4):169-175

[63] Lacroix D, Sonnier M, Moncion A, Cheron G, Cresteil T. Expression of CYP3A in the human liver—Evidence that the shift between CYP3A7 and CYP3A4 occurs immediately after birth. European Journal of Biochemistry. 1997;**247**(2):625-634

[64] Williams JA, Ring BJ, Cantrell VE, Jones DR, Eckstein J, Ruterbories K, et al. Comparative metabolic capabilities of CYP3A4, CYP3A5, and CYP3A7. Drug Metabolism and Disposition. 2002;**30**(8):883-891

[65] Yamaori S, Ebisawa J, Okushima Y, Yamamoto I, Watanabe K. Potent inhibition of human cytochrome P450 3A isoforms by cannabidiol: Role of phenolic hydroxyl groups in the resorcinol moiety. Life Sciences. 2011;**88**(15-16):730-736

[66] Burchell B, Coughtrie M, Jackson M, Harding D, Fournel-Gigleux S, Leakey J, et al. Development of human liver UDP-glucuronosyltransferases. Developmental Pharmacology and Therapeutics. 1989;**13**(2-4):70-77

[67] Hryhorowicz S, Walczak M, Zakerska-Banaszak O, Slomski R, Skrzypczak-Zielinska M. Pharmacogenetics of cannabinoids. European Journal of Drug Metabolism and Pharmacokinetics. 2018;**43**(1):1-12

[68] Hayton WL. Maturation and growth of renal function: Dosing renally cleared drugs in children. AAPS PharmSci. 2000;**2**(1):E3

[69] Wolking S, Schaeffeler E, Lerche H, Schwab M, Nies AT. Impact of genetic polymorphisms of ABCB1 (MDR1, P-glycoprotein) on drug disposition and potential clinical implications: Update of the literature. Clinical Pharmacokinetics. 2015;**54**(7):709-735

[70] Chadwick B, Miller ML, Hurd YL. Cannabis use during adolescent development: Susceptibility to psychiatric illness. Frontiers in Psychiatry. 2013;**4**:129

[71] Volkow ND, Compton WM, Weiss SR. Adverse health effects of marijuana use. The New England Journal of Medicine. 2014;**371**(9):879

[72] Barbour AM, Fossler MJ, Barrett J. Practical considerations for dose selection in pediatric patients to ensure target exposure requirements. The AAPS Journal. 2014;**16**(4): 749-755

[73] Knibbe CA, Melenhorst-de Jong G, Mestrom M, Rademaker CM, Reijnvaan AF, Zuideveld KP, et al. Pharmacokinetics and effects of propofol 6% for short-term sedation in paediatric patients following cardiac surgery. British Journal of Clinical Pharmacology. 2002;**54**(4):415-422

[74] Moore TJ, Weiss SR, Kaplan S, Blaisdell CJ. Reported adverse drug events in infants and children under 2 years of age. Pediatrics. 2002;**110**(5):e53

[75] Geffrey AL, Pollack SF, Bruno PL, Thiele EA. Drug-drug interaction between clobazam and cannabidiol in children with refractory epilepsy. Epilepsia. 2015;**56**(8):1246-1251

[76] Nadulski T, Pragst F, Weinberg G, Roser P, Schnelle M, Fronk EM, et al. Randomized, double-blind, placebo-controlled study about the effects of cannabidiol (CBD) on the pharmacokinetics of Delta9-tetrahydrocannabinol (THC) after oral application of THC verses standardized cannabis extract. Therapeutic Drug Monitoring. 2005;**27**(6):799-810

[77] Robson P. Therapeutic aspects of cannabis and cannabinoids. The British Journal of Psychiatry. 2001;**178**:107-115

Chapter 11

Cannabis for Pediatric and Adult Epilepsy

Richard James Huntsman, Richard Tang-Wai and
Jose Tellez-Zenteno

Additional information is available at the end of the chapter

http://dx.doi.org/10.5772/intechopen.85719

Abstract

Epilepsy is a chronic disease of the central nervous system characterized by recurrent unprovoked seizures. Up to 30% of patients continue to have seizures despite treatment with appropriate anticonvulsant medications. The presence of abnormal oscillatory events within neural networks is a major feature of epileptogenesis. The endocannabinoid system can modulate these oscillatory events and alter neuronal activity making the phytocannabinoids found in *Cannabis* a potential therapeutic option for patients with treatment resistant epilepsy. Many in vitro and in vivo studies have demonstrated the anticonvulsant effects of several phytocannabinoids including Δ^9-tetrahydrocannabinol (Δ^9-THC) and Cannabidiol (CBD). Several small observational studies demonstrated a favorable response to cannabis herbal extracts (CHE) containing high concentrations of CBD in children with treatment resistant epilepsy. Two large double blinded clinical trials assessing the efficacy of pharmaceutical grade CBD have also been performed in children with treatment resistant seizures in Dravet syndrome and Lennox-Gastaut syndrome. Both studies demonstrated an improvement in seizure reduction in children taking CBD as compared to the placebo groups. To date there is very limited data regarding the use of cannabis based products to treat adult patients with treatment resistant epilepsy with only one randomized double blinded placebo controlled clinical trial underway.

Keywords: epilepsy, endocannabinoid system, cannabis, tetrhydrocannabinol, cannabidiol

1. Introduction

Recently, there has been renewed interest in the use of cannabis in patients with treatment resistant epilepsy. This has, in large part, been driven by a public perception that cannabis offers a safe and natural alternative to conventional anticonvulsant therapies. However, the phytocannabinoids found in the cannabis plant do offer some very unique anticonvulsant pharmacological properties that warrant further exploration.

In this chapter the authors will provide a brief review of epilepsy and epileptogenesis followed by a review of how the endocannabinoid system can alter the processes involved in the propagation and suppression of epileptic seizures. This is then followed by a review of the phytocannabinoids and their anticonvulsant mechanisms of action. Finally, the authors provide a historical background on the use of cannabis to treat patients with epilepsy and a review of the most recent clinical trials.

2. Epilepsy

Epilepsy is a chronic disease characterized by recurrent unprovoked seizures. It is defined as a disease of the brain in which the patient has either (1) two or more unprovoked seizures occurring more than 24 hours apart or (2) one unprovoked seizure and a probability of further seizures to be greater than 60% [1]. The prevalence of epilepsy worldwide is estimated to be between 4 and 10/1000 people with epilepsy accounting for up to 0.5% of the global burden of disease [2, 3]. There is significant geographic variation with prevalence rates of epilepsy prevalence rates being much higher in the developing world [4].

Most children and adults with epilepsy respond well to anticonvulsant therapy with approximately 50% of adults and 70% of children becoming seizure free with their first anticonvulsant medication [5, 6, 7]. Up to 30% of patients with epilepsy can be considered to be drug resistant which is defined by the International League Against Epilepsy as having failed two or more appropriate anticonvulsant treatments at an appropriate dosage [8, 9].

In patients who have failed two appropriate anticonvulsants the likelihood of seizure freedom with the addition of further anticonvulsant therapies is low. Treatment options for patients with drug resistant epilepsy include further trials of anticonvulsants, resective surgery, neural pathway stimulation with receptive or vagal nerve stimulation and dietary therapies [10]. Further trials of anticonvulsants in adults will result in 16% of patients who had failed their first two medications becoming seizure free [11]. In pediatric patients while the likelihood of achieving remission for 1 year or more with further medication trials is higher at 57%, many will continue to have relapses over time [12]. Resective surgery success rates (as defined as obtaining Engel Class 1 seizure freedom) in pediatric and adult patients with surgically amenable epileptogenic lesions range from 34 to 90% depending on the nature and extent of the lesion [10, 13].

A full review of the processes that result in brain abnormalities causing seizures (epileptogenesis) is beyond the scope of this chapter. However, in order to understand how cannabinoids can have potential in treating epilepsy it is worth knowing the basic principles of these processes. One of the major hallmarks of epilepsy is the presence of abnormal oscillatory events within neuronal networks in the form of recurrent interictal spikes and high frequency oscillations within the epileptic zones of the patients' brain [14]. These abnormal oscillations then result in excessive synchronous firing of neurons causing an epileptic seizure with alteration in the patient's behavior, motor activity or sensorium. Epilepsy can result from injury (either ischemic or traumatic) to cortical brain structures or genetic, inflammatory, structural and metabolic disturbances within the brain. The main components of the development of the abnormal oscillations within neuronal networks and epileptogenesis (seizure development) are (a) neuronal hyperexcitability—the ability of neurons to generate abnormal intrinsic burst discharges (b) a loss of GABA mediated interneuron neuronal inhibition that would normally prevent these discharges from spreading to adjacent neurons and (c) neuronal hypersynchrony in which excessive synaptic enhancement of neighboring neurons through the development of excitatory pathways allows these bursts to spread in a synchronous manner within a group of neurons [15]. Neuronal hyperexcitability can arise from abnormalities in excitatory or inhibitory neurotransmitter receptors resulting in a loss of the normal balance between neuronal excitation and inhibition. Of particular interest in epileptogenesis are the excitatory glutamatergic N-methyl-D-aspartate (NMDA) and α-amino-3-hydroxy-5-methyl-4-isoxazole propionate (AMPA) receptors [16]. Alterations in ion channel function as is seen in the channelopathy associated epilepsies such as Dravet syndrome also lead to neuronal hyperexcitability [17].

3. The endocannabinoid system and epilepsy

The endocannabinoid system comprises the two endogenous endocannabinoid receptors (CB1R and CB2R) their two endogenously produced endocannabinoids; anandamide (*N*-arachidonyl-ethanolamide) and 2-AG (2-arachadonoylglycerol) which act as endogenous CBR ligands as well as the enzymes involved in endocannabinoid production and breakdown. Of the endocannabinoids produced in the human brain, 2-AG is produced in much higher concentrations and plays the most significant role in regulation of oscillatory networks [18]. For a full review of the endocannabinoid system please refer to this book's introduction and the review article by Ligresti et al. [19] CB1R is one of the most abundant G protein-coupled receptors (GPCR) within the mammalian brain and is expressed on the presynaptic axon terminal. In response to activation of the postsynaptic neuron, anandamide (a partial CB1R agonist) and 2-AG (a full CB1R agonist) are both produced within and released by the postsynaptic neuron. Activation of the presynaptic CB1R receptors by the endocannabinoids then results in a temporary suppression in voltage gated Ca^{2+} channels and activation of K^+ channels resulting in suppression of further neurotransmitter release from the presynaptic neuron [20].

Although CB1R is one of the most abundantly expressed GPCRs in the brain, its expression is concentrated within certain groups of neurons. For example, in the hippocampus, CB1R expression is concentrated on the axon terminals of inhibitory GABAergic CA1 region interneurons and Schaffer collaterals arising from CA3 pyramidal cells [22]. These interneurons play a key role in the formation and maintenance of normal oscillatory behavior in the hippocampus essential for memory formation [18]. The effect of stimulation of CB1R is very localized within neuronal networks both from a spatial and temporal point of view. This is achieved by the production of monoacylglycerol lipase (MAGL) by astrocytes and nerve terminals which breaks down 2-AG in the synaptic cleft. This temporal and spatial control allows for precise regulation of oscillations within neuronal networks by the endocannabinoid system [18].

During an epileptic seizure there is excessive glutamate release from presynaptic excitatory neurons. In rodent models of epilepsy this has been shown to cause increased production of both 2-AG and anandamide that in turn active CB1R on the glutamatergic axon terminals to decrease the release of further excessive glutamate. This prevents further neuronal hyperexcitability which may play a role in terminating seizures. The increased anandamide is felt to play a role in preventing seizure induced excitatory neurotoxic effects [18, 21].

Temporal lobe epilepsy secondary to mesial temporal sclerosis (scarring of the hippocampi) is a common cause of epilepsy in adults that is often amenable to surgical resection of the mesial temporal structures. Pathological examination of surgically resected specimens has shown alterations in expression of CB1R of neurons within the hippocampi that provide insight into how disruption of the endocannabinoid system could predispose to epileptogenesis. In resected hippocampi there is a downregulation of CB1R expression on the axon terminals of excitatory (glutamatergic) neurons within the inner molecular layer of the dentate gyrus and an upregulation of CB1R expression on inhibitory (GABAergic) axon terminals within the dentate molecular layer [18]. These changes in CB1R expression result in both a loss of the normal inhibition of excessive glutamate release and increased suppression of GABAergic activity both of which result in increased neuronal hyperexcitability and subsequent seizure generation [22]. In patients with chronic epilepsy, there is also a decrease in the amount of anandamide and 2-AG released with excessive neuronal activation further contributing to a loss of the endocannabinoid mediated inhibition of excessive neuronal activation [18].

The growing body of evidence demonstrating the role the endocannabinoid system plays in the brains' mechanisms in regulating neuronal network oscillations and preventing excessive neuronal hyperexcitability coupled with alterations in the endocannabinoid receptors seen in epileptogenic tissue make the endocannabinoid system an attractive therapeutic target in the treatment of epilepsy. Modulation of the endocannabinoid system would provide a potential novel anticonvulsant mechanism not provided by other anticonvulsant therapies.

4. Phytocannabinoids and epilepsy: mechanisms of action and preclinical studies

The phytocannabinoids are a class of cannabinoids that are produced by plants of the cannabis species. The phytocannabinoids are C_{21} aromatic compounds consisting of an aromatic isoprenyl terpenophenolic core and resorcinyl side chain. Based on the structure of the oxygen bond between the isoprenyl and resorcinyl moieties the phytocannabinoids can be placed into 6 main families. Within each family, variations of the R-chain on the resorcinyl moiety differentiate each individual cannabinoid [23]. To date, over 140 different phytocannabinoids have been identified in *C. sativa.* While there is a high degree of structural preservation among the

http://dx.doi.org/10.5772/intechopen.85719

phytocannabinoids, they appear to display widely different effects on the mammalian central nervous system. The structural and stereochemical requirements for biological activity of the cannabinoids have been well established. Most biologically active cannabinoids (with a few exceptions) have a hydroxyl group on the C_1 and an alkyl group on the C_3 aromatic positions. As well, naturally occurring cannabinoids are biologically active in the trans (−) enantiomer [24]. Following the first isolation of the cannabinoids it did not take long for their anticonvulsant properties to be recognized [25]. Of the cannabinoids produced by the *C. sativa* the most comprehensively studied in the field of epilepsy are Δ^9-tetrahydrocannabinol (Δ^9-THC) and cannabidiol (CBD).

Initial research focused on the anticonvulsant effects of Δ^9-THC and other CB1R agonists such as anandamide. Through their activation of CB1R, anandamide and the synthetic cannabinoid WIN 55,212-2 were able to block the production of postsynaptic neuronal spiking and excitatory post synaptic potential production. Both compounds were also able to suppress the production of abnormal burst activity in neurons placed in Mg_2^+ depleted solution. Depletion of Mg^{2+} in solution allows activation of NMDA receptors at normal resting potentials without the usual prerequisite neuronal depolarization. This effect was abolished when CB1R antagonists were added, suggesting that the effect was secondary to activation of CB1R by these agents [26]. Δ^9-THC is a major phytocannabinoid in *C. sativa*. It is a high affinity partial agonist of both CB1R and CB2R that is competitive with both anandamide and 2-AG. The direct activation of CB1R by Δ^9-THC is responsible for its psychoactive effects [19]. Numerous studies have assessed the anticonvulsant activity of Δ^9-THC and its metabolites with conflicting results. These studies showed that Δ^9-THC and its metabolites showed both anticonvulsant and proconvulsant activity depending on the dosage, animal species and seizure model used. In Maximal Electroshock (MES) and Maximal Electroshock Threshold (MEST) mouse models which mimic generalized onset convulsive seizures both Δ9-THC and its metabolites showed anticonvulsant activity by blocking or increasing the latency to hind limb extensor seizures [27]. In other studies Δ^9-THC was also shown to potentiate the effects of several anticonvulsants [28]. In models that showed an anticonvulsant effect of Δ^9-THC, all three of its metabolites including 11-OH-Δ^9-THC showed anticonvulsant effect. The anticonvulsant effect of 11-OH-Δ^9-THC was more potent than its parent compound by almost 1 order of magnitude suggesting that much of the anticonvulsant activity attributed to Δ^9-THC may in fact come from its metabolites [27].

In a rat model of electrically induced limbic seizures Δ^9-THC increased the threshold of electrically induced after discharges at the site of electrode implantation in the left subiculum. However, Δ^9-THC increased the duration of cortically recorded after discharges in electrodes remote from the site of stimulation. This suggested that Δ^9-THC may have both anticonvulsant and proconvulsant effects in focal onset epilepsies [27]. In the cobalt model of focal epilepsy in rats Δ^9-THC increased the frequency of epileptic potentials at the site of the cobalt-induced lesion. This was not seen with Δ^9-THC's main metabolite 11-OH-Δ^9-THC. Both Δ^9-THC and 11-OH-Δ^9-THC seemed to increase generalized cortical excitation as seen by the production of brief intermittent cortically recorded after discharges [27]. Similar findings were seen in a rat model using iron to induce a seizure focus. While both Δ^9-THC and 11-OH-Δ^9-THC both caused increased cortical excitability, only Δ^9-THC provoked clinical seizures. As well, the dose of Δ^9-THC required to induce seizures was much higher than that required to induce electrographic changes in keeping with cortical excitation [29]. In mice, Δ^9-THC has also been shown to induce kindling of a second epileptic focus in response to both electroconvulsive therapy as well as pentylenetetrazol (PTZ) and picrotoxin induced seizures [30]. When administered to rabbits with a genetic mutation causing audiogenic seizures Δ^9-THC caused signs of neurotoxicity but prevented seizures when the rabbits were stimulated with a sound stimulus above their normal seizure threshold range. Conversely, in another breed of rabbits, injection with Δ^9-THC induced both neurotoxicity and behavioral seizures in a dosage dependent manner [31].

The results of these studies show that Δ^9-THC and its metabolites display anticonvulsant activity in animal models using seizure models with rapidly evoked tonic discharges which mimics certain types of generalized onset seizures in humans. However, in models mimicking focal onset seizures, Δ^9-THC and its metabolites seem to display a proconvulsant effect. This is manifested by increasing the activity at the site of the focal lesion and increasing generalized cortical activity [27]. A proconvulsant effect is also seen in models mimicking genetic based generalized epilepsies and absence seizures. Δ^9-THC and its metabolites seem to induce hypersynchrony with slowly propagating epileptic discharges [32]. While Δ^9-THC showed some potential as an anticonvulsant agent the potential to increase seizure activity along with its neurotoxic and psychotropic side effect profile limited its potential benefit in patients with epilepsy.

CBD is a low affinity negative allosteric modulator of CB1R with no psychotropic side effects due to the fact it does not cause activation of CB1R. It modulates the influx of both Ca^{2+} and Na^+ into neurons by binding to human T-type voltage gated Ca^{2+} channels, Melastatin and Vanilloid type Transient Receptor Potential membrane receptors (TRPM and TRPV) and voltage gated Na^+ channels [19]. This decreases neuronal excitability in response to stimulation. CBD has also been shown to inhibit intrasynaptic re-uptake of adenosine as well as activation of neuronal Serotonin, Glycine and Vanilloid receptors [33, 34]. The anticonvulsant effect of CBD is felt to be independent of activation of the endogenous CBR pathways. While the exact mechanism of anticonvulsant activity of CBD remains uncertain it appears to have a polypharmacological effect on modulating neuronal excitability.

In the Cobalt induced focal epilepsy rat model CBD had no effect on focal discharges at the lesion site but decreased the frequency of seizures. CBD also blocked the proconvulsant effects in of Δ^9-THC [27, 35]. In the limbic seizure rat model CBD decreased the frequency, duration and amplitude of electrically induced after discharges at the site of stimulation in the left subiculum but did not prevent the spread of after discharges from the site of focal stimulation to distal electrodes. It had no apparent effect on generalized cortical excitability. This suggests that in focal models of epilepsy, CBD acts directly on the site of focal seizure onset [27].

Other animal studies continued to show the anticonvulsant effect of CBD in both transcorneal electroshock, drug induced and lesional epilepsies. This anticonvulsant effect was seen when a single intraperitoneal (i.p.) dose of CBD was administered alone but like Δ^9-THC it also potentiated the effects of several anticonvulsant medications [33, 36, 37]. While CBD had potent anticonvulsant effect against tonic seizures its effect against clonic seizures was minimal. Consroe et al. hypothesized that this effect was due to the fact that tonic seizures are spread rapidly throughout the brain from a focal lesion via post-tetanic stimulation. Unlike Δ^9-THC, CBD suppressed tetanic potentiation in isolated bullfrog ganglia [27]. This coupled with the fact that CBD is effective in preventing 3-Mercaptoproprionic acid (3-MPA) induced seizures suggested that some of the anticonvulsant effect of CBD may result from its ability to increase production of GABA in presynaptic GABAergic neurons [36]. Unlike Δ^9-THC, the brain concentrations of CBD correlated well with its anticonvulsant effect in several animal models. This suggests that the anticonvulsant effect of CBD is due to the parent compound and not its metabolites [27].

In summary, CBD was shown to display broad spectrum anticonvulsant activity in a wide range of animal models of epilepsy including generalized seizures caused by electroshock and GABA inhibiting drugs and focal seizures induced by placement of toxic metals on the cortex. It however had no effect on models of generalized absence seizures [38]. CBD also blocked kindling of a second epileptic focus [36]. Even at high doses it failed to cause any behavioral or cognitive side effects in test animals. This would suggest that CBD is a potent anticonvulsant with limited cognitive side effects, making it an attractive potential anticonvulsant in the pediatric population [33, 37].

4.1. Other cannabinoids and terpenes

In addition, Δ^9-THC and CBD several other cannabinoids have been evaluated for the potential anticonvulsant activity. These include Δ^9-tetrahydrocannibivarin (Δ^9-THCV) and cannabidivarin (CBDV) which have been shown to have anticonvulsant effects. Δ^9-THCV is a non-psychoactive cannabinoid that acts as a CB1R antagonist. In a Mg^{2+} depleted solution Δ^9-THCV decreased the amplitude and duration of abnormal neuronal burst activity. Δ^9-THCV potentiated the effects on neuronal bursting of both phenobarbital and valproic acid. In a PTZ rat model Δ^9-THCV did not decrease the severity or duration of seizures or seizure mortality. However significantly fewer rats exposed to PTZ that were treated with Δ^9-THCV displayed seizures compared to those that were given PTZ alone [39]. Like CBD, CBDV is believed to exert its effects via CB1R independent mechanisms and has limited neurotoxicity [40]. CBDV has been shown to decrease the amplitude and duration of abnormal bursting in mouse and rat hippocampal slices in in both Mg^{2+} depleted solution and solution to which 4-aminopyridine (4-AP) has been added. CBDV also significantly decreased the number of seizures seen in in vitro MES and audiogenic seizure models in mice and PTZ induced seizures in rats. Unlike CBD, CBDV also prolonged the latency of seizure induction in a dose dependent manner. Administration of CBDV had no effect on motor performance in mice regardless of the ode administered [41]. The terpenes, which are another class of compounds found in cannabis, also possess a wide range of pharmacological activity on the mammalian nervous system at very low concentrations. Individually, these terpenes have not been assessed in patients with epilepsy [42, 43].

The combinatorial effect of the chemical components of cannabis has been postulated wherein cannabis whole plant extracts may benefit from 'entourage' effects to yield greater effectiveness than treatment with a purified cannabinoid [42, 44]. This is supported by preclinical studies. In the *in vitro* oxotremorine-M mouse model of epilepsy, excessive neuronal bursting activity can be suppressed with Δ^9-THC, but not CBD, while a standardized cannabis extract containing both Δ^9-THC and CBD can abolish the abnormal bursting activity faster than purified Δ^9-THC alone [45]. In another study, both purified Δ^9-THC and CBD can increase intracellular Ca^{2+} in rat hippocampal neuronal and glial cells. This effect is compounded when the two compounds are mixed together, with the greatest effect occurring with whole plant extract containing both Δ^9-THC and CBD [46]. These preclinical data support the hypothesis that the 'entourage' effects between the various cannabinoids provide therapeutic benefit of cannabis whole plant extract, benefit that exceeds the activity of a single purified cannabinoid. This remains to be demonstrated in the human clinical context.

5. Early clinical experience with cannabis for the treatment of epilepsy

The use of cannabis as a treatment for a variety of ailments in eastern and Mediterranean cultures over the last several millennium has been well documented [47]. The first description of the use of cannabis to treat seizures came from Dr. W. O'Shaugnessy who while working in India reported its successful use to treat seizures in an infant [48]. Following this, cannabis extracts became widely used throughout Europe and North America as an accepted treatment for epilepsy [49]. Following prohibition and with the introduction of other anticonvulsants, cannabis fell out of use as a treatment for epilepsy in western cultures.

During the mid-twentieth century, several reports on the effect of recreational cannabis consumption surfaced with contrasting effects. Several case reports described patients having decreased seizure frequency following the consumption of cannabis [50]. Cannabis consumption was also shown to be protective against first unprovoked seizures. In adult males who smoked cannabis in the last 90 days, the odds of having a first unprovoked seizure was 0.38 compared to adult males who never consumed cannabis [51]. Conversely, a patient with a history of epilepsy who had been seizure free for several months on medication was reported to have had an exacerbation of seizures following the consumption of cannabis [52].

In 1978, Mechoulam et al. reported their double blinded placebo-controlled study of CBD used as an add-on therapy in patients with refractory focal onset seizures. Of the four patients who took CBD two were seizure free for the 3 months of the study while another had partial improvement. None of the five patients who took placebo had any improvement in their seizures [53]. Cunha et al. reported the results of their study investigating the potential of CBD in patients with refractory temporal lobe epilepsy. In the first phase of the study, healthy adult volunteers were randomized to receive either placebo or CBD at 3 mg/kg/day for 30 days. Of 8 volunteers receiving CBD, 2 reported somnolence otherwise no adverse effects were reported. In the second phase, 15 adult patients with drug-resistant temporal lobe epilepsy were randomized to receive either placebo or CBD (up to 300 mg/day) for a period of 18 weeks in a double-blinded manner. Four of 8 patients dosed with CBD had complete improvement while three had partial improvement. No adverse effects were noted in patients given CBD [54].

http://dx.doi.org/10.5772/intechopen.85719

Two further studies showed no significant difference in seizure reduction with the addition of CBD as an adjunctive therapy. However, in one study patients were given CBD at a dose of 300 mg/day and their plasma CBD levels were maintained at 20–30 ng/ml. Subsequently one participant who had no difference in their seizure frequency was placed on CBD at a higher dose of up to 1200 mg/day. CBD plasma levels were higher averaging 150 ng/ml. This patient had a significant decrease in their seizure frequency suggesting that higher doses of CBD (and higher plasma levels) were required for seizure control [55].

6. Recent clinical trials and experience

In recent years there has been a public perception that cannabis is a potent, natural, and safe alternative therapy for epilepsy. This has driven the demand for and use of cannabis and its derived products to treat epilepsy especially in those patients whose seizures are medically intractable. Coupled with the media exposure showing examples of the apparent miraculous effects of CBD oil in select epileptic patients, treating physicians have struggled to balance the patient demand for cannabis products and the need for studies to determine their, efficacy, dosing, side-effect profile, and indication. To that end, there have been multiple studies, predominantly in children, looking into these clinical questions. Unfortunately, the overwhelming majority of these studies have been retrospective, unblinded, and uncontrolled resulting in their being hampered by various forms of bias and potential placebo effect. Despite the plethora of published research on this topic, questions still remain on the use of cannabis in epilepsy.

In this section, we will review the limitations of the studies, the studies using artisanal and CBD enriched cannabis herbal extracts (CHE), the studies using highly purified pharmaceutical grade CBD, and a meta-analysis of the CBD studies.

6.1. Limitations of the studies

The widespread use of cannabis and the effect of bias are highlighted in various published surveys. McLachlan performed a survey in London, Ontario, Canada, in which more than 60% of patients declared that cannabis was effective for their seizures and stress levels [56]. Ladina et al. reported a case series of 18 patients who all found medicinal cannabis very helpful for seizure control and improvement of mood disorder [57]. By contrast, Press had reported a significant discrepancy in reported responder rate between preexisting Colorado residents and those who moved to Colorado to obtain cannabis to treat their child's epilepsy (22 vs. 47%) suggesting there is a significant perception bias among these children's caregivers as to the therapeutic benefits of cannabis [58]. Physician bias may also play a role as a recent survey by Mathern showed contrasting opinions about CBD between neurologists and the general public. In his study, a minority of epileptologists and general neurologists said that there were sufficient data safety (34%) and efficacy data (28%) and only 48% would advise using medical cannabis and only in severe cases of epilepsy. Conversely, nearly all patients and the general public responded that there was sufficient safety (96%) and efficacy (95%) data, and 98% would recommend cannabis in cases with severe epilepsy [59].

Given the present approved indications for medical coverage, the high cost of pharmaceutical grade CBD products, and the illegal status of cannabis in some countries and US states, the overwhelming majority of patients will at this time be using CBD oil extracts or artisanal products. In many jurisdictions these products are unregulated and therefore their content and consistency are uncertain and can vary. In Australia, where medical use of cannabis is highly restricted, Suraev reported that in parents treating their children with "illicit" cannabis extracts, the majority of extract samples used by the families contained low concentrations of cannabidiol, while Δ^9-THC was present in nearly every sample [60]. These findings highlighted the profound variation in the illicit cannabis extracts being used. Studies examining the use of artisanal and CBD oil extracts therefore could have had uncertain and inconsistent amounts of cannabinoids. This inconsistency in combination the inherent problems of retrospective studies, make the findings of these studies questionable; moreover, none of published studies included serum CBD levels.

To date, there are few prospective, double blind, placebo-controlled studies which all only examined the use of the highly purified, pharmaceutical grade CBD (Epidiolex). None involved artisanal CBD or the CBD oil extracts.

6.2. The artisanal and CBD oil extracts

While keeping the limitations of the studies examining artisanal and CBD oil extracts in epilepsy in mind, most of these studies did find that CBD oil extracts are effective in reducing seizures and improving quality of life.

Tzadok reported out of 74 children being treated with a 20% CBD and 1% Δ^9-THC CHE, 89% reported reduction in seizure frequency with only 43% of patients having a >50% reduction in seizures. Five patients reported aggravation of seizures leading to withdrawal from the study. Improvement in behavior and alertness, language, communication, motor skills and sleep were noted. Adverse reactions included somnolence, fatigue, gastrointestinal disturbances and irritability leading to withdrawal of cannabis use in five patients. The CBD dosing ranged from 1 to 20 mg/kg/day with 83% taking <10 mg/kg/day [61].

Similarly, Porcari retrospectively studied the efficacy of artisanal CBD preparations in children with epilepsy. The study also included a subgroup comparison to determine if the addition of clobazam was related to any beneficial effects of CBD. Overall, the addition of CBD resulted in 39% of patients having a >50% reduction in seizures, with 10% becoming seizure-free. The difference in effect between CBD alone and CBD with clobazam was not statistically significant. Increased alertness and improved verbal interactions were reported in 14% of patients in the CBD group and 8% of patients in the CBD and clobazam group. The average dose of CBD was 2.9 mg/kg/day in the CBD group and 5.8 mg/kg/day in the CBD and clobazam group [62].

McCoy et al. performed a prospective open label study using a 2:100 Δ^9-THC:CBD CHE in 20 children with Dravet syndrome. The dose of CBD ranged from 7 to 16 mg/kg/day (mean 13.3 mg CBD/kg/day). They reported that during the 20-week intervention period the median monthly reduction in motor seizures was 70.6%. The CHE also resulted in improvements in quality of life measures and spike index on electroencephalogram (EEG). Adverse events during the titration period included somnolence, anorexia and diarrhea [63].

The Cannabinoid Research Initiative of Saskatchewan is currently conducting a Canadian, multicenter, prospective, open-label, dose-escalation phase 1 trial entitled Cannabidiol in Children with Refractory Epileptic Encephalopathy (CARE-E). The source of the CBD oil is consistent with a single batch of 1:20 Δ^9-THC:CBD CHE used for all study participants. Concentrations of the cannabinoids in the CHE were confirmed through Health Canada Quality Assurance and Good Manufacturing Practices (GMP) certification [64]. Preliminary data showed that all 6 participants had improvements in seizure frequency, Quality of Life in Childhood Epilepsy (QOLCE) and EEG rating scores—with three participants showing continued improvements in these measures after the oil extract was discontinued. In addition, serum CBD levels suggested linear dose independent pharmacokinetics in all but one participant. In most participants, serum Δ^9-THC concentrations remained lower than what would be expected to cause intoxication even at the maximum dose of oil extract. None of the participants displayed any evidence of Δ^9-THC intoxication clinically throughout the study. Preliminary data suggests that an effective and well-tolerated CBD initial target dose of 5–6 mg/kg/day is effective and well tolerated when a 1:20 Δ^9-THC:CBD CHE is used. In addition, the serum concentration of CBD follows dose-independent linear pharmacokinetics for most participants, although non-linear pharmacokinetics might occur but requires confirmation. Continued improvement in seizure frequency and QOLCE following the discontinuation of CHE suggest a possible enduring anticonvulsant effect [65].

6.3. The highly purified, pharmaceutical grade CBD products

With the production of a highly purified, pharmaceutical grade CBD (Epidiolex), studies could now be performed with a CBD source of greater reliability. Although potential bias remained, better clinical studies had been performed.

Devinksy published an open label trial in patients aged 1–30 with severe, intractable, childhood-onset, drugs resistant epilepsy. All patients were receiving their regular anti-epileptic drugs. Patients were given CBD at 2–5 mg/kg/day, titrated over a period of 2 weeks till intolerance or to a maximum dose of 25 mg/kg to 50 mg/kg/day. The main objective of the study was to establish safety and tolerability of CBD and the primary end point was the median percentage in the mean monthly frequency of motor seizures at 12 weeks. This study included mainly patients with Dravet and Lennox-Gastaut syndromes. One hundred and sixty-two patients were enrolled. A significant high rate of adverse events was reported in 128 patients (79%). The most common were somnolence (n = 41 [25%]), decreased appetite (n = 31 [19%]), diarrhea (n = 31 [19%]) and fatigue (n = 21 [13%]). This high rate of side effects (many of which were seen during the titration period) suggests that too rapid a titration rate may predispose toward side effects. The median monthly frequency of motor seizures was 30·0 (IQR 11·0–96·0) at baseline and 15·8 (5·6–57·6) at 12 weeks of treatment. The median reduction in monthly motor seizures was 36·5% (IQR 0–64·7) [66].

From this same cohort, Rosenberg et al. reported that caregivers of 48 patients indicated an 8.2–9.9-point improvement in overall patient QOLCE ($p < 0.001$) following 12 weeks of CBD. Subscores with improvement included energy/fatigue, memory, control/helplessness, other cognitive functions, social interactions, behavior, and global quality of life (QOL). Interestingly, these differences were not correlated to changes in seizure frequency or adverse events. The results suggest that CBD may have beneficial effects on patient QOL, distinct from its seizure reducing effects [67].

Devinsky et al. later performed a double blind, placebo-controlled trial in patients with Dravet syndrome including 120 children and young adults using Epidiolex with a CBD dosage of 20 mg/kg/day. The median frequency of convulsive seizures per month decreased from 12.4 (baseline) to 5.9 with CBD, as compared with a decrease from 14.9 (baseline) to 14.1 with placebo (adjusted median difference between cannabidiol vs. placebo was −22.8% points [CI], −41.1 to −5.4; p = 0.01). The percentage of patients who had at least a 50% reduction in convulsive seizure frequency was 43% with cannabidiol and 27% with placebo (odds ratio, 2.00; 95% CI, 0.93–4.30; p = 0.08). This study shows an overall benefit of CBD over placebo but also a large placebo effect in the control group [68].

Another trial that assessed the efficacy of Epidiolex in reducing atonic seizures in patients with Lennox-Gastaut syndrome. In this double blind, placebo-controlled trial, a total of 225 patients were enrolled, 76 patients were assigned to a treatment group (20 mg/kg/day CBD) and 76 to the placebo group. The median percent reduction from baseline in monthly atonic seizure frequency during the treatment period was 41.9% in the treatment group vs. 21.8% in the placebo group. As with the other studies assessing Epidiolex, the most common adverse events among the patients in the treatment groups were somnolence, decreased appetite, and diarrhea [69].

A recent systematic review assessed the safety and efficacy of pharmaceutical grade CBD in pediatric onset drug resistant epilepsy with outcome measures including 50% seizure reduction, complete seizure freedom, improved QOL. A total of 36 studies were identified including 6 randomized controlled trials and 30 observational studies. Overall CBD at a dose of 20 mg/kg/day was more effective than placebo in reducing seizure frequency by 50% (Relative Risk 1.74: 1.24–2.43). For one patient to achieve a 50% reduction in seizures the number of patient needed to treat was 8. In pooled data of 17 of the observational studies CBD at 20 mg/kg/day resulted in 48.5% of patients achieving a 50% reduction in seizures (95% CI: 39.0–58.1%) while pooled data from 14 observational studies showed 8.5% of patients became seizure free (95% CI: 3.8–14.5%). Quality of life improved in 55.8% of patients (95% CI: 40.5–70.6%) while serious adverse events related to treatment with CBD was very low at 2.2% of patients (95% CI: 0.0–7.9%). From this data, the authors concluded that pharmaceutical grade CBD may reduce seizure frequency but other randomized controlled trials examining a more diverse group of epilepsy syndromes and other cannabinoids was needed [70].

To date, the evidence to support the use of cannabis in adults is minimal. STAR 1 is a phase 2A, randomized, double blind, placebo-controlled study that evaluated the safety and efficacy of synthetic transdermal CBD in adult patients with focal epilepsy. In this study 174 patients were randomized to receive either 195 mg CBD, 390 mg CBD or placebo via a transdermal patch. Patients who completed the 12-week study were able to continue into the 24-month open-label extension STAR 2 study (n = 171). In as of yet published data from these trials there was an increase in efficacy of transdermal CBD over 18 months. Median percentage change in seizure rates was −25% at 3 months, −40% at 6 months, −48% at 9 months, −52% at

http://dx.doi.org/10.5772/intechopen.85719

12 months, −57% at 15 months and −55% at 18 months. The transdermal patch was well tolerated. Serious adverse events were as follows: seizures (n = 2) and increased anxiety (n = 1); one death was reported after the 15 month visit. In addition, no significant elevations in alanine aminotransferase and aspartate aminotransferase levels >3 times upper limit of normal were seen [71].

In comparing cannabis derived treatments to standard therapies, it is worthwhile to note that the STICLO group examining the effects of stiripentol in Dravet patients in a double blind randomized placebo controlled study showed that 15 (71%) patients had >50% seizure reduction (including nine free of clonic or tonic-clonic seizures) compared to only one (5%) on placebo (none were seizure free; stiripentol 95% CI 52.1–90.7 vs. placebo 0–14.6). Stiripentol's responder rate is therefore suggested to be superior to Epidiolex with a far lower placebo responder rate [72]. Similarly, in a double-blind, randomized, placebo-controlled trial of the anti-epileptic drug rufinamide in patients with Lennox-Gastaut syndrome, the median percentage reduction in total seizure frequency was greater in the rufinamide therapy group than in the placebo group (32.7 vs. 11.7%, $p = 0.0015$). There was also a difference ($p < 0.0001$) in tonic-atonic ("drop attack") seizure frequency with rufinamide (42.5% median percentage reduction) vs. placebo (1.4% increase). These findings are comparable with the results with Epidiolex. One also has to keep in mind that the median reduction of atonic seizures in the placebo group was markedly higher with the Epidiolex study suggesting potential bias [73].

Of note, the results from the study by McCoy et al. and the preliminary data from CARE-E study showed a much higher responder rate than those with pharmaceutical grade CBD. This apparent superiority of a CHE containing Δ^9-THC would be in keeping with the proposed entourage effect in which the various cannabinoids can act synergistically with one another [42, 44].

7. Conclusion

The cannabinoids found in cannabis appear to offer a unique pharmacological mode of action in the treatment of epilepsy. This, combined with the apparent low risk of serious side effects, makes cannabis and an attractive potential option for patients with treatment resistant epilepsy.

Currently, there is a large public perception that cannabis products are superior to and safer than conventional anti-epileptic medications especially in treating patients with Dravet syndrome and other pediatric onset epileptic encephalopathies. Based on interpretation of the available data, the authors feel that cannabis based therapies show promise in the treatment of children with treatment resistant epilepsies. While the studies to date assessing cannabis based therapies for the treatment of epilepsy have been encouraging, they should be interpreted with caution. At this time, the long-term adverse effects, the indicated epilepsy and seizure types suitable for treatment with cannabis, the dosing of CBD and other cannabinoids, remain unknown. Also, there is minimal data regarding the pharmacokinetics of the cannabinoids especially in children and when used in patients with multiple concomitant medications. Moreover, the existing studies are limited with the majority of them being retrospective and subject to bias, possible placebo effect, and other limitations.

As such, further studies assessing the safety and efficacy of cannabis based therapies in both adults and children are urgently needed. The authors recommend that these studies start with well-designed dose finding studies that include age stratified pharmacokinetic analysis followed by larger scale clinical trials. When faced with physicians that are reluctant to authorize cannabis based products due to a lack of high quality safety and efficacy data, parents who are desperate to help their children are then forced to turn to unregulated suppliers of cannabis. This puts their children at risk of harm and themselves in legal jeopardy.

Author note

Purpose statement: This chapter explores the role of cannabis-based therapies in the treatment of children and adults with epilepsy.

Author details

Richard James Huntsman[1,2*], Richard Tang-Wai[1,3] and Jose Tellez-Zenteno[1,4]

*Address all correspondence to: rjh762@mail.usask.ca

1 Cannabinoid Research Initiative of Saskatchewan (CRIS), University of Saskatchewan, Saskatoon, Canada

2 Department of Pediatrics, Division of Pediatric Neurology, University of Saskatchewan, Royal University Hospital, Saskatoon, Saskatchewan, Canada

3 Department of Pediatrics, Division of Child Neurology, Loma Linda University, Loma Linda, California, USA

4 Department of Medicine, Division of Neurology, University of Saskatchewan, Royal University Hospital, Saskatoon, Saskatchewan Canada

References

[1] Fisher RS, Avacedo C, Arzimanoglou A, Bogacz A, Cross JH, Elger CE, et al. A practical clinical definition of epilepsy. Epilepsia. 2014;**55**(4):475-482

[2] World Health organization. Fact Sheet: Epilepsy. 2018. Available from: http://www.who.int/news-room/fact-sheets/detail/epilepsy

[3] Dua T, Garrido Cumbrera M, Mathers C, Saxena S. Global burden of neurological disorders: Estimates and projections. In: Neurological Disorders: Public Helath Challenges. Geneva: World Health Organization Press. 2006

[4] Newton CR, Garcia HH. Epilepsy in poor regions of the world. Lancet. 2012;**380**:1193-1201

[5] Schmidt D, Schacter SC. Drug treatment of epilepsy in adults. British Medical Journal. 2014;**348**:g2546

[6] Brodie MJ, Barry SJE, Bamagouse GA, Norrie JD, Kwan P. Patterns of treatment response in newly diagnosed epilepsy. 2012;**78**(20):1548-1554

[7] Arhan E, Serdaroglou A, Kurt ANC, Aslanyavrusu M. Drug treatment failures and effectivity in children with newly diagnosed epilepsy. Seizure. 2010;**19**(9):553-557

[8] Kwan P, Brodie MJ. Early identification of refractory epilepsy. The New England Journal of Medicine. 2000;**342**(5):314-319

[9] Kwan P, Arzimanoglou A, Berg AT, et al. Definition of drug resistant epilepsy: Consensus proposal by the ad hoc task force of the ILAE commission on therapeutic strategies. Epilepsia. 2010;**51**(6):1069-1077

[10] Nair DR. Management of drug-resistant epilepsy. Continuum. 2016;**22**(1):157-172

[11] Luciano AL, Shorvon SD. Results of treatment changes in patients with apparently drug-resistant chronic epilepsy. Annals of Neurology. 2007;**62**(4):375-381

[12] Berg AT, Levy SR, Testa FM, D'Souza R. Remission of epilepsy after two drug failures in children: A prospective study. Annals of Neurology. 2009;**65**(5):510-519

[13] Jobst BC, Cascino GD. Resective epilepsy surgery for drug-resistant focal epilepsy. Journal of the American Medical Association. 2015;**313**(3):285-293

[14] Bragin A, Wilson CL, Almajano J, Mody I, Engel J. High frequency oscillations after status epilepticus, epileptogenesis and seizure genesis. Epilepsia. 2004;**45**:1017-1023

[15] Najm I, Ying Z, Janigro D. Mechanism of epileptogenesis. Neurologic Clinics of North America. 2001;**19**(1):237-250

[16] Benke TA, Brooks-Kayal AR. Experimental Models of Seizures and Mechanisms of Epileptogenesis. In: Wyllie's Treatment of Epilepsy: Principles and Practice. 5th ed. Lippincott Williams & Wilkins; 2011

[17] Catterall WA. Forty years of sodium channels: Structure, function, pharmacology and epilepsy. Neurochemical Research. 2017;**42**(9):2495-2504

[18] Soltesz I, Alger BA, Kano M, Lee S-H, Lovinger DM, Ohno-Shosaku T, et al. Weeding out bad waves: Towards selective cannabinoid circuit control in epilepsy. Nature Reviews. Neuroscience. 2015;**16**(5):264-272

[19] Ligresti A, De Petrocellis L, Di Marzo V. From phytocannabinoids to cannabinoid receptors and endocannabinoids: Pleiotropic physiological and pathological roles through complex pharmacology. Physiological Reviews. 2016;**96**:1593-1659. DOI: 10.1152/physrev.00002.2016

[20] Sugaya Y, Kano M. Control of excessive neural circuit excitability and prevention of epileptic seizures by endocannabinoid signalling. Cellular and Molecular Life Sciences. 2018;**75**:2793-2811

[21] Marsicano G, Goodenough S, Monory K, Hermann H, Eder M, Cannich A, et al. CB1 cannabinoid receptors and on demand defense against neurotoxicity. Science. 2003;**302**: 84-88

[22] Lupica CR, Hu Y, Devinsky O, Hoffman A. Cannabinoids as hippocampal network administrators. Neuropharmacology. 2017;**124**:25-37

[23] Hanus LO, Meyer SM, Muñoz E, Taglialatela-Scafati O, Appendino G. Phytocannabinoids: A unified critical inventory. Natural Product Reports. 2016;**33**:1357-1392

[24] Mechoulam R, Devane WA, Glaser R. Cannabinoid geometry and biological activity. In: Nahas GG, Sutin KM, Harvey DJ, Agurell S, editors. Marihuana and Medicine. Totowa: Humana Press; 1999

[25] Garriott JC, Forney RB, Hughes FW, Richards AB. Pharmacological properties of some cannabis related compounds. Archives Internationales de Pharmacodynamie et de Thérapie. 1968;**171**(2):425-434

[26] Ameri A, Wilhelm A, Simmet T. Effects of endogenous cannabinoid, anandamide, on neuronal activity in rat hippocampal slices. British Journal of Pharmacology. 1999;**126**:1831-1839

[27] Karler R, Turkanis SA. Cannabis and epilepsy. In: Nahas GG, WDM P, editors. Marihuana Biological Effects: Analysis, Metabolism, Cellular Response, Reproduction and Brain: Proceedings of the Satellite Symposium of the 7th International Congress of Pharmacology, Paris 22-23 July 1978. Oxford: Pergamom Press; 1978

[28] Karler R, Turkanis SA. The antiepileptic potential of the cannabinoids. In: Cohen S, Stillman R.C. eds. The Therapeutic Potential of Marihuana. 1976. Springer, Boston

[29] Turkanis SA, Karler R. Central excitatory properties of Δ^9-tetrahydrocannabinol and its metabolites in iron induced epileptic rats. Neuropharmacology. 1982;**21**:7-13

[30] Karler R, Calder LD, Sangdee P, Turkanis SA. Interaction between delta-9-tetrahydrocannabinol and kindling by electrical and chemical stimuli in mice. Neuropharmacology. 1984;**23**:1315-1320

[31] Schneiderman Fish B, Consroe P, Fox RR. Convulsant-anticonvulsant properties of delta-9-tetrahydrocannabinol in rabbits. Behavior Genetics. 1983;**13**:205-211

[32] Feeney DM. Marihuana and epilepsy: Paradoxical anticonvulsant and convulsant effects. Advances in Bioscience and Biotechnology. 1978;**22-23**:643-657

[33] Jones NA, Hill AJ, Weston SE, Burnett MDA, Stephens GJ, Whalley BJ, et al. Cannabidiol exerts anticonvulsant effects in animal models of temporal lobe and partial seizures. Seizure. 2012;**2**:344-352

[34] Gaston TE, Friedman D. Pharmacology of cannabinoids in the treatment of epilepsy. Epilepsy & Behavior. 2017;**70**:313-318

[35] Chiu P, Olsen DM, Borys HK, Karler R, Turkanis SA. The influence of cannabidiol and Δ^9-tetrahydrocannabinol on cobalt epilepsy in rats. Epilepsia. 1979;**20**:365-375

[36] Consroe P, Benedito MAC, Leite JR, Carlini EA, Mechoulam R. Effects of cannabidiol on behavioral seizures caused by convulsant drugs or current in mice. European Journal of Pharmacology. 1982;**83**:293-298

[37] Jones NA, Hill AJ, Smith I, Bevan SA, Williams CA, Whalley BJ, et al. Cannabidiol displays antiepileptiform and antiseizure properties in vitro and in vivo. The Journal of Pharmacology and Experimental Therapeutics. 2010;**332**:569-577

[38] Devinsky O, Gordon E. Marihuana: Effects on neuronal excitability and seizure threshold. In: Nahas GG, Sutin KM, Harvey DJ, Agurell S, editors. Marihuana and Medicine. Totowa: Humana Press; 1999

[39] Hill AJ, Weston SE, Jones NA, Smith I, Bevan S, Williamson EM, et al. Δ^9-Tetrahydrocannibivarin suppresses in vitro epileptiform and in vivo seizure activity in adult rats. Epilepsia. 2010;**51**:1522-1532

[40] Hill TDM, Cascio M-G, Romanao B, Duncan M, Pertwee RG, Williams CM, et al. Cannabidivarin-rich cannabis extracts are anticonvulsant in mouse and rat via a CB1 receptor-independent mechanism. British Journal of Pharmacology. 2013;**170**:679-692

[41] Hill AJ, Mercier MS, Hill TDM, Glynn SE, Jones NA, Yamasaki Y, et al. Cannabidivarin is anticonvulsant in mouse and rat. British Journal of Pharmacology. 2012;**167**:1629-1642

[42] Russo EB, Taming THC. Potential cannabis synergy and phytocannbinoid-terpenoid entourage effects. British Journal of Pharmacology. 2011;**163**:1344-1364

[43] Russo EB, Marcu J. Cannabis pharmacology: The usual suspects and a few promising leads. Advances in Pharmacology. 2017;**80**:67-134

[44] Williamson EM. Synergy and other interactions in phytomedicines. Phytomedicine. 2001;**8**:401-409

[45] Wilkinson JD, Whalley BJ, Baker D, Pryce G, Constanti A, Gibbons S, et al. Medicinal cannabis: Is delta9-tetrahydrocannabinol necessary for its effects? The Journal of Pharmacy and Pharmacology. 2003;**55**:1687-1694

[46] Ryan D, Drysdale AJ, Pertwee RG, Platt B. Differential effects of cannabis extracts and pure cannabinoids on hippocampal neurons and glia. Neuroscience Letters. 2006;**408**:236-241

[47] Hanus LO. Pharmacological and therapeutic secrets of plant and brain (endo)cannabinoids. Medicinal Research Reviews. 2009;**29**(2):213-271

[48] O'Shaughnessy WB On the preparations of the Indian Hemp or Gunjah. Transactions of The Medical and Physical Society of Bengal 1838-1840;**8**:421-461

[49] Gowers WR. Epilepsy and Other Chronic Convulsive Diseases. London: Churchill; 1881. p. 283

[50] Ellison JM, Gelwan E, Ogletree J. Complex partial seizure symptoms affected by marijuana abuse. Journal of Clinical Psychiatry. 1990;**51**:439-440

[51] Brust JC, Ng SK, Hauser AW, Susser M. Marijuana use and the risk of new onset seizures. Transactions of the American Clinical and Climatological Association. 1992;**103**:176-181

[52] Keeler MH, Reifler CB. Grand mal convulsions secondary to anticonvulsant use. Diseases of the Nervous System. 1967;**28**:474-475

[53] Mechoulam R, Carlini EA. Toward drugs derived from cannabis. Die Naturwissenschaften. 1978;**65**:174-179

[54] Cunha JM, Carlini EA, Pereira AE, Ramos OL, Pimental C, Gagliardi R, et al. Chronic administration of cannabidiol to healthy volunteers and epileptic patients. Pharmacology. 1980;**21**:175-185

[55] Trembly B, Sherman M. Double-blind clinical study of cannabidiol as a secondary anticonvulsant. In: Presented at: Marijuana '90. International Conference on Cannabis and Cannabinoids. Crete. July 8-11 1990

[56] Massot-Tarrus A, McLachlan RS. Marijuana use in adults admitted to a Canadian epilepsy monityoring unit. Epilepsy & Behavior. 2016;**63**:73-78

[57] Ladino LD, Hernandez-Ronquillo L, Tellez-Zenteno JF. Medical marijuana for epilepsy: A case series. The Canadian Journal of Neurological Sciences. 2014;**41**:753-758

[58] Press C, Knupp K, Chapman K. Parental reporting of response to oral cannabis extracts for treatment of refractory epilepsy. Epilepsy & Behavior. 2015;**45**:49-52

[59] Mathern GW, Beninsig L, Nehlig A. Fewer specialists support using medical marijuana and CBD in treating epilepsy patients compared with other medical professionals and patients: Result of Epilepsia's survey. Epilepsia. 2015;**56**:1-6

[60] Suraev A, Lintzeris N, Stuart J, Kevin RC, Blackburn R, Richards E, et al. Composition and use of Cannabis extracts for childhood epilepsy in the Australian community. Nature: Scientific Reports. 2018;**8**:10154. DOI: 10.1038/s41598-018-28127-0

[61] Tzadok M, Uliel-Siboni S, Linder I, Kramer U, Epstein O, Menascu S, et al. CBD enriched medical cannabis for intractable pediatric epilepsy: The current Israeli experience. Seizure. 2016;**35**:41-44. DOI: 10.1016/j.seizure.2016.01.004

[62] Porcari GS, Fu C, Doll ED, Carter EG, Carson RP. Efficacy of artisanal preparations of cannabidiol for the treatment of epilepsy: Practical experiences in a tertiary medical center. Epilepsy & Behavior. 2018;**80**:240-246

[63] McCoy B, Wang L, Zak M, Al-Mehmadi S, Kabir N, Alhadid K, et al. A prospective open-label trial of a CBD/THC cannabis oil in Dravet syndrome. Annals of Clinical and Translational Neurology. 2018;**5**(9):1077-1088. DOI: 10.1002/acn3.621

[64] Reithmeier D, Tang-Wai R, Seifert B, Lyon AW, Alcorn J, Acton B, et al. The protocol for the Cannabidiol in children with refractory epileptic encephalopathy (CARE-E) study: A phase 1 dosage escalation study. BMC Pediatrics. 2018;**18**:221. DOI: 10.1186/s12887-018-1191-y

[65] Huntsman RJ, Tang-Wai R, Alcorn J, Vuong S, Acton B, Corley S, et al. Dosage related efficacy and tolerability of Cannabidiol in children with treatment resistant epileptic encephalopathy: Preliminary results of the CARE-E study. In: American Epilepsy Society Annual Meeting. 2018 Available from: https://www.aesnet.org/annual_meeting/abstract_search#/sortDate_na_dt/DESC/0/tang~wai/

[66] Devinsky O, Marsh E, Friedman D, Thiele E, et al. Cannabidiol in patients with treatment-resistant epilepsy: An open-label interventional trial. Lancet Neurology. 2016;**15**:270-278. DOI: 10.1016/S1474-4422(15)00379-8

[67] Rosenberg EC, Louik J, Conway E, Devinsky O, Friedman D. Quality of life in childhood epilepsy in pediatric patients enrolled in a prospective, open-label clinical study with cannabidiol. Epilepsia. 2017;**58**(8):e96-e100

[68] Devinsky O, Cross JH, Laux L, Marsh E, et al. Trial of cannabidiol for drug-resistant seizures in the Dravet syndrome. New England Journal of Medicine. 2017;**376**:2011-2020. DOI: 10.1056/NEJMoa1611618

[69] Thiele EA, Marsh ED, French JA, Mazurkiewicz-Beldzinska M, et al. Cannabidiol in patients with seizures associated with Lennox-Gastaut Syndrome (GWPCARE4): A randomized, double blind, placebo controlled phase 3 trial. Lancet. 2018;**391**:1085-1096. DOI: 10.1016/S0140-6736(18)30136-3

[70] Stockings E, Zagic D, Campbell G, Weier M, Hall WD, Nielsen S, et al. Evidence for cannabis and cannabinoids for epilepsy: A systematic review of controlled and observational evidence. Journal of Neurology, Neurosurgery, and Psychiatry. 2018;**89**:741-753. DOI: 10.1136/jnnp-2017-317168

[71] O Brien T, Berkovich SF, French J, Messenheimer J, Bonn-Miller MO, Gutterman D. Synthetic transdermal cannabidiol for the treatment of focal epilepsy in adults. In: American Epilepsy Society Annual Meeting; 2018

[72] Chiron C, Marchand MC, Tran A, Rey E, d'Athis P, et al. Stiripentol in severe myoclonic epilepsy in infancy: A randomised placebo-controlled syndrome-dedicated trial. STICLO study group. Lancet. 2000;**356**:1638-1642

[73] Glauser T, Kluger G, Sachdeo R, Krauss G, Perdomo C, Arroyo S. Rufinamide for generalized seizures associated with Lennox-Gastaut syndrome. Neurology. 2008;**70**:1950-1958